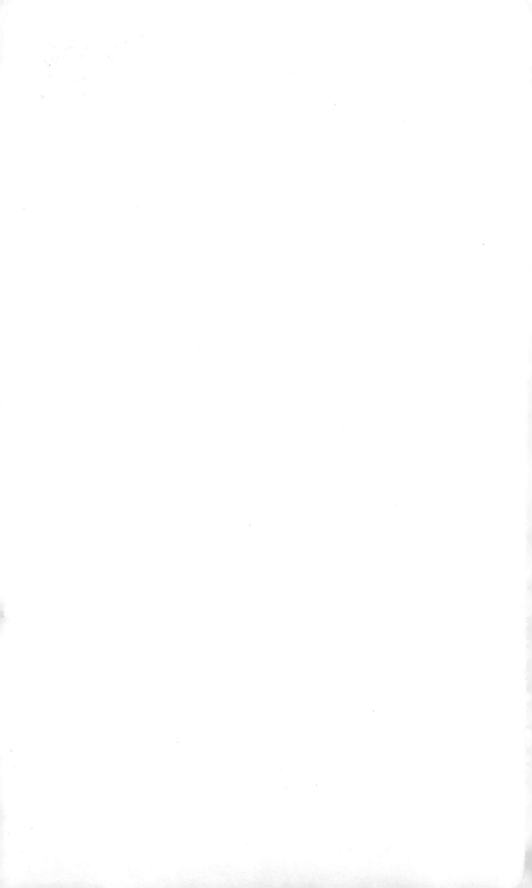

Breast Cancer

Collaborative Management

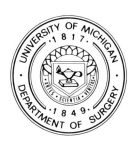

Edited by
Jay K. Harness
Harold A. Oberman
Allen S. Lichter
Dorit D. Adler
Robert L. Cody

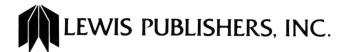

LEWIS PUBLISHERS, INC.

Library of Congress Cataloging-in-Publication Data

Breast cancer.

   Includes bibliographies and index.
   1. Breast – Cancer.   I. Harness, Jay K. (Jay Kenneth),
1942-   .   [DNLM: 1. Breast Neoplasms – therapy.
2. Patient Care Team. WP 870 B8233]
RC280.B8B666   1988   616.99′449   87-31125
ISBN 0-87371-106-8

LEWIS PUBLISHERS, INC.
121 South Main Street, P.O. Drawer 519, Chelsea, Michigan 48118

PRINTED IN THE UNITED STATES OF AMERICA

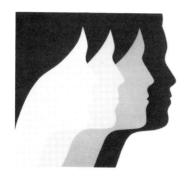

JAY K. HARNESS, MD
Clinical Associate Professor, Department of Surgery
Director, Breast Care Center
University of Michigan Medical Center
Ann Arbor, Michigan

HAROLD A. OBERMAN, MD
Professor and Head, Section of Clinical Pathology
Department of Pathology
University of Michigan Medical School
Ann Arbor, Michigan

ALLEN S. LICHTER, MD
Professor and Chairman
Department of Radiation Oncology
University of Michigan Medical Center
Ann Arbor, Michigan

DORIT D. ADLER, MD
Assistant Professor and Director
Division of Mammography
Department of Radiology
University of Michigan Medical School
Ann Arbor, Michigan

ROBERT L. CODY, MD
Instructor, Division of Hematology/Oncology
University of Michigan Medical School
Ann Arbor, Michigan

MARY L. HARPER
Research Editor
Department of Surgery
University of Michigan
Ann Arbor, Michigan

Preface

Breast Cancer: Collaborative Management has been assembled and written from the viewpoint that the contemporary management of breast (or any) cancer requires the partnership of physicians, nurses, social workers, and all others whose special training and talents should be combined and integrated in treating the whole patient. Like the treatment of so many other diseases, the management of breast cancer continues to undergo evolutionary change, and the twentieth century has witnessed the most rapid progress and change.

This book is based on the experience of the University of Michigan Breast Care Center, and was compiled at a conference sponsored by the Breast Care Center in May 1987 called The Collaborative Management of the Patient with Breast Cancer. Participating in that conference were some of the prominent specialists in various aspects of treatment of the patient with breast cancer, and each was asked to prepare a chapter addressing a specific aspect of breast cancer.

Dr. Richard Margolese outlines (Chapter 2) the process of change, from Halsted's important contributions and concepts on the spread of breast cancer to a contemporary biologic concept of the behavior of the disease. He notes the importance of systemic and local factors in treatment. Throughout human history, female breasts have been symbols of femininity, sexuality, and maternity. As the apparent equal outcome of less radical procedures gained recognition, strong voices could be heard urging women and their doctors to seriously consider breast-sparing procedures. Ms. Rose Kushner has been one of the strongest advocates, not only for breast preservation, but also in urging health professionals to work in an understanding way to help women cope better with breast cancer and with the entire process of diagnosis, treatment, and follow-up (Chapter 3). So strong has been the impact of the women's movement on the subject of breast conservation that laws mandating women be given treatment options before beginning breast cancer therapy have been enacted in one-fourth of the states. Attorney Edward Goldman (Chapter 5) has clearly summarized this recent legal trend and its implications for the future.

The epidemiology and costs of treating breast cancer are major areas of concern. Patients in the United States, Canada, the countries of Europe, and other industrialized countries of the world most often present with Stage I or II disease, while Stage III disease remains the most typical form of presentation in other countries. Epidemiologist Dr. David Schottenfeld has studied current concepts on the origins and risks of breast cancer and has outlined these in Chapter 6. Therapy for breast cancer, the most common cancer of women, continues to consume its share of total health care expenditures in the United States. The experience of one large insurance company, Blue Cross and Blue Shield of Michigan, is presented by Dr. George Gerber. Whether breast conservation is employed or not, the costs of diagnosis, therapy, reconstruction, and follow-up are substantial.

The contemporary management of patients with breast cancer has raised many new concerns. First are the issues of diagnosis and evaluation of breast masses. Second are the issues of integrated management of breast cancer, especially the unusual presentation and difficult cases. Finally, the recognition of psychosocial and "wellness" issues is the key to treating the "whole" patient. Each of the remaining sections of the book addresses and analyzes all of these important issues.

All physicians need an integrated approach to evaluating breast masses. Dr. William Donegan outlines his concepts and concerns in Chapter 7. Mammography and fine needle aspiration have evolved as key procedures in the diagnosis of breast lesions. Drs. Pennes, Adler, and Naylor point out the strengths and weaknesses of these procedures in their chapters. Fundamental to breast conservation and local control of breast cancer is the proper performance of surgical excisional biopsies and lumpectomies. Dr. Richard Margolese reviews the National Surgical Adjuvant Breast Project's (NSABP) experience with the technique of segmental mastectomy in Chapter 10. Key in this process is the role of the pathologist in interpretation of excised tissue and in noting subtle but important changes of atypia and carcinoma in situ. Dr. Harold Oberman clearly outlines these important areas in Chapter 11.

The management of breast cancer was relatively simple in Halsted's era, with radical mastectomy as the only effective method of therapy. Contemporary management, with or without breast conservation, requires many colleagues working in concert. These varied approaches to treatment are addressed by Drs. Coon, Lichter, Cody, Wicha, East, McLeod, Guice, and Oldham. Following mastectomy, reconstruction of the operative site and augmentation of the remaining breast are now accepted standards of treatment for the breast cancer patient. Dr. Thomas Stevenson discusses the subject in Chapter 15. Exciting new concepts and methods of breast (and other) cancer management are actively being pursued in research labs around the world. Most research is focusing at the cellular level in an attempt to understand the concepts of cancer cell growth and possible regulation of that process. The use of monoclonal antibodies for imaging and therapy offers a promising future. Drs. John Niederhuber and Stephen Desiderio present an overview of these horizons in Chapter 19.

Historically, little attention has been given to the psychosocial impact of the diagnosis, therapy, and follow-up of breast cancer in the patient. The contemporary management of breast cancer has begun to address these issues in a way that should have application to the treatment of all cancer patients. These issues range from how a breast care center should be organized to minimizing stress to the issues of the impact of the diagnosis on family, work, and sexuality. Coping during these stressful times requires the sensitivity and cooperation of all members of a treatment team, including the social worker. Special intervention skills are of paramount importance. Peer counseling and support groups along with specific rehabilitation and exercise programs are key elements in successful coping and recovery. Patients are now becoming aware of the possible impact of their own wellness on their long-term quality of life and survival. All of these important issues are addressed in Chapters 20 through 27.

Chapter Authors

DORIT D. ADLER, MD
    Assistant Professor and Director, Division of Mammography, Department of Radiology, University of Michigan Medical School

MARY ANNE BORD, RN, MN, OCN
    Manager, Clinical Nursing Services, Department of Ambulatory Care Nursing, University of Michigan Medical Center

KATHLEEN A. CALZONE, RN, BSN
    Clinical Nurse II, Division of Hematology/Oncology, Department of Internal Medicine, University of Michigan Medical Center

ROBERT L. CODY, MD
    Instructor, Division of Hematology/Oncology, University of Michigan Medical School

WILLIAM W. COON, MD
    Professor and Division Chief, Division of Surgical Oncology, Section of General Surgery, Department of Surgery, University of Michigan Medical School

STEPHEN V. DESIDERIO, MD, PHD
    Assistant Investigator, Howard Hughes Medical Institute, and Assistant Professor, Department of Molecular Biology and Genetics, Johns Hopkins University Medical School, Baltimore, Maryland

WILLIAM L. DONEGAN, MD
    Professor of Surgery, Medical College of Wisconsin, Chief of Surgery, Mt. Sinai Medical Center, Milwaukee, Wisconsin

MARY K. EAST, MD
    Instructor, Section of General Surgery, Department of Surgery, University of Michigan Medical School

GEORGE R. GERBER, MD, MBA
    Medical Director, Health Care Network, Southfield, Michigan

EDWARD B. GOLDMAN, JD
    Hospital Attorney, University of Michigan Hospitals

KAREN S. GUICE, MD
Assistant Professor, Section of General Surgery, Department of Surgery, University of Michigan Medical School

JAY K. HARNESS, MD
Clinical Associate Professor, Department of Surgery, and Director, Breast Care Center, University of Michigan Medical Center

CLAUDIA W. KRAUS, MSW, ACSW
Social Worker, Ambulatory Care Social Work, Division of Hematology/Oncology, Department of Internal Medicine, University of Michigan Medical Center

ROSE KUSHNER
Executive Director, Breast Cancer Advisory Center, and Co-Founder, National Alliance of Breast Cancer Organizations

ALLEN S. LICHTER, MD
Professor and Chairman, Department of Radiation Oncology, University of Michigan Medical Center

MICHAEL K. McLEOD, MD
Assistant Professor, Section of General Surgery, Department of Surgery, University of Michigan Medical School

RICHARD G. MARGOLESE, MD
Professor of Surgery, McGill University, and Associate Director, McGill Cancer Center, and Director of Oncology, Jewish General Hospital, Montreal, Quebec, Canada

BERNARD NAYLOR, MD
Professor, Department of Pathology, and Director, Cytopathology Laboratory, University of Michigan Medical School

JOHN E. NIEDERHUBER, MD
Professor, Department of Surgery, Department of Oncology, Department of Molecular Biology and Genetics, Johns Hopkins University Medical School, Baltimore, Maryland

SHARON J. NOFFSINGER, RN, MSN
Clinical Nurse Specialist, Department of Radiation Oncology, University of Michigan Medical Center

HAROLD A. OBERMAN, MD
Professor and Head, Section of Clinical Pathology, Department of Pathology, University of Michigan Medical School

KEITH T. OLDHAM, MD
Assistant Professor, Section of Pediatric Surgery, Department of Surgery, University of Michigan Medical School

CARL E. ORRINGER, MD
Medical Director of Cardiac Programs, University of Michigan MedSport

DAVID R. PENNES, MD
Assistant Professor, Department of Radiology, University of Michigan Medical School

PENNY F. PIERCE, PHD, RN
Clinical Specialist, Department of Internal Medicine, University of Michigan Medical Center, and Assistant Research Scientist, Center for Nursing Research, University of Michigan School of Nursing

LEE K. ROSENBLUM, BA
Social Worker, Hospital Social Work, University of Michigan Medical Center

PATRICIA A. SARAN, RN, BSN
Clinical Care Coordinator, Division of Surgical Oncology, Section of General Surgery, Department of Surgery, University of Michigan Medical Center

GORDON A. SAXE, MPH
Graduate Student Teaching Assistant, Department of Epidemiology, School of Public Health, and Graduate Student Research Assistant, Department of Surgery, University of Michigan

WENDY S. SCHAIN, EDD
Medical Care Consultant, National Institutes of Health, and Adjunct Clinical Professor, Georgetown Medical School, Washington, DC

DAVID SCHOTTENFELD, MD
John G. Searle Professor and Chairman, Department of Epidemiology, School of Public Health, and Professor, Department of Internal Medicine, University of Michigan Medical School

DIANE K. SOMMERFIELD, RN, BSN
Clinical Nurse III, Hematology/Oncology Consulting Service, University of Michigan Medical Center

THOMAS R. STEVENSON, MD
Assistant Professor, Section of Plastic and Reconstructive Surgery, Department of Surgery, University of Michigan Medical School

MARY M. WAKEFIELD, BA, PT
Staff Physical Therapist II, Division of Physical Therapy, Department of Physical Medicine and Rehabilitation, University of Michigan Medical Center

DAVID K. WELLISCH, PHD
Associate Professor of Medical Psychology, Department of Psychiatry, University of California at Los Angeles Medical School, Los Angeles, California

MAX S. WICHA, MD
Associate Professor and Chief, Division of Hematology/Oncology, Department of Internal Medicine, Director, Simpson Memorial Institute, and Interim Director, University of Michigan Cancer Center, University of Michigan Medical School

Contents

SECTION ONE

Past and Present Trends in the Management of the Patient with Breast Cancer

1. Organizing for Collaborative Management: What Are the Options?

JAY K. HARNESS

The contemporary management of breast cancer is interdisciplinary and collaborative. The treatment of this disease requires a process that addresses the impact on the whole patient of diagnosis, therapy, and follow-up. Greater specialization has led to greater fragmentation. The need now is for greater integration and a focus on the entire human being.

New strategies have emerged for organizing and coordinating the necessary services. This chapter will analyze these new approaches and describe the more traditional ways patients have been evaluated, treated, and followed for breast disease.

PHYSICAL EXAMINATION AND BREAST SELF-EXAMINATION

Still fundamental to the diagnosis of any pathologic condition of the breast is the physical examination. It should be performed routinely by primary health care providers as part of any periodic health appraisal. Physical examination of the breasts also has emerged as an integral component of the performance of screening or diagnostic mammography. Many centers, such as departments of radiology in hospitals, or freestanding clinics, employ nurses to perform physical examination in conjunction with mammography. Radiologists may also perform physical examination for better clinical correlation with mammographic findings, and before performing procedures such as ultrasound and fine needle aspirations of the breast.

Breast self-examination (BSE) should be performed by all women and men on a routine basis after age 16. The importance of this technique is stressed elsewhere in this book. Historically, there have been no meaningful incentives for women to detect breast cancer early because the discovery of a malignant lesion would usually mean the surgical loss of the involved breast. With the increasing use of breast-sparing procedures (e.g., partial mastectomy and radiation therapy) for the primary treatment of breast cancer, women should be more highly motivated toward early detection, since the smaller the cancer (i.e., 2–3 cm or less) the greater the chance that breast sparing procedures can be utilized. This new approach to patient motivation should be emphasized by all health care providers teaching BSE. Those patients treated by partial mastectomy (lumpectomy) and radiation therapy will also use BSE for the detection of recurrent disease in the ipsilateral breast and new disease in the contralateral breast.

DIAGNOSTIC ORGANIZATIONS

The technical aspects of mammography are discussed elsewhere in this textbook (Chapter 8). Several methods have emerged recently for organizing mammographic services. Such units can be freestanding or be part of a hospital-based radiology department. Mammograms may be performed in either of these settings with or without correlating physical examinations done by either trained nurses, technicians, or radiologists. While mammography is the best diagnostic procedure currently available for the detection of breast cancer, it has limitations. Mammograms can be normal with a palpable breast cancer. Knowing there is a palpable abnormality helps both the radiologist and X-ray technicians to ensure that the mammographic views of that area are detailed and clear. Clinical correlation in the interpretation of any diagnostic procedure, especially by the radiologist, is always superior to simply performing the procedure and providing uncorrelated results.

Freestanding or hospital-based mammographic centers may offer additional diagnostic services. Ultrasound and fine needle aspiration (or core) biopsies are important adjuncts in the diagnosis of breast lesions. Performing such studies as part of the mammographic evaluation speeds up the diagnostic process considerably. Some freestanding breast diagnostic units have added equipment to perform bone and liver-spleen scans so that these preoperative diagnostic studies can be performed at one location. Freestanding breast units can be so "freestanding" that they move on wheels to the patients! One Ohio manufacturer has designed diagnostic motorcoaches ranging from 22 to 35 feet in length in which mammography, film developing, and ultrasound can be performed. Such units could be used for breast screening at the work place, at health care units such as nursing homes, or at high-density living units. The future of such mobile units remains to be seen.

Highly skilled and experienced mammographic radiologists are a key component in the collaborative management of patients with either benign or malignant breast disease. A close working relationship with the surgeon is particularly critical in the performance of wire or needle localizing biopsies for nonpalpable lesions. Freestanding mammographic units find it more difficult to provide such services. Hospital-based units, especially those located next to outpatient departments, ambulatory surgical units, or hospital operating rooms, have a clear advantage in providing such necessary coordinated services.

Hospital-based units also have better access to pathology departments for the rapid evaluation of fine needle or core biopsy specimens. The removal and pathologic evaluation of nonpalpable lesions requires a high degree of coordination between pathologist, radiologist, and surgeon. Excised wire or needle localized specimens, especially those with microscopic calcifications, should be radiographed prior to being sent to the pathology laboratory to ensure removal of the suspicious area. The radiologist is able to place an additional needle in the excised specimen to ensure that the pathologist evaluates the correct spot. Tissue must be handled quickly to permit prompt fixation of the specimen and to allow for determination of hormonal receptors when there is sufficient neoplastic tissue for such assays.

The importance of the mammographic unit in the accurate and rapid diagnosis of breast cancer is evident. What about the role of such units in the follow-up care of the patient with breast cancer? With the greater use of breast sparing procedures, routine follow-up mammograms are an integral component for detecting recurrent cancer in the treated breast and new cancer in the contralateral breast. High quality mammographic X-ray equipment, processors, and technicians are needed to ensure the production of films of such clarity that the most subtle changes suggestive of recurrent or new disease can be detected early. Again, the use of X-ray guided fine needle aspirations, and of needle, or hook-wire localization biopsies are important factors in the coordinated follow-up of breast cancer patients.

THE PROCESS—DIAGNOSIS AND TREATMENT

Elsewhere in this book there are detailed discussions of the diagnosis and management of breast masses and the treatment options for breast cancer (Chapters 7, 10, 12, 13, 14). Many steps are involved in both the diagnostic and the treatment processes, especially if breast-sparing therapy is the goal. In most settings, the patient moves from one physician specialist to another. Communication between physicians is accomplished by phone or letter. There are often delays in arranging for diagnostic tests and evaluations by other specialists, such as surgeons, radiation oncologists, and medical oncologists. The entire process may take up to two weeks, and often there is no one physician who is acting as "captain" of the team.

What happens to the patient during this process? Most patients express both fear and an urgent desire to learn of the diagnosis once a breast mass is detected. They want an answer quickly about the nature of the mass and also want the potential threat to their lives removed as rapidly as possible. Anxiety follows the patient through every step of the process and often clouds the patient's decision-making ability. Physicians and all other health care personnel who have contact with these patients need to be very sensitive to their fearful state and must do their best to communicate openly and provide emotional support at every step of the diagnostic and treatment process.

The process can be accelerated if there is prompt communication between specialists. The finding of a suspicious mass on physical examination should prompt performance of mammography and, perhaps, fine needle (or core) biopsy at the initial visit. Often the radiologist is skilled in these techniques and may perform them after taking the initial mammograms. Radiologists also may perform X-ray guided fine needle aspiration on non-palpable lesions found at screening mammography. If either the initial provider or the radiologist has not performed any definitive diagnostic test, then the patient should be referred to a general surgeon for fine needle (or core) biopsy and subsequent excisional biopsy (lumpectomy).

The general surgeon plays a key role in informing the patient of treatment options once a diagnosis of cancer is made. For a patient to be fully informed, she (or he) should be evaluated, and if the likelihood of regional metastasis is high, discuss available treatment options with a radiation oncologist and a medical oncologist. Once the patient is apprised of all the therapeutic options, she must make the final selection of treatment. Patients are particularly vulnerable during this time and can be swayed by a strong and articulate physician as to which option that physician prefers. It is best that all the specialists involved agree on the most medically appropriate treatment plan so that the patient is not caught in the middle of a "treatment dispute." One of the specialists should assure the patient that he or she will be the primary physician to ensure coordination of both the treatment of the primary breast cancer as well as the long-term follow-up. It has been our experience at the University of Michigan Breast Care Center that such needs and considerations of our referred patients have not always been met.

The problems of the diagnostic and treatment process just outlined have been remedied to some extent when patients are evaluated and treated in group practice settings such as large hospital-based groups, health maintenance organizations (HMOs), preferred-provider associations (PPAs or PPOs), and other such organizations. In these settings, there is an established network of other specialists, which can enhance communication and shorten delay. There may, however, be the problem of who will be the captain of the team for both the short-term treatment needs and long-term follow-up. Also, the structure may not be in place in this setting to provide emotional support for the patient and her (his) family. Overall coordination and collaboration is enhanced, but may not be optimal.

THE COMPREHENSIVE BREAST CARE CENTER

The contemporary treatment of most cancers requires a comprehensive, multidisciplinary approach. Cancer therapy is less and less a one-modality program, but increasingly involves two or more disciplines and treatment methods. Surgery, radiation therapy, and medical oncology are the three treatment specialities involved in breast cancer therapy. All three are often required in the initial phase of treatment, and all three require their own follow-up of patients for many years. The treatment of recurrent disease may involve one, two, or all three of the disciplines. Multimodality, comprehensive, collaborative treatment of breast cancer has become the "state of the art" in the 1980s. This concept has best been exemplified by the National Cancer Institute (NCI) of the National Institutes of Health (NIH).

In most medical settings in the United States, the collaborative management of patients with breast cancer occurs on an informal basis between locally based referring specialists. This process works well to a greater or lesser degree, depending on the willingness of the specialists to work together, their current state of knowledge of contemporary management of breast cancer, and the ability of one of them to serve as coordinator of the short-term and long-term management needs of the patient. Several difficulties exist with this typical model, including potential breakdown in physician communications; delays in the timing of the diagnostic and treatment process; lack of uniformity in patient treatment plans; lack of coordination in treatment phasing, for example chemotherapy and radiation therapy; increased patient anxiety; and lack of uniform long-term follow-up. Other less important problems may also be encountered with this model, including potentially higher treatment costs because of a lack of efficiency and duplication of tests and services.

The comprehensive center approach solves virtually all of the problems outlined as well as having additional benefits. In a comprehensive center, not only are all necessary services provided at one location, but also they are administratively organized in a way to ensure maximum efficiency and timeliness. The diagnostic and treatment process is organized to ensure complete coordination between the various services (e.g., radiology, surgery, pathology, radiation oncology, medical oncology, and social work). Communication between providers is done in person, and the medical records are uniform. Difficult or controversial cases are managed by specialists meeting in organized conferences or in the clinical examining area. Such meetings produce a consensus opinion on diagnostic, treatment, and follow-up methods so that the patient is not caught in a dispute between specialists.

One of the greatest benefits of a comprehensive center is the pooling of knowledge of all of the specialists involved. New information is constantly evolving in all specialty areas, and it is difficult for specialists in one area to keep up with new knowledge in other specialities. Comprehensive centers are often part of regional or national study groups, for example, the Southwest Oncology Group and the National Surgical Adjuvant Breast Project, and are involved in ongoing prospective protocols. Trends or results from these studies usually are available earlier to the cooperating centers, and this information is often shared and implemented sooner by the local centers. Patients seeking their care at such centers are the beneficiaries. The treatment of breast, or any, cancer is an active and dynamic process. The collaborative sharing of knowledge enhances that process and also serves as a catalyst to push all the providers involved to higher degrees of excellence. This, in turn, gives patients greater confidence and less anxiety, resulting in a positive influence during an extremely stressful time.

Organized protocols for long-term follow-up should ensure uniform and efficient data gathering and timely periodic evaluations of patients. Early detection and treatment of recurrent disease or discovery of new cancers should improve patient outcomes. The careful collection and reporting of such data by comprehensive centers will increase overall knowledge of the biology of breast cancer in all age groups.

The benefits of a comprehensive breast center are clear. The concept of a single center for the treatment of both benign and malignant breast disease began to emerge at The University of Michigan Medical Center in 1984, and the Breast Care Center began operation in early 1985. The details on the workings of this center are discussed in Chapter 20. Both provider and patient satisfaction with the Breast Care Center remains extremely high. It is anticipated that the center will soon be treating in excess of 300 new cases of breast cancer per year.

The concept of a comprehensive center for the treatment of breast cancer appears to be gaining momentum across the United States. While data on the exact numbers of such centers is incomplete, the National Consortium of Breast Centers, organized in 1986, has a national directory listing 60 breast centers, of which 20 appear to work on the comprehensive model.[1] From the telephone calls and letters directed to The University of Michigan Breast Care Center, it is apparent that many more institutions are considering or developing comprehensive centers. Many hospitals and medical centers are realizing not only the medical advantages of such centers, but also the marketing advantages. In this day of increased competition for patients, the opening of a comprehensive center may well increase a hospital's market share and bed occupancy. These forces alone will undoubtedly increase the numbers of comprehensive breast centers in the United States.

Throughout the United States, group practices in small and large clinics are increasing. With administrative organization and dedication of resources to a program for breast cancer, the group practice setting can function like a comprehensive center. With such efforts, the group practice setting may provide many, if not all, of the benefits of a comprehensive center. Competitive and economic forces, as well as the increasing supply of physicians, are pushing these changes. The offer of programs in a variety of areas, including complete breast care, will be necessary for private practice groups to remain competitive. The extent of care that can be provided will vary with the size of the group practice.

SUMMARY

The provision of breast care is undergoing significant change. Radiologists, who once only interpreted X-rays of breasts, now are actively organizing centers for the "complete" diagnosis of benign and malignant disease of the breast. With large scale mammographic breast screening, the radiologist is rapidly becoming a "primary" care physician for breast disease. Such operations may be freestanding, affiliated with a hospital or medical center, or part of such entities. The linkage of mammographic radiologists to surgeons, group practices, or comprehensive breast centers is the next important step in the collaborative management of patients with breast disease. Surgeons, radiation oncologists, medical oncologists, pathologists, radiologists, and others can be further linked in an informal referral system in a group practice or in a comprehensive center. The contemporary treatment and follow-up of patients with breast cancer requires an organized approach. Of all of the options discussed, it appears that the comprehensive center offers the most efficient and coordinated opportunity for state-of-the-art management of breast cancer patients. Such centers should and will increase in number.

REFERENCE

1. Directory of Breast Centers, National Consortium of Breast Centers, New Brunswick, NJ, 1986.

2. Management of Primary Breast Cancer: A Biologic and Therapeutic Review

RICHARD G. MARGOLESE

One of the great surgical controversies of the twentieth century has been the choice of operation for primary breast cancer. For fifty years there was virtually unanimous agreement in favor of the Halsted radical mastectomy. The last twenty years has been a period of considerable uncertainty, from which has developed a trend for less radical surgical intervention.

THE HALSTED ERA

The Halsted operation was an elegant and scientific answer to the problem as it was conceived in that day. Cancer was thought to be a process which extended along lymphatic pathways directly, not by a process of embolization. It was believed that bloodborne metastases did not occur.[9] If this premise was true, then en bloc removal of adjacent tissue and nodes was a logical surgical solution to the problem.

The Halsted mastectomy quickly became widely practiced because local recurrence rates improved, even though overall survival rates were not affected (Table 1). Survival rates eventually did improve, largely because patients presented with earlier tumors. When these improvements could not be extended further, some dissatisfaction with the Halsted operation arose.

The fact that the first experiments with other procedures ranged from extended and super-radical operations at one extreme to simple mastectomy or biopsy and radiation at the other indicates that this change was more a result of dissatisfaction with the Halsted procedure and less a result of logical scientific thinking. Several early clinical trials were con-

Table 1. Comparative Results: Halsted versus Contemporaries[11]

Study Group	Local Recurrence (%)	10-year Survival (%)
Halsted	26	12
Comparative Group	80	9

ducted.[2,3,10,12-14] These trials tested extended mastectomy, radical mastectomy, and simple mastectomy, with or without the addition of regional radiotherapy. One can see a thrashing about for new ideas, but one does not see a scientific pattern for a test of a single hypothesis. One hypothesis did emerge, however, and led to a substantial change in surgical practice for the treatment of breast cancer.

THE FISHER HYPOTHESIS

The alternate hypothesis, developed over a fifteen-year period by Fisher,[8] suggested that cancer was a systemic disease almost from its inception. This does not mean that all patients will show metastases, but that the possibility exists, and depends on a complex interplay of biologic factors, including tumor aggressiveness and host defenses. Prompt treatment will benefit some patients, but many will require systemic treatment. Focusing on variations of local or regional treatments does not allow one to fully appreciate the scope of the problem.

The Halsted hypothesis was widely accepted and taught to generations of surgeons as tradition and heritage, though it had never been subjected to scientific testing in the laboratory. The Fisher hypothesis departed from the anatomical basis for cancer spread and presented a more biologic view, based on many laboratory observations. Among these were the demonstration of lymphatico-hematogenous connections: tumor cells injected into the venous or lymphatic system would be found within minutes in the other circulation. It was also shown that regional lymph nodes are not barriers to tumor cell dissemination as had been thought since the days of Virchow.[4] The hypothesis resulting from these observations could be tested by a prospective randomized clinical trial and provide a scientific basis for accepting or rejecting this new concept.

Surgical Trials

Surgical investigators had been preoccupied for decades with minor technical variations on the basic radical operation. Concern for features such as the "apical node" and levels of involvement took precedence over the larger question of the biologic importance of these nodes. In two separate and related studies to test these concepts and validate the Fisher hypothesis, the National Surgical Adjuvant Breast Project (NSABP) has evaluated radical mastectomy, modified radical mastectomy, and segmental mastectomy in Protocols B-04 and B-06.

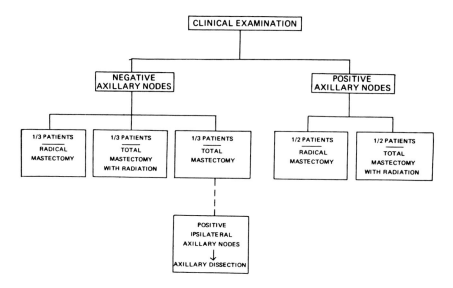

Figure 1.   Schema for Protocol B-04. Evaluation of radical mastectomy or total mastectomy with or without radiation.

Protocol B-04

The first protocol, B-04, was begun in 1971 to evaluate the importance of lymph node treatment. The objectives of that trial were to determine the usefulness of surgical or radiation treatment of axillary lymph nodes in comparison with no treatment or delayed treatment if recurrences arose.

One thousand seven hundred sixty-five patients were randomly allocated to groups to be treated with radical mastectomy; total mastectomy with irradiation; or total mastectomy alone in patients with clinically negative nodes. If a patient in the latter group developed axillary tumor involvement at any future time, an axillary dissection was then done. Patients with positive nodes were randomized to be treated with either radical mastectomy or total mastectomy plus radiation therapy (Figure 1).

Ten-year results indicate no significant difference in recurrence rates or survival rates between any of the treatment groups[7] (Figure 2). In other words, removing the nodes by traditional surgical dissection did not help the patient and leaving the nodes untreated did not harm the patient. Positive nodes are a sign of a poor prognosis, but the nodes are not the source of metastases — they are themselves only one of the metastatic sites.

Although the use of radiotherapy decreased the incidence of chest wall and supraclavicular node recurrence, survival was not altered. Even for patients with lesions in the inner quadrants, radiation therapy was of no benefit (Figure 3). This sheds further biologic light on the futility of the treatment of lymph nodes for prevention of the dissemination of cancer. It is well known that patients whose primary tumors are in the medial or

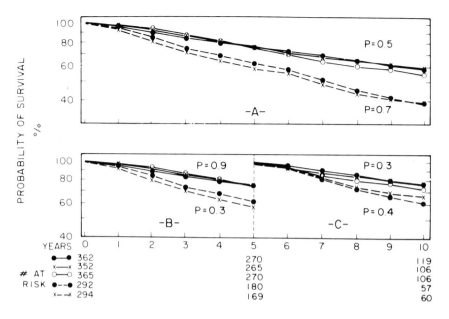

Figure 2. Results of Protocol B-04. Survival through 10 years (A), during the first 5 years (B), and during the second 5 years for patients alive at the end of the fifth year (C). Patients were treated by radical mastectomy (solid circle), total mastectomy and radiation (X), or total mastectomy alone (open circle). There were no significant differences among the three groups of patients with clinically negative nodes (solid line) or between the two groups with positive nodes (broken line).

central part of the breast have a higher likelihood of internal mammary node metastases, yet when these patients were compared with patients with laterally placed tumors, there was no difference in any of the three end points, regardless of whether the patients were treated by radiation therapy or by either of the surgical techniques. Again, this shows the lack of benefit of treating nodes that may harbor a metastasis, demonstrating that the nodes are only an indicator that disseminated disease is present. Therefore, the Halstedian view that cancer is an anatomical and regional problem is no longer tenable. A more modern biologic view of cancer is that it is a systemic problem and that metastases may be present at any time. The word "early" refers to a biologic state and not a time frame.

Protocol B-06

The second NSABP protocol, B-06, was designed to compare segmental mastectomy with total mastectomy. Axillary dissection was done in all cases (Figure 4).

There was an intentional congruency between Protocols B-04 and B-06. In B-04, the lymph nodes were being evaluated by three treatments: surgical removal, radiation, and observation. In Protocol B-06, it is the surrounding

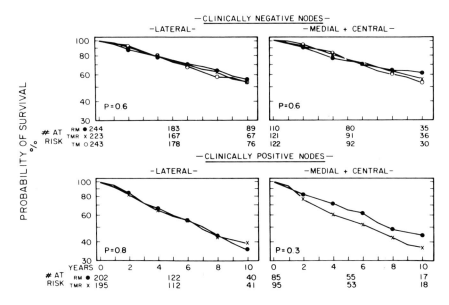

Figure 3. No benefit demonstrated with internal mammary node radiation, regardless of tumor site. Radical mastectomy (solid circle), total mastectomy and radiation (X), total mastectomy alone (open circle).

breast parenchyma that is subjected to the same three treatments. In addition, all patients with positive axillary nodes were subjected to a standard two-drug adjuvant chemotherapy program consisting of 5-fluorouracil and L-phenylalanine mustard. The use of this three-arm plan provides biologic insight as well as statistical and numerical answers.

Analysis of the findings in 1843 patients, with an average follow-up of 39 months, indicates no difference in disease-free survival, distant disease-free survival, or overall survival for any of the three treatment arms.[5]

Because one half of the patients treated with segmental mastectomy did not receive radiation therapy, we will be able to determine the effects of surgical therapy and radiation therapy on the problem of multicentric neoplasia. Within the segmental mastectomy groups, there is evidence that radiation therapy prevents local recurrence to a considerable extent. Patients who had segmental mastectomy alone had a 28% local recurrence rate compared with 8% for those treated with segmental mastectomy plus radiation therapy[5] (Figure 5).

Patients with positive nodes had a 36% local recurrence rate if radiotherapy was not given and a 2% recurrence rate if radiotherapy was given. This freedom from local recurrence in patients with positive nodes is surprisingly better than that for the patients with negative nodes. As those with positive nodes all received chemotherapy, it is reasonable to speculate that there may

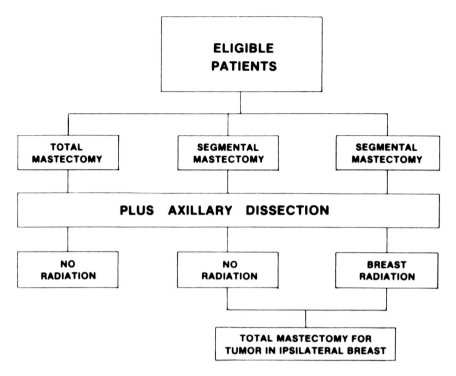

Figure 4.   Schema for Protocol B-06. Evaluation of total mastectomy versus segmental mastectomy with or without radiation.

be an additive or even a synergistic effect between these two modalities that helps to diminish the incidence of local recurrence in this group of patients.

This difference in local recurrence rate, however, has no impact on disease-free survival, distant disease-free survival, or overall survival. These end points are the same for all three treatment arms (Figure 6). These findings support and extend the original hypothesis. It is disseminated disease and not the primary tumor that causes ultimate failure. Therefore, an integral part of breast cancer treatment must be systemic therapy.

Adjuvant Chemotherapy Studies

Beginning in 1972, the NSABP instituted Protocol B-05, which was a series of trials of systemic adjuvant therapy with a single drug, L-phenyl-alanine mustard. The group of patients receiving this treatment was compared with a group receiving standard surgical treatment and placebo. Early analysis showed a delay in recurrence in drug-treated patients.[6] Following this, a series of second generation protocols was undertaken, in a stepwise process, to evaluate several two- and three-drug combinations. Results of these various studies indicate a distinct and significant advantage for certain

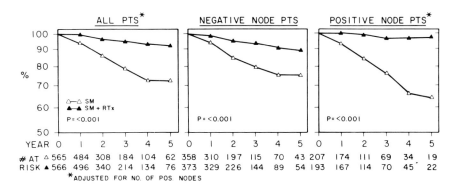

Figure 5. Percentage of patients remaining free of breast tumor after segmental mastectomy (SM) or segmental mastectomy with breast irradiation (SM + RTx).

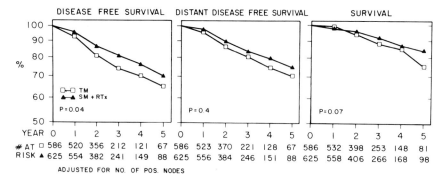

Figure 6. Disease-free survival, distant disease-free survival, and overall survival of patients treated by total mastectomy (TM) or by segmental mastectomy plus radiation (SM + RTx).

groups of women who receive adjuvant chemotherapy.[8] The advantage is most clearly displayed in those patients who are less than 49 years old with fewer than four lymph nodes involved. Ten-year results show a 64% reduction in mortality for this group.[8]

When compared with the results from other studies, the trends seem to be fairly consistent.[1] The natural history of breast cancer has been altered, and particular survival advantages are detected amongst younger women with small lymph node tumor burdens. While these results are encouraging, the process is still evolving, and further studies will be necessary in order to extend these gains.

SUMMARY

The current biologic concept of the behavior of breast cancer indicates that both systemic and local treatment factors are important. Radical and en bloc operations do not provide improved survival. Tests of various local and regional therapies (radical mastectomy, total mastectomy plus radiation therapy, total mastectomy alone, segmental mastectomy, and segmental mastectomy plus radiation therapy) all have equivalent outcomes. Improved survival rates will come only from the combination of adequate locoregional procedures and effective systemic treatments. The ongoing adjuvant studies of the NSABP and others are aimed at this goal.

REFERENCES

1. Bonadonna G, Valagussa P: Adjuvant systemic therapy for resectable breast cancer. J Clin Oncol 3:259–275, 1985.
2. Butcher HR, Seaman WB, Eckert C, et al.: Assessment of radical mastectomy and postoperative irradiation therapy in treatment of mammary cancer. Cancer 17:480–485, 1964.
3. Crile G: Treatment of breast cancer by local excision. Am J Surg 109:400–403, 1965.
4. Fisher B: Laboratory and clinical research in breast cancer — A personal adventure. The David A Karnofsky Memorial Lecture. Cancer Res 40:3863–3874, 1980.
5. Fisher B, Bauer M, Margolese R, et al.: Five-year results of a randomized clinical trial comparing total mastectomy and segmental mastectomy with or without radiation in the treatment of breast cancer. N Engl J Med 312:665–673, 1985.
6. Fisher B, Carbone P, Economou SG, et al.: L-phenylalanine mustard (L-PAM) in management of primary breast cancer: Report of early findings. N Engl J Med 292:117, 1975.
7. Fisher B, Redmond C, Fisher E, et al.: Ten-year results of a randomized clinical trial comparing radical mastectomy and total mastectomy with or without radiation. N Engl J Med 312:674–681, 1985.
8. Fisher B, Redmond C, Fisher E, et al.: *Systemic Adjuvant Therapy in Treatment of Primary Operable Breast Cancer: National Surgical Adjuvant Breast and Bowel Group Experience.* NCI Monographs, 35:44, 1986.
9. Halsted WS: The results of radical operations for the cure of carcinoma of the breast. Ann Surg 56:1–19, 1907.
10. Kaae S, Johansen H: Breast cancer. Comparison of results of simple mastectomy with postoperative roentgen irradiation by McWhirter method with those of extended radical mastectomy. Acta Radiol [Suppl] (Stockh) 188:155–161, 1959.
11. Lewis D, Rienhoff WF: A study of results — Johns Hopkins Hospital 1889–1931. Ann Surg 95:336, 1932.

12. McWhirter R: Simple mastectomy and radiotherapy in treatment of breast cancer. Br J Radiol 28:128–139, 1955.
13. Paterson R, Russell MH: Clinical trials in malignant disease. III. Breast cancer: Evaluation of postoperative radiotherapy. J Fac Radiol 10:175–180, 1959.
14. Urban JA, Baker HW: Radical mastectomy in continuity with en bloc resection of internal mammary lymph node chain; new procedure for primary operable cancer of breast. Cancer 5:992–1008, 1952.

3. *Coping with Breast Cancer: What Health Professionals Can Do to Help*

ROSE KUSHNER

Ask any woman what disease she dreads most, and she will say "breast cancer." Mammary carcinoma is now epidemic in the United States: The American Cancer Society and the National Cancer Institute predict that about 123,000 new cases were diagnosed in 1986. This means almost one of ten American women can expect to develop breast cancer at some time in her life. It accounts for 28% of all female cancers. And mammary carcinoma is a lethal disease. An estimated 40,200 women, treated in previous years, will die of breast cancer in 1986.[1]

All grave illnesses cause changes in lifestyle; many result in disability and disfigurement; some cause economic hardship; all are accompanied by some psychological trauma. But the mammary gland is not merely another organ of a woman's body: It is the foremost visible symbol of her femininity, sexuality, and maternity. To women of all past and current cultures, losing a breast — or even to be threatened with its loss — is devastating.

While many people believe "breast worship" is a twentieth-century, American, *Playboy/Penthouse* phenomenon, this is not so. The ancient Greek historian, Herodotus, chronicled that Atossa, daughter of the Persian king Cyrus the Great and wife of Darius I, concealed her breast tumor from everyone until it ulcerated and could no longer be hidden from her husband. In many countries of the world, women remember St. Agatha, the patron saint of breasts, on the fifth of February every year in honor of the young Roman virgin whose breasts were torn off by giant pincers because she refused to share her bed with the governor of Sicily.

Dr. Edward F. Lewison, of the Johns Hopkins Hospital Breast Cancer Clinic in Baltimore, said breast worship is eternal and universal:

> It is a revealing commentary to note that throughout the annals of history women have never outlived their vanity. Cosmetic considerations and false

21

modesty have hindered the early diagnosis and timely treatment of breast cancer from the dawn of humanity until today. Since the breast has always been an aesthetic symbol of fertility and womanhood, amputation of the breast provoked mutilation of the mind as well as the body.[12]

In 1986, it seems as if "coping with breast cancer" — in the sense of having constant anxiety about developing the disease — is an everyday factor that affects every woman in the western world throughout her entire adult life. Fear of breast cancer, as a matter of fact, often begins much earlier: Young girls who have seen mothers, aunts, or other relatives endure its treatment start worrying as soon as the two small bumps on their preadolescent chests begin to sprout. Even if they never actually develop breast cancer, they are nonetheless "coping" with the disease.[2]

There have been numerous studies of women's emotional suffering after having one or two mastectomies, and there has also been some retrospective research to study women after diagnosis and treatment. For example, "avoidance," "delay," "lagtime," etc., (patients' *and* physicians') between women's discovery of a symptom and its eventual diagnosis have been analyzed extensively.[5,13,16,18] Other work compared anxiety levels before and after a biopsy to see if women who were found to have cancer had higher anxiety levels than those who did not.[9] There have also been studies of the avoidance behaviors (denial) of asymptomatic women, behaviors that prevent them from dealing with breast cancer in any way.[4,7,8]

But no research has been done to even try to estimate the emotional price healthy women pay as they wait, watch, and worry that the sword of Damocles will fall. The only clue about this psychological trauma may be the increasing use of prophylactic mastectomy to prevent breast cancer: The Breast Cancer Task Force of the National Cancer Institute, in two separate conferences, heard data suggesting that as many as 10,000 women agreed to have their healthy breasts amputated and replaced with implants in 1982![3]

Therefore, annual incidence rates cannot and do not mirror the magnitude of the emotional pain of the long disease process known as breast cancer, because they ignore the vital prediagnostic and pretreatment intervals: (1) the anxiety and distress of the tens of millions of women who dread the disease for personal reasons and who are constantly reminded of it by publicity urging them to examine their breasts regularly; and (2) the pain suffered (and money spent) by millions of women who do find lumps, thickenings, or other symptoms of breast cancer, who must endure countless examinations, tests, and biopsies — but who never develop mammary carcinoma at all.[11]

PRECLINICAL ANXIETY

The suffering that women *without* breast cancer endure can be described by the term "preclinical anxiety," a period whose severity will never be quantified. Obviously, since so many women are affected, it is impossible to measure their emotional pain before they are diagnosed to have breast cancer.

Denial

While more and more women are examining their breasts routinely as part of their personal wellness and fitness plans, all surveys indicate that no more than 25% of women ever do so regularly. Many do not want to look for something they do *not* want to find and refuse to examine their breasts or have their doctors examine them. Health care providers can do little about their obsessive fears except to try to give the time and effort to reassure them. Whatever their reasons for refusal may be, these women are also "coping with breast cancer."[10,17] These women suffer in silence, and their attitudes are also never calculated, tabulated, and recorded.

However, the second and third intervals of preclinical anxiety can be measured and can even be staged, just as the disease itself is staged.[11]

Discovery of a Symptom

About 90% of all breast cancers are found by women themselves during deliberate self-examination or accidentally. In addition, partners frequently discover them while making love. Although some women request a professional examination immediately, most wait weeks—or even months—or more to see if the symptom disappears. And while they wait, they worry.[3]

Professional Examination

Most women who find breast cancer symptoms eventually call their physicians for professional examinations and must then wait for seemingly endless weeks for office visits where they are palpated, light-scanned, thermographed, sonographed, mammographed, and aspirated.

The vast majority of them, of course, will be told the symptom was harmless and to stop worrying. But about a half million women in the United States—more than 1,000 every day—will be wheeled into operating rooms for biopsies, and will learn, two or three harrowing days later, that "it" was a lipoma, fibroadenoma, papilloma, or that ubiquitous umbrella diagnosis, "benign fibrocystic disease."[10]

Since such lesions are not malignant, the ordeals these women endure are not included in biostatisticians' incidence tables and charts. Yet the women who *never* develop mammary carcinoma, but experience considerable emotional pain, are also "coping with breast cancer."[11]

A Scenario: Mrs. A, Mrs. B, and Mrs. C

One way to illustrate the emotional costs of preclinical anxiety is to follow three women, who do examine their breasts, as they travel along the tortuous road of waiting, watching, and worrying.

Mrs. A represents women who do breast self-examination regularly and never find a symptom. Every month, as BSE time approaches, Mrs. A is frightened and apprehensive that she will certainly discover a lump this time. But she never does.

Before and during her annual professional examinations, Mrs. A is petrified that her doctor will find something. But this too never happens.

Afterward, she breathes a sigh of relief . . . until next time. Mrs. A is also coping with breast cancer.

Mrs. B represents women who find symptoms but do nothing about them. Like "deniers" who refuse to examine their breasts, women represented by Mrs. B never enter the health care "pipeline" at all. Obviously, there can be two outcomes: If the lesion is carcinoma, it may grow, metastasize, and cause her death; or, benign or malignant, it may never create any life-threatening problem. As she waits, worries, and watches, silent and symptomatic, Mrs. B is coping with breast cancer.

Mrs. C represents most American women who find a symptom. While some "self-refer" immediately to a surgeon, they are exceptions: Ninety per cent of American women who see any doctor at all consider their OB/GYNs or family doctors to be their primary care physicians.

Premenopausal women who find a lesion often wait for two or three menstrual cycles before calling their doctors to see if "it goes away"; postmenopausal women are less likely to wait as long before calling their doctors. But all are frantic with fear as they count the waiting days on their calendars. Usually, they make their initial visit alone, telling no one about the symptom.[2]

Some OB/GYNs, family practitioners, and primary care providers know enough about breast disease to be able to determine that a symptom is a harmless fluid-filled cyst by aspirating it. If the mass is solid, however, primary care providers—too often—tell patients to "watch it" for a few months and return for another examination. This medical habit, almost routine for women under age 40, is, happily, changing as more and more health professionals are learning more and more about breast cancer and are referring symptomatic women of all ages to radiologists for mammography or directly to surgeons as quickly as possible.

Everyone who cares for women during this emotionally critical stage must realize how painful and traumatic the many inevitable waiting periods are to their patients. First, women must wait for the initial examination; then, for appointments for mammography, ultrasonography, or other detection tests; next, for the films to be read, for the report to be dictated, typed, and mailed. Finally, women must wait for the primary physician to tell them that the examinations showed nothing.

Health care professionals can ease the pain and reduce the anxiety by instructing their office staffs to find time for women complaining of breast problems as quickly as possible. If this cannot be done, physicians can usually calm terrified women via telephone by explaining that breast cancer is never a medical emergency and that the warning "don't delay" refers to weeks and months, not to a few days.

Open Surgical Biopsy

Regardless of age, risk status, or the results of any detection modality, a woman whose breast symptom persists, who began by visiting an OB/GYN, surgeon, or family physician—after months of watching, waiting, and worrying (and perhaps hundreds of dollars)—will eventually end her odyssey on an operating room table. This means more dreadful days of calendar watching for an empty slot on the operating schedule, either as an out- or inpatient.

While fewer women must suffer through this part of preclinical anxiety, the total is still impressively high: To discover the 123,000 new cases of breast cancer estimated for 1986, more than a half-million women will undergo a surgical biopsy. Until the mid-1970s, most women admitted to hospitals for breast biopsies were required to sign a form granting the surgeon permission to perform an immediate mastectomy if cancer is found on frozen section. Of course, the vast majority of breast lesions are not malignant, but each woman endured the same anguish of going to sleep without knowing if she would wake up with one breast or with both.

In June 1979, the National Institutes of Health recommended that breast biopsies be separated from treatment (by mastectomy or any other surgery) in what has become known as the "two-stage procedure." Women, in general, welcomed this NIH recommendation, because it gives them time to adjust to the frightening knowledge that they have "The Big C," to get second opinions on the diagnosis, and to investigate treatment alternatives other than mastectomy.[14]

But the two-stage procedure does have disadvantages. In addition to enduring another anxious period of waiting, women facing surgical biopsies must choose between several "forks" they will encounter in the tortuous road from BSE to definitive treatment. When such therapy immediately follows a frozen section diagnosis of carcinoma, these decisions are usually made for her. These women, of course, have the right to ask about being inpatients or outpatients; whether the anesthetic will be local or general; or if the vital estrogen and progesterone receptor assays will be done. As a rule, however, these decisions are made for them by their surgeons.

Waiting for the Diagnosis

Women who choose the two-stage procedure and have biopsies performed separately must undergo yet another waiting period of preclinical anxiety: two or three days for the pathologist's permanent section diagnosis.

During the last two decades, psychosocial researchers have studied the emotional trauma of breast cancer as if women's psychic suffering begins only at the moment of diagnosis or mastectomy.[4,17,18,19] Yet the preceding events, which comprise the long interval of preclinical anxiety, have nothing to do with the emotional trauma of breast cancer treatment. Preclinical anxiety subjects the hundreds of thousands of lucky women who do *not* have cancer to the same anguish as the unfortunate fraction who do.[2]

CLINICAL ANXIETY

Staging

While the women who had benign lesions go home to have happy champagne celebrations, their less fortunate sisters must brace themselves for staging, the first phase of the most stressful time, "clinical anxiety."

Will the tests show that the disease has already spread to other organs? Was the breast tumor discovered "too late"? The terrifying word "inoperable" is in every patient's thoughts as she is shunted from department to department for X-rays, scans, and laboratory workups.

More waiting, watching and worrying.

Of course, women who have one-stage biopsy/immediate-treatment procedures should be staged to rule out the presence of disseminated disease before any definitive therapy is performed.

Choosing Definitive Treatment

Although the classical Halsted radical mastectomy is no longer routine in the United States, the majority of surgeons in this country were trained to believe amputating the breast is the only safe treatment for mammary carcinoma. Most women, however, thanks to newspapers, magazines, television, and radio, are well aware of various kinds of breast-conservation procedures in which the tumor and axillary lymph nodes are removed but the breast is left relatively intact. Regardless of age, thousands of women want to investigate treatments other than mastectomy. Indeed, by October 1986, more than a dozen states had enacted "informed decision" legislation requiring that physicians tell women diagnosed to have breast cancer about the various treatment options available to them.[11]

Actually, there are only four viable choices, if the archaic Halsted radical is omitted: (1) most important, but rarely suggested, is participating in a controlled clinical trial in which patients are randomly assigned to a specific procedure; (2) the modified mastectomy (also known as total mastectomy plus an axillary dissection); (3) some kind of partial mastectomy (known variously as quadrantectomy, wedge resection, segmental resection, lumpectomy, tylectomy, wide excision, local excision, etc.) followed by radiotherapy to the preserved breast; and (4) a partial surgical procedure *without* postoperative irradiation.

Regardless of the treatment given to the breast, experts generally agree that at least a sampling of ten or a dozen axillary lymph nodes must be excised to stage the patient for extent of the disease.[6]

Health professionals should (must!) begin to add their crisis intervention techniques to this difficult period of clinical anxiety, because each of the procedures has risks as well as benefits, disadvantages as well as advantages.

Since mastectomy has been the "gold standard" for the past century, its physical and psychological sequelae are well known. But doctors and patients are still learning the problems that may accompany partial breast surgery, especially procedures that are followed by radiotherapy. By asking a few questions, health care providers can help women unravel the tangled knot of confusion and contradiction they face at this time:

1. What size is the tumor in relation to the breast? Because the main purpose of conservation surgery is cosmesis, excising a cancer plus an adequate margin of healthy tissue can leave a small breast unattractive. A woman whose brassiere cup size is AAA would probably be happier with a modified mastectomy followed by reconstructive plastic surgery.

2. Can the patient "live with uncertainty"? Does she believe breast conservation procedures are not as safe as mastectomy? Does she worry that her family and friends will think she is vain "to play Russian roulette" with a still, to many, unproved therapy?

   For women who are considering partial surgery followed by irradiation, there are other questions whose answers will help their decision making:

3. Is she afraid of radiation, in general? Does she worry about accidents in nuclear power plants or about the dozens of X-rays taken of her feet in shoe stores when she was a child? If so, radiotherapy may not be for her.

4. Does her medical insurance policy cover radiation as a primary therapy for breast cancer? Some third party carriers still consider breast-conservation procedures to be "experimental," and since five weeks of irradiation can cost as much as $5,000, inability to pay could rule this option out immediately.

A woman's fiscal status can be just as important as her physical status when treatment options are considered.

5. Can the patient visit a radiotherapist every day for five weeks? If, for example, she has small children and cannot afford to hire a baby-sitter or if she would lose her job, these are "risks" of breast-conservation procedures that must be taken into account.

6. Is there a trained, qualified, and experienced radiation oncologist, with appropriate equipment for treating the intact breast, near her home? The American Society of Therapeutic Radiation Oncologists has a membership of about 2,000 certified radiotherapists, and most work in medical centers in large cities. If no such specialist is conveniently located, this factor has a profound effect on a breast cancer patient's "available" treatment options.

Women who opt for the higher-risk procedure that includes partial surgery *without* irradiation must be carefully followed for at least the first three postoperative years. According to data from numerous studies, these women have a 20% to 25% higher incidence of local breast recurrences. Frequent and diligent monitoring is imperative to detect and treat such second tumors as early as possible. For these women, there are other questions:

7. Does she practice regular BSE? Is she confident that she would be able to find and recognize a new growth, or any other change?

8. Is she financially and logistically able to see the doctor as often as might be necessary during the first five postoperative years?

Problems in breast cancer patients' decision making are compounded by the fact that each of these alternatives has other suboptions women may need to explore, with the assistance of an informed health professional. For example, if a woman chooses mastectomy because she believes it is safer, does she want to have the lost breast reconstructed?

Does her surgical oncologist know a board-certified plastic surgeon? If so, can the reconstructive surgery be done at the time of mastectomy? Must there be a delay? What kind of implant should be used? Is she at such high risk (e.g., because of a strong family history) that she should seriously consider having a prophylactic mastectomy on her contralateral breast? If so, would this be done at the same time as the initial surgery, or later?

If segmental surgery and radiation are chosen, this procedure also has suboptions. Should a boost of radiation be applied to the tumor site? If so, will it be electron beam therapy or interstitial implants? If a woman has a medial lesion, should her internal mammary and supraclavicular nodes be irradiated?

The list of questions to be asked and answered is literally endless. Thus, health care professionals, especially those involved with crisis intervention, must have the medical and surgical knowledge to help patients understand their options enough to assist in making such treatment decisions, if they wish.

Controlled Clinical Trials

Participating in a clinical trial was mentioned earlier as one of the four primary treatment options that health professionals should offer women with newly diagnosed breast cancer. Until January 31, 1984, this was a vital "first alternative" that was widely available to patients in the United States and Canada. The National Surgical Adjuvant Breast Project (NSABP), chaired by Dr. Bernard Fisher, had been actively recruiting and randomizing women into Protocol B-06, a clinical trial to compare total mastectomy with axillary dissection (modified radical mastectomy) with segmental surgery with and without postoperative radiotherapy.[6]

Although this international trial has accrued all the patients it needed, there is another that can still be offered: The National Cancer Institute (NCI) in Bethesda, Maryland, has been conducting a two-armed trial to compare mastectomy with lumpectomy (removal of the tumor *only*) since 1979 and is still recruiting.

All detection, diagnostic, and therapeutic procedures are performed at no cost to the patients, and women randomized to mastectomy may also have reconstructive mammoplasty free of charge. For those randomized to lumpectomy and radiation, the NCI will provide financial assistance for travel and hotel expenses.[11] The value of lifetime follow-up care, an important part of this trial, cannot be underestimated.

Health professionals should tell interested women about the NCI's Early Breast Cancer Trial and give them the telephone number of the director of the protocol, Dr. Judith Bader: (301) 496-5457.

In early 1986, the NSABP began a randomized trial to compare lumpectomy alone with lumpectomy plus irradiation for the primary treatment of intraductal carcinoma in situ. About 3,000 women will be needed to obtain statistically significant data. Mary Ketner ([412] 648-9720), coordinator of all NSABP trials, will be happy to provide complete information about eligibility criteria for enrollment in this, or any, NSABP trial.

In addition, there are numerous trials sponsored locally or regionally by individual cancer centers, and health professionals who cannot tell their patients details about relevant clinical trials are not really offering them all available options. To keep current, doctors, nurses, and other health care providers must become familiar with the NCI's Physician Data Query (PDQ) "on-line" information system. It might also be valuable to patients for health care providers to learn what information the nearest office of the Institute's national toll-free Cancer Information Service (CIS) hotline, 1–800–4-CAN-CER, gives women who call with questions about breast cancer. Since the various CIS offices are independent contractors to the NCI, the information they give often differs from area to area around the country.

Waiting for Pathology Reports

When a woman has a symptom of breast cancer, she is most anxious about what is to be done to her breast, but physicians are more concerned about her nodal status because of the disease's invasive potential. At this time, the presence or absence of cancer in the axillary lymph nodes is the only way they can even guesstimate which women are most likely to experience recurrence and/or develop metastases in other organs. It has been proved that premenopausal women are being helped by adjuvant chemotherapy, while adjuvant endocrine therapy, using tamoxifen, has increased disease-free intervals for postmenopausal women.

Deciding on appropriate adjuvant therapy, of course, is the time when the results of the estrogen and progesterone receptor assays are imperative for informed decision making: Women whose tumors were "rich" (or positive) in receptors are treated differently from those whose cancers were "poor" (or negative). So regardless of the local treatment performed, all breast cancer patients must once again wait anxiously for two or three days while pathologists examine their nodes, measure receptors, dictate a report, have it typed, and finally send it to the woman's surgeon. Patients treated by mastectomy who are node-negative and hormone-positive can breathe sighs of relief and begin making plans for breast reconstruction if they wish. Women who had partial mastectomy and are node-negative can begin radiotherapy as soon as possible

But if cancer is found in a single node of a premenopausal woman, all plans for mammoplasty to replace the lost breast must wait at least six months until adjuvant chemotherapy is completed. Premenopausal women found to have positive axillary nodes after segmental mastectomy are usually given one course of adjuvant chemotherapy before the radiotherapy begins. Afterward, a schedule of "interdigitation" is planned for the five weeks of radiation treatments.

If a woman is Stage II, postmenopausal and hormone receptor–positive, her adjuvant therapy will probably be the antiestrogen tamoxifen, and she can proceed with reconstructive mammoplasty or radiotherapy as if she were Stage I.

Coping with Adjuvant Chemotherapy

Health professionals who want to help women solve their psychosocial problems must also know the answers to medical questions about the whys and wherefores of adjuvant therapy for this interval of "crisis intervention." Sensitive and knowledgeable health professionals can play most important roles before and during the interval of clinical anxiety when breast cancer patients at high risk of recurrence are being prescribed adjuvant regimens of various types.

While there are only four options for primary treatment of breast cancer, there are so many adjuvant therapies in use that newly diagnosed Stage II patients need an IBM mainframe computer to learn the hundreds of permutations and combinations of anticancer agents available to them.

And there are so many conflicting and confusing data about their usage that a Consensus Development Conference, sponsored in September 1985 by the National Institutes of Health, recommended that *all patients and their physicians are strongly encouraged to participate in controlled clinical trials.*[15]

By following this NIH recommendation, health professionals can give women the most valuable assistance possible. The data reported to the Consensus Conference proved that "optimal" adjuvant therapy is still unknown. There is, at this time, no combination of drugs whose dosage, sequencing, and duration have been shown to be superior to any other.

Thus, all women assigned to any adjuvant regimen are being treated with investigational therapies; all are essentially acting as guinea pigs. While about 50,000 women will be found to have Stage II disease in 1986, only a maximum of 6% of them will be treated in the setting of a controlled clinical trial.[15] The other 90% will be using physicians who do not belong to any oncology group; their experiences and outcomes are not reported to any central computer where they would help future generations of breast cancer patients. The other 90% will be using physicians who report their data only to their patients' medical insurance company.

Any attempts at "crisis intervention" during this time must stress the importance of being treated within the setting of an approved, controlled, randomized clinical trial. And health professionals should help women find appropriate trials for their age and stage of disease by calling the PDQ or the CIS.

Afterward, they should turn their attention to assisting patients with the routine problems of managing the side effects of chemotherapy. Many cancer patients of both genders have reported alopecia to be more psychologically painful than losing a limb or an organ. To help women during this time, there are many ways health care providers can be of service. For example, they might put together a list of places where wigs can be bought at reasonable prices or even borrowed. Instructions for designing and making attractive turbans are also helpful. Medications for nausea, vomiting, diarrhea, and mouth sores are available, but oncologists may neglect these "tolerable" problems because patients often believe they must develop a "red badge of courage" attitude that they are having no trouble.[9]

Health professionals, especially nurse oncologists, must be aware of women's reluctance to complain and take the time and make the effort to draw out details about unreported side effects. Because many financial costs of breast cancer—travel, housekeepers, baby-sitters, parking fees, some medications, etc.—are not reimbursed, worries about money may also be plaguing patients. In addition, sensitive doctors and nurses can help women by referring them for psychiatric or psychological counseling if and when they need more than a shoulder to cry on.

POSTCLINICAL ANXIETY: LIVING WITH FEAR

Statistically, about 25% of node-negative women will develop metastatic disease in spite of the absence of cancer in their axillas; those who had positive nodes and received adjuvant therapy have, of course, a higher risk of recurrence. So all women treated for breast cancer face added years of waiting, watching, and worrying about unusual bone pain, hoarseness, coughing, and digestive problems. Moreover, women who have had cancer in one breast have a higher risk of developing another in the remaining breast. Periodic follow-up examinations, with all their accompanying anxieties, become new patterns of their lives.

The lucky hundreds of thousands whose lumps were benign also face years of anguish and anxiety, because they are now in the high-risk category. Some will deny; some will opt for prophylactic mastectomies. All of these women — after suffering through weeks or months of waiting, multiple examinations, and finally, diagnostic surgery — will again face the harrowing ordeal of "coping with breast cancer" from the beginning.

Health professionals must understand that coping with breast cancer is a lifetime problem and that the standard definition of crisis intervention must be changed to include giving their patients knowledge to make intelligent and informed decisions about their treatment. By learning all they can about the medical and surgical aspects of breast cancer treatment, psychiatrists, psychologists, social workers, and other mental health professionals can help women make such informed decisions.

An excellent slogan is that a woman's rehabilitation from the trauma of breast cancer begins the moment her disease is diagnosed.

REFERENCES

1. American Cancer Society: *1986 Cancer Facts and Figures.*
2. Breast Cancer Advisory Center Data Bank: Kensington, MD (1975–86).
3. Breast Cancer Task Force, National Cancer Institute, Bethesda, 1984.
4. Buls JG et al.: Women's attitudes to mastectomy for breast cancer. Med J Aust, 2:336–38, 1976.
5. Cameron A, Hinton J: Delay in seeking treatment for mammary tumors, Cancer 21: 1121–26, 1968.
6. Fisher B, Bauer M, Margolese R, et al.: Five-year results of a randomized clinical trial comparing total mastectomy and segmental mastectomy with or without radiation in the treatment of breast cancer. N Engl J Med 312:665–73.

7. Gallup Organization, Inc. Women's attitudes regarding breast cancer. American Cancer Society, New Jersey, 1973.
8. Greer S, Morris T: Psychological attributes of women who develop breast cancer. J Psychosom Res 19:147-53.
9. Henry J: *Surviving the Cure*. Cleveland, Cope, Inc., 1984.
10. Ingall J: *Hope versus Fear—Action versus Inaction*. London, ISPO, 1980.
11. Kushner R: *Alternatives: New Developments in the War on Breast Cancer*. Warner Books, New York, 1986.
12. Lewison EF: *Breast Cancer and Its Diagnosis and Treatment*. Baltimore, Williams & Wilkins, 1955.
13. Magary J, Todd P: Breast loss and delay in breast cancer: Behavioral science in surgical research. Aust NZ J Surg, 46:391-93, 1976.
14. National Institutes of Health, Consensus Development Conference Recommendations: *Primary Treatment of Breast Cancer*, 1979.
15. National Institutes of Health, Consensus Development Conference Recommendations: *Adjuvant Chemotherapy for Breast Cancer*, 1985.
16. Opinion Research Corp: *Breast Cancer: A Measure of Progress in Public Understanding*. National Cancer Institute, 1980.
17. Rosser JE: The interpretation of women's experience: a critical appraisal of the literature on breast cancer. Soc Sci Med [E] 15:257-65, 1981.
18. Stoll BA: *Coping with Cancer Stress*. Dordrecht/Boston/Lancaster, Martinus Nijhoff, 1986.
19. Worden JW, Weisman AD: Psychosocial components of lagtime in cancer diagnosis. *J Psychosom Res* 19:69-79, 1975.

4. Payments for Breast Cancer During 1985: The Michigan Blue Cross/ Blue Shield Experience

GEORGE R. GERBER

Breast cancer is a costly disease both in the toll it takes on human lives and in the portion of the health care dollar that it consumes. This year 130,000 women will receive a diagnosis of breast cancer—one in ten women in the United States, according to the latest statistics from the American Cancer Society. In the same time period, approximately 41,000 will die from the disease.[1]

Only a few previous studies have specifically addressed the monetary costs of breast cancer. Using Blue Cross/Blue Shield records from the year 1980, Long and colleagues ascertained the costs during the last year of life of 1,054 people with terminal cancer.[4] Of these, 235 had breast cancer. The mean expenditure for these breast cancer patients during their last year of life was $14,545/patient. This included charges for inpatient hospitalization, physician's services, hospital outpatient services, and other services, which covered some major medical and prescription drugs and claims for nonhospital services, such as home care and extended care facilities.[2]

This review presents the Blue Cross/Blue Shield payments for the diagnosis and treatment of breast cancer in one statewide population. As pressures for cost-effective treatment and limitations on hospital stays mount, detailed and accurate information will become more important. While these data are preliminary, and by no means exhaustive, they represent a necessary early step in portraying the financial burden this disease.

METHODOLOGY

Data from the 1985 Michigan Blue Cross/Blue Shield files were run against the ICD9CM codes for three types of diagnostic mammography;

Table 1. Mammographies with All Diagnoses, 1985

Type	ICD9CM Code	Number of Procedures	Total BC/BS Payments	Payment per Procedure
Unilateral	76090 (7565)	2,601	$ 104,825	$40.30
Bilateral	76091 (7655)	48,211	3,065,963	63.59*
Xerography	76150 (7573)	56,734	525,664	9.27†
TOTAL		107,546	$3,696,452	

*weighted average payment = $62.39
†additional amount over mammography whether bilateral or unilateral

five procedures for the surgical treatment of breast cancer; therapeutic radiation for breast cancer; and chemotherapy for breast cancer.

Information retrieved included: payments for diagnostic mammography; payments for inpatient treatment; payments for professional fees; number and type of surgical procedures performed; total and average payments for each procedure; and average costs for radiation therapy and chemotherapy. The latter was run on a random sample of 15 patients rather than the entire Michigan cohort, as was the case for the surgical procedures.

TOTAL PAYMENTS

In 1985, Michigan Blue Cross/Blue Shield paid out $9,488,752.83 in charges for diagnosis and treatment of breast cancer. Of this total, $6,641,837.30 was for inpatient charges and $2,846,915.53 for professional fees. These by no means represent all the costs incurred by patients or payers. For example, breast reconstruction (unless done at the time of mastectomy), physical therapy, prostheses, and psychotherapy, although reimbursable by the Blues, are not included in these figures. Other costs, such as prescription drugs and follow-up office visits, which the patient or other third-party payers bore, are also excluded.

The inpatient charges represent a total of 1822 patients spending 12,076 days in the hospital. This constitutes an average length of stay of 6.63 days/ patient. The total charges incurred were $8,703,298.50, some $2 million beyond what was paid by Blue Cross. The average payment per case was $3645.36 resulting in a per diem average payment of $550.00.

Table 1 shows the number of procedures, overall Blues payments, and the average cost of each of three types of diagnostic mammography. These data were not run against a specific diagnosis of cancer, but rather represent the total number of diagnostic mammograms performed. Of the 107,546 mammograms, only a small percentage of the patients actually had cancer. The maximum Blue Cross payment for a mammogram is $88.00, while the weighted average Blue Cross payment for mammography is $62.39.

The payments for selected surgical procedures performed for a diagnosis of cancer are outlined in Table 2. The average payment made was $834.92. It is interesting to note that the costs for a radical, modified radical, and partial mastectomy are very close. This valuation indicates that the surgical skill and time needed for each type of operation did not differ greatly.

Professional charges include chemotherapy and radiation therapy as well as surgeon's fees. Total payments reported for chemotherapy were $419,647. Radiation therapy charges totalled $1,178,904. The average cost of a course of radiation therapy was $1354.55. Chemotherapy netted an average charge of $30/treatment. Assuming an average course of 15 treatments, the cost for a course of chemotherapy was $450.

Reconstruction, when performed at the time of mastectomy, added between $150 to $500 to the bill; nipple reconstruction was the most expensive. Immediate insertion of a prosthesis added about $300. The number of immediate reconstructions reflected in the 1985 Michigan data was low, only 21. Complete information on delayed reconstruction was not obtained in this data run, perhaps because delayed reconstruction was not submitted to Blue Cross/Blue Shield under the cancer diagnosis codes. The average payment for the 160 delayed breast reconstructions reported was $1358.

Payment Profile

Based on the data obtained, we developed a Blue Cross/Blue Shield payment profile for a patient with carcinoma of the breast. Typical costs break down as follows:

Preoperative office visit	$ 35.00
Diagnostic bilateral mammogram	88.00
Needle aspiration	46.00
Incisional biopsy (not including anesthesia)	260.00
Inpatient charges ($550/day, 6.63 days)	3646.50
Anesthesia	60.00
Modified radical mastectomy	838.77
Radiation therapy	1355.00
Chemotherapy ($30/visit, 15 visits)	450.00
TOTAL	$6779.27

As mentioned before, numerous other costs are not included in this figure, both those payable by the Blues and those that are not. It is safe to say that at least 20% more should be added onto the bill to cover those costs, giving an estimated total of $8072.72 charge for surgical excision and follow-up radiotherapy and chemotherapy.

Table 2.   Surgical Procedures for Breast Cancer, 1985

Type of operation	ICD9CM Code	Number of Procedures	BC/BS Payments	Payment per Procedure
Radical mastectomy	19200 (0483,0485)	120	$ 90,764	$ 756.37
Radical mastectomy with internal mammary nodes	19220 (0484)	16	18,746	1,171.63
Modified radical mastectomy	19240 (0486)	1,049	879,871	838.77
Partial mastectomy with axillary nodes	19162	1	813	813.00
Partial mastectomy	19160	570	240,540	422.00
TOTAL		1,756	$1,230,734	

COMPARATIVE COSTS OF MASTECTOMY VS LUMPECTOMY

One of the issues of debate in regard to treatment of breast cancer is whether breast-sparing procedures such as partial mastectomy (also known as quandrantectomy and lumpectomy) are preferable to the more traditional methods of radical mastectomy and modified radical mastectomy.

Munoz and colleagues of New York reported on a series of 79 patients with Stage I or Stage II disease treated during 1983 and 1984.[6] Mean total charges per patient for lumpectomy with axillary sampling and postoperative irradiation were $14,176 ± $4262 and for mastectomy and radiation were $10,345 ± $3134. Although hospital inpatient fees were significantly less for lumpectomy ($5741) than for mastectomy ($7238), mean total physician fees (including surgeon and radiation oncologist) were substantially higher for lumpectomy ($4505) than mastectomy (surgeon only, $3016). Substantial radiation therapy outpatient charges postoperatively ($5015) made the mean total charges for lumpectomy significantly higher than for mastectomy.[6]

Since our data are too sparse for comparison with those of Munoz—only one patient with lumpectomy and axillary node sampling was reported in 1985—we can only speculate on the universality of his findings. Logic tells us, however, that since the costs for the actual surgical procedure for a partial mastectomy and a modified radical mastectomy are not that far apart, and since it is obvious that partial mastectomy patients will need considerably more radiotherapy and chemotherapy, the breast-sparing procedure could end up being considerably more expensive, at least in the first year of treatment. On the other hand, costs for reconstruction for patients with more breast and muscle tissue removal could tend to even out the expenditures.[2] Also possible is the fact that patients losing a whole breast will need more support from physical therapists and psychotherapists, which increases the overall costs again. Over the long run, we can speculate that from the third-party payers' point of view, the breast-sparing procedures and the traditional operations will cost about the same in dollars and cents.

Our 1985 data indicate that physicians in Michigan still favored the traditional approach over the breast-sparing methods by a substantial margin. Since physicians and hospitals are often very slow to report their information to Blue Cross/Blue Shield, we may be seeing a lag of a year or so in the actual years of treatment represented. Wider advocacy of breast-sparing procedures within medical centers probably began about 1983 or 1984. Therefore, we need to reexamine these same data for the next few years to see if different trends emerge.

THE ROLE OF SCREENING MAMMOGRAPHY

A related issue springs forth from the information generated by this report: the costs and advisability of widespread diagnostic mammographic screening for breast cancer. Without question, mammography is the most important tool we have in the detection of breast cancer, yet it is a very expensive diagnostic procedure at $88/screen. Blue Cross/Blue Shield of Maryland has estimated that supplementary screening mammography coverage costs each of its subscribers $1.14/month.[5] Blue Cross/Blue Shield of Michigan does not currently pay for a screening mammogram. A complaint must be diagnosed if the Blues are to pay for mammograms. Even so, more than $3.5 million were paid out for this procedure in 1985.

Considering the nearly epidemic proportions of breast cancer, should screening mammography be made more widely available to the public? Some authors feel this is necessary and possible.[3,7,8] They recommend streamlining imaging and operational procedures, batch-processing of films, computerization of records, payment at the time of examination, and utilization of mobile vans.[7] If cheap and accessible screening methods can be developed, we believe that mass screening would be appropriate and would save enough lives and dollars to be worth the effort of setting up a program.

RELIABILITY OF THE DATA

While these 1985 Michigan data begin to give us a picture of the trends and costs in carcinoma of the breast, our feeling is that many of the numbers may be too low. Blue Cross/Blue Shield can only produce data as good as that which is given us. There are several explanations for the data being less accurate than we would like:

1. Physicians either fail to update their profiles or take a very long time to do so, thus, we may not have current fee ranges on file for charge data.
2. Incorrect code numbers are used for billing.
3. Incorrect diagnoses are reported.
4. Payments made by Blue Cross/Blue Shield may be less than the actual costs, depending on the type of plan under which the patient is covered or whether the patient has other insurers covering her medical costs.
5. A confounding factor involves the fact that in 1985 Blue Cross/Blue Shield initiated a coding changeover, and not all payment data have been converted to the new coding system for retrieval.

Reports like these can be of major service to physicians, hospitals, and consumers, but physician cooperation is necessary to make them accurate. Let me issue a plea to caregivers to report your data to us as promptly and accurately as you can, so we in turn can give them accurate cumulative information, report trends, and ultimately help to contain costs insofar as that is possible. I also recommend a carefully designed, ongoing, year-to-year study be initiated so that we can get a truer picture of what is going on with the treatment of this major disease. This is especially important because of the changing philosophy in regard to breast-sparing procedures.

REFERENCES

1. American Cancer Society. Cancer Facts and Figures for 1987.
2. Elias D, in discussion, Munoz E, Shamash F, Wise L, et al.: Lumpectomy vs mastectomy. Arch Surg 121:1301, 1986.
3. Feig SA: Assessment of the hypothetical risk from mammography and evaluation of the potential benefit. Radiol Clin North Am 21:173, 1983.
4. Long SH, Gibbs JO, Crozier JP, et al.: Medical expenditures of terminal cancer patients during the last year of life. Inquiry 21:315, 1984.
5. Maryland insurers pay for screening. ACR Bull, July, 1986, p5.
6. Munoz E, Shamash F, Wise L, et al.: Lumpectomy vs mastectomy. Arch Surg 121:1301, 1986.
7. Sickles EA, Weber WN, Galvin HB, et al.: Mammographic screening: How to operate successfully at low cost. Radiology 160:95, 1986.
8. Wertheimer MD, Costanza ME, Dodson TF, et al.: Increasing the effort toward breast cancer detection. JAMA 255:1311, 1986.

5. *Legal Requirements of Informed Consent for Treatment of Breast Cancer: Telling It All*

EDWARD B. GOLDMAN

Since 1980, several states have passed laws regulating consent for patients receiving treatment for breast cancer. These laws do not apply to all cancer patients but are strictly limited to breast cancer. The laws are probably a response to patients who consented to biopsies and allegedly were anesthetized, had positive biopsies, and then had that surgical procedure extended to radical mastectomy. The laws seek to avoid traumatizing women who have mastectomies without prior notice and preparation.

The laws are basically of two types. First, there are laws requiring that a specific consent form be executed prior to treatment. These laws typically provide patients with the option of consenting solely to biopsy or consenting to a biopsy and whatever added surgery is determined by their physician to be appropriate. Second, there are laws that mandate specific information be provided describing the advantages, disadvantages, and risks involved in medically appropriate treatment alternatives. This chapter will consider the rules of consent, specific laws concerning consent for breast cancer, and the implications of these laws.

THE RULES OF INFORMED CONSENT

General Rules

The term "informed consent" is a misnomer. This area of the law should more properly be called "informed choice." Why? Because the legal theory is that the health care professional should provide adequate information to allow the patient to be fully informed. The informed patient then makes a choice of treatments. The patient's choice can be documented, and treatment can then occur. Documentation is not essential unless mandated by

41

law, but it is useful to prove later that the exchange of information and the informed choice by the patient occurred.

The general rule is that absent a life-threatening emergency, no patient should be treated without receiving a clear explanation of his or her condition and of the proposed procedure to be carried out. The explanation should include the possible benefits of the treatment, possibilities of any substantial risks of serious side effects involved in the treatment, and medically significant alternative forms of treatment, and should be provided to a competent patient. The patient then chooses a treatment. Assuming that the treatment selected is agreed to by the physician and can be provided by the physician, treatment proceeds. If the treatment is medically appropriate but cannot be provided by the physician, a referral is necessary.

Rules Concerning Research

The rules concerning research will not be extensively discussed in this chapter. For a thorough discussion see Robert J. Levine, *Ethics and Regulation of Clinical Research*, Urban and Schwarzenberg, 1986.

Research is governed by specific federal law, which essentially says that no patient should be subjected to human experimentation without the patient's prior knowledge and approval. The patient must be given information regarding the experimental treatment, specifically including: (1) a fair explanation of the procedures to be followed including an identification of those which are experimental, (2) a description of the discomforts and risks, (3) a description of the potential benefits, (4) a disclosure of appropriate alternative procedures, (5) an offer to answer any questions concerning the procedures, and (6) notification that the subject is free to withdraw consent and discontinue participation in the project at any time without any loss of benefits to which the subject is otherwise entitled (Department of Health and Human Services Rules and Regulations 45CFR46 Section 46.116).

If a proposed treatment for breast cancer is experimental, then the process of obtaining institutional review board approval and acting in strict accordance with the federal regulations must occur.

The Elements of Consent

Consent must be voluntarily obtained from a competent patient. Voluntary is defined as a patient making a free choice without coercion. Competent patients are those who understand the nature and benefits of their actions. They do not have to make a choice preferred by the health care professional, but they do have to make a choice with a full understanding of the results of their choice. For example, a competent patient could say, "I understand the alternatives, and I choose not to seek treatment even though this will result in my death. I do this because I have carefully considered my situation in life, and I feel nontreatment is preferable to treatment with its attendant side effects and minimal likelihood of remission." Although the health care professional may disagree with this particular patient's choice, the patient is acting in a competent fashion.

The competent, voluntary patient must be told the nature of the procedure, the possible benefits, the possible risks, and the medically significant alternative forms of treatment. In explaining the procedure, the explanation should include any inconveniences the patient will encounter. For example, the procedure could include multiple return visits for radiation oncology or chemotherapy and involve restraints on normal activities following the procedure. The risks are the possible harmful effects which a reasonable person would wish to know. These risks include medically significant risks, as well as known side effects. For example, the chemotherapy may cause nausea, vomiting, hair loss, and other side effects. The benefits to be described are always potential benefits. There should never be a guarantee of cure.

The alternatives can include current as well as experimental treatment. One possible alternative is always no treatment, in which case other types of health care such as a hospice should be described. It is not necessary to describe medically ineffective treatments such as Laetrile.

Why Do Consent Requirements Exist?

Assault and Battery

Historically, informed consent comes from the notion that no one can be touched without the person's prior permission. Thus, doing a surgical procedure on someone first requires the person's consent. There are some historical cases where patients have received surgical treatment which results in a substantial enhancement of their condition, but nonetheless they sue, claiming that they did not give permission to have the procedure done. As Justice Benjamin Cardozo said, "every human being of adult years and sound mind has a right to determine what shall be done with his own body . . ." (*Scholendorff v Society of New York Hospital*, 211NY 125, 105NE 92 [1914]).

Avoiding Treating a Patient as a Passive Victim

The modern theory of consent is that it is negligent to provide treatment without prior permission. The word "victim" in the title of this section was chosen to emphasize the thrust behind the patients' rights movement. Patients feel that they can be victimized by having treatment without full knowledge and explanation of the treatment. In response to these feelings, many states have passed laws concerning patients' rights. For example, in Michigan the Public Health Code, at Section MCLA 333.20201 (2)(e), says that a patient is entitled to receive information about the proposed course of treatment in terms that the patient can understand.

This modern theory is especially relevant in the area of breast cancer treatment. Here patients have felt victimized and are seeking laws that require physicians to provide adequate and appropriate information prior to treatment.

Who Must Obtain Consent?

As a general rule, the physician performing or in charge of the treatment shall ensure that the patient is properly informed regarding the treatment. The discussion concerning the available treatments should occur between the physician or a member of the physician's team knowledgeable about the treatments and licensed to carry out the treatments. Consent is not an area to delegate to someone without adequate knowledge of the procedures. The patient's choice should then be documented by the person who provided the information.

When Should Consent Be Obtained?

In some instances there are specific laws about when consent should be obtained. For example, under the federal Medicare program, consent to sterilization must be obtained 30 days prior to the procedure. In general, consent should be obtained within 30 to 60 days before the treatment will be performed or whenever the course of treatment will be substantially altered. Many hospitals have their own internal rules for timing of consent. The hospital procedure manual should be consulted for those rules.

From Whom Should Consent Be Obtained?

Competent adult patients give their own consent for treatment. If an adult patient is not competent, that individual's legally authorized representative should grant or withhold consent. An individual can be legally authorized by being a guardian or by specific state law provisions. For example, many states have laws saying that a patient's spouse can consent on behalf of the incompetent patient.

If the patient is a minor, the legally authorized representative must grant or withhold consent for treatment. This is typically the minor's parent or legal guardian. In some cases, state and federal law allows a minor to consent. For example, under Michigan law minors may consent to medical advice or treatment for substance abuse or venereal disease without parental consent. The state law says a treating physician may, but is not obligated to, inform the parents as to treatment. See MCLA 333.5257 and MCLA 333.6121.

The Process of Consent

It is important to not confuse the consent process with the documentation that the process has occurred. The process is the time when the health care professional sits and discusses the procedure, its risks, possible benefits, and alternatives with the competent patient or the representative of the incompetent patient. The patient than has an opportunity to ask questions. Once the health care professional and the patient are comfortable that the patient is fully informed, the patient makes a choice.

Documentation of Consent

Once the patient has made a choice, the health care professional has several options. First, the procedure can proceed at that point. Second, a brief note can be made in the medical record stating "Procedure discussed, patient consented." Third, a more extensive note can be made describing the process in more detail and perhaps listing the risks, benefits, and alternatives. Fourth, a consent form can be filled out. These forms are generally supplied by the hospital and specifically document risks, benefits, and alternatives. Finally, since the items in the above list are not mutually exclusive, the health care professional could make a note in the record and fill out a form.

Documentation of consent is useful to prove that the process occurred. Some state laws on breast cancer specifically require documentation. Even in the absence of state law, it is simply easier to prove at trial what occurred if it is written down than if a health care professional is asked to remember several years after the fact what occurred. This proof issue is why oral agreements are reduced to written contracts.

It is always a good idea to use both a consent form and a brief note in the medical record. Notes written in the record are seen by juries as valid, truthful, and accurate since they were created before any injury or lawsuit. Of course, notes should never be altered following initiation of a lawsuit.

SPECIFIC LAWS CONCERNING TREATMENT
FOR BREAST CANCER

Law can be developed both through the courts and through the legislatures. Law made in court is called common law. Law made by legislatures is called statutory law. This section will discuss both common law and statutory law requirements.

Common Law

There have been a few court cases requiring physicians to disclose information in breast cancer treatment cases. For example, in *Truan v Smith* 578 SW 2nd, 73 (TN, 1979), a patient noticed a change in the size and firmness of her left breast. She discussed this with her family physician. He did not make an examination. She returned 45 days later complaining of numbness and pain. The physician did an examination and told her to return the following month. He did not mention the possibility of cancer. Her symptoms did not change, so she called the doctor's office to see if she should set up a return appointment. He did not call back. She then went to a specialist and obtained a diagnosis of metastatic breast cancer. She ultimately underwent radical mastectomy, chemotherapy, and other adjunct treatment. She sued the family physician, and the court found that the physician was negligent for not informing the patient of the possibility of cancer as a cause for her complaint. This case is a typical example of informed consent.

In an earlier California case, a woman agreed to undergo biopsy. She signed a consent to the biopsy. Biopsy was done, and the initial frozen section report came back positive for cancer of the breast. Before the surgeons could proceed with mastectomy, a second report was received saying that the first report was erroneous, and a correct diagnosis was either lymphoma or Hodgkin's disease. Despite this report, the surgeons performed a radical right mastectomy. The court held that the consent document did not authorize the additional operation and, therefore, the woman had a claim against her physicians. See *Valdez v Percy*, 35 Cal App. 2nd, 485, 96 P 2nd 142 (1939).

The California case makes it clear that the physician must have the patient's permission to go from biopsy to mastectomy. Physicians should not extend the scope of an operative procedure beyond that authorized by the patient.

Statutory Law

So far, the states of California, Florida, Kentucky, Massachusetts, Maryland, Michigan, New Jersey, Pennsylvania, and Virginia have passed laws concerning treatment for breast cancer.

The laws are of two types: laws requiring that certain information be provided to patients before treatment, and laws requiring written consent before treatment. Each law will be briefly discussed.

California

The California 1980 law was the first to be enacted. It states that the failure of a physician to inform a patient (by means of a standardized written summary as developed by the California Department of Public Health on recommendation of the Cancer Advisory Council), in layman's language understood by the patient, of alternative efficacious means of treatment which may be medically viable, including surgical, radiological, or chemotherapeutic treatment or combination thereof, when the patient is being treated for any form of breast cancer constitutes unprofessional conduct. A standardized written summary in lay language given to the patient constitutes compliance with the law (California Health and Safety Code Section 1704.5).

The California law does several things:

1. It requires the Public Health Department to develop a standardized summary in consultation with an advisory council.
2. It requires the summary to be in layman's language.
3. It requires the summary to describe all the medically appropriate alternative forms of treatment for breast cancer.
4. It requires a physician to provide this information to the patient or be liable for a charge of unprofessional conduct.

Thus, the law mandates specific disclosure of materials. Although the law has been in effect since 1980, there have been no court cases construing this law. In fact, so far no court has construed any of these laws.

Florida

The Florida law was enacted in 1984 and is essentially similar to the California law. It has some additions and changes. It requires that both actual and high-risk breast cancer patients be informed. It also requires the Florida Cancer Control and Research Advisory Board to develop educational programs as well as booklets to inform citizen's groups about early detection and treatment of breast cancer. The board has 26 members, including physicians, nurses, health department personnel, tumor registry personnel, representatives from teaching hospitals, and consumers. See Florida Statutes Annotated, Vol. 14A, Section 381.3812 (m). Florida law at Section 458.324 says that medically viable treatment alternatives are those generally considered by the medical profession to be within the scope of current acceptable standards. Physicians treating patients who either have or are at high risk of developing breast cancer must be informed of the medically viable treatment alternatives so the patient can make a prudent decision concerning treatment options. The informing can occur orally or by providing a copy of the board-prepared booklet. In providing the information, the physician is told to "take into consideration the emotional state of the patient, and the patient's ability to understand the information." The physician must document on the record that the information was provided. Finally, the physician may recommend any mode of treatment felt to be best for the individual patient. Violation of Section 458.324 is a misdemeanor.

Kentucky

The Kentucky law was enacted in 1984 and requires development of a booklet on the advantages, disadvantages, risks, and nature of procedures for all medically efficacious and viable alternatives for the treatment of breast cancer. The booklet must be distributed to all licensed physicians. Upon receipt of the booklet, any physician providing treatment to a breast cancer patient must provide the summary to the patient (Kentucky Revised Statutes, Vol. 1, Section 311.935).

Massachusetts

In 1985, Massachusetts amended its patients' rights law to state that patients suffering from breast cancer have the right to "complete information on all alternate treatments which are medically viable." The law simply codifies common law and does not require any group to develop standardized information. The law took effect in April of 1986. See Annotated Laws of Massachusetts, Chapter 111, Section 70E (h).

Maryland

The Maryland law was passed in 1986 to become effective July 1, 1987. It requires that patients be educated concerning alternative methods of treatment that may be medically practical. The Department of Health is to provide a booklet, which should be updated annually. The booklet is to be distributed to hospitals and physicians. Maryland is the only state that has a requirement that the booklet be developed and annually updated.

A physician is in compliance with Maryland law so long as the booklet is given to the patient, and the patient signs a statement acknowledging receipt of the booklet. The booklet must be provided "within five days of the start of treatment." This is a curious requirement, since treatment can already have been started, and informed consent should be obtained prior to the start of treatment.

Finally, the law creates an exception if immediate treatment is necessary "to save the life of the patient." Again, this is a curious requirement, since breast cancer is not a life-threatening emergency in the way that trauma from a motor vehicle accident is. There should always be time to explain the procedure and alternatives to the patient (Annotated Code of Maryland Health – General, Section 20–113).

Michigan

The Michigan law was passed July 8, 1986. It is part of the disciplinary code for physicians. The law says that beginning in November of 1986, physicians must provide information "orally and in writing" about alternative methods of treatment for breast cancer. The Department of Public Health, in cooperation with the Chronic Disease Advisory Committee, should develop a brochure. The physician can use that brochure or a brochure containing information substantially similar. Patients are required to sign a form indicating that they have received a copy of the brochure. That form shall be included in each patient's medical record.

The Michigan law says the duty to inform does not require disclosure of information "beyond what a reasonably well qualified physician" would be expected to know. A patient who signs a form is barred from bringing a claim based on failure to obtain informed consent in regard to information pertaining to alternative forms of treatment of breast cancer and the advantages, disadvantages, and risks of each method. The law has a sunset provision so that it repeals July 1, 1989. This makes it clear that the state is going to evaluate the usefulness of the law. Violation of the Michigan law is grounds for the department to investigate the licensee for a determination of whether discipline is appropriate (Michigan Compiled Laws Annotated, Sections 333.16221, 333.17013, and 333.17513).

New Jersey

The New Jersey law took effect November 14, 1984, and simply states that before operating on a patient for a tumor of the breast, a physician shall obtain written consent on a form which allows the patient to give consent only for biopsy, or give consent for any necessary operation including breast removal if the tumor is malignant, or give consent to biopsy and any added procedure that may be necessary.

The New Jersey law does not mandate an explanation of risks, benefits, and alternatives, but simply gives the patient a choice between having a biopsy and then having a separate consent process, or having the biopsy and going directly ahead with additional surgery. Penalty for violating the law is that a physician is liable for action by the State Board of Medical Examiners (New Jersey Statutes Annotated, Title 45:9-22.2 and 45:9-22.3).

Pennsylvania

The Pennsylvania law took effect February 1985, and is essentially similar to the New Jersey law except that the consent form must have language that says "I have been informed of the currently medically accepted alternatives to radical mastectomy." Thus, before a physician operates on a patient with a breast tumor the patient must sign a form permitting biopsy and, if the patient wishes, additional surgery including breast removal after having been informed about medically acceptable alternatives to radical mastectomy. Penalty for violation can be both a civil suit by the patient and disciplinary action by the State Licensing Board (Laws of Pennsylvania, Act. 1984−213; PL 10−68). While the law specifically mentions civil suit as a remedy, this mention is unnecessary, since it is always possible for the patient to sue for lack of informed consent.

Virginia

The 1985 Virginia law says that before operation a consent form shall be executed including permission for biopsy and/or surgery "including breast removal." Thus, Virginia, like Pennsylvania and New Jersey, simply has a consent form requirement. These laws do not specify details about alternatives to surgery. They make no indication as to the type of discussion that should occur between physician and patient, and they seem to diminish the notion of consent by leaving it in the hands of the physician to decide what is necessary. It is likely that the common law in each of these states would have required the physician to discuss alternatives and obtain consent for a specific procedure from the patient. If that is true, then these laws may have restricted rather than expanded the consent process. These laws are examples of requiring consent forms instead of forcing provision of specialized information.

Is There a Need for Statutory Enactments?

The laws that simply require a particular consent form may not expand a patient's rights. See the discussion of the Virginia, Pennsylvania, and New Jersey laws above. To the extent that the laws simply require a form, they do not seem to fully address the breast cancer patient's concern that she get all the facts. These laws should be contrasted to the informational laws, which seek to require that the patient be provided with adequate information to make a reasonable choice (see, for example, Michigan, California, and Florida).

Even though the laws do not really change the common law consent requirements, they are symbolic of a concern that patients be informed of treatment alternatives. The mere existence of the laws may result in behavior changes by health care professionals. So, even though the laws do not change preexisting requirements, they do reflect a concern that health care professionals may not be telling all. By highlighting this concern, the laws could provide a benefit in the form of better communication from health care professional to patient.

IMPLICATIONS OF THE BREAST CANCER TREATMENT LAWS

Should Such Laws Be Limited
to Breast Cancer? Slippery Slope Arguments

Is it reasonable to single out breast cancer for special consideration? Should there be laws for other treatments, or is this simply a response to a particular concern of breast cancer patients? The slippery slope argument is that if the legislature writes laws in one area, they have then embarked on a slippery slope, where other interest groups will also want specific laws covering their particular concerns. For example, why should breast cancer be distinguished from treatment of the developmentally disabled, the senile, patients with other forms of cancers, etc.? Has the legislature started on a never-ending cycle of laws mandating certain types of practice by health care professionals?

Electrocortical Shock Treatment and Psychosurgery

As a result of Ken Kesey's book *One Flew over the Cuckoo's Nest* and other concerns, many states have passed laws regulating the use of shock treatment and psychosurgery. In Michigan, for example, patients shall not have surgery or be the subject of electroconvulsive therapy (ECT) unless consent is obtained from the patient, if competent, or the guardian if the patient is incompetent. Here, as with breast cancer, there is substantial concern that patients may be inappropriately treated.

Autopsy

Many states have laws with detailed requirements that the physician make explanations to the next of kin before an autopsy can be performed.

Abortion

Many state legislatures have passed laws requiring that women be given specific information before they can consent to an abortion. In some cases the information includes graphic descriptions of fetal development and statements that the fetus can feel pain. The laws have required provision of information through words and pictures. So far, these laws have been challenged in courts and determined to be unconstitutional. See, for example, *Planned Parenthood of Central Missouri v. Danforth*, 428 U.S. 52 (1976), where the United States Supreme Court said informed consent means telling the woman "just what would be done and to require more might put the physician in a straitjacket." After the *Danforth* decision, many states enacted legislation saying in great detail what information should be provided. For example, the city of Akron, Ohio, required that the attending physician inform the women of the fact that the unborn child is a human being from the moment of conception and that fetuses have ability to experience pain. This ordinance was held unconstitutional by the United States Supreme Court, which said that the government should not decide what specific information the woman must be given, but rather it was the responsibility of the physician "to insure that appropriate information in conveyed to his patient, depending on her particular circumstances" (*City of Akron v The Akron Center for Reproductive Health, Inc.* 103 Sup. Ct. 2481, 2500 [1983]).

Maternity Patients

Massachusetts has a clear example of special interest legislation. Each hospital must provide maternity patients with information on its annual rate of cesarean sections, annual percentage of birthing room deliveries, annual percentage of cases when only external monitoring was used, percentage of epidural anesthesia, and the percentage of women breastfeeding on discharge from the hospital.

This is clearly a law designed to help pregnant patients choose a preferred hospital for delivery. A logical extension, currently being pursued by peer review organizations and the Medicare Program, is to publish hospital mortality rates for the public's information.

Are Laws Written in Stone?

The law is not static but rather is flexible and based on societal concerns. It is interesting that no one has challenged the breast cancer treatment laws under the theories used in the abortion laws discussed above. The abortion cases clearly state that government cannot mandate what specific information must be given to patients. If this is true, then the same theory could be used to invalidate the breast cancer treatment laws. Of course, the important distinction is that the laws were intended to bring about different consequences. The abortion informed consent laws were intended to make it more difficult for a woman to obtain an abortion. The breast cancer laws are intended to be sure that patients have adequate information before consenting to treatment for their condition. In other words, the invalidated abortion laws attempted to talk women out of an abortion while the breast cancer treatment laws attempt to protect women from unnecessary operations. Thus, the abortion consent laws interfere with the woman's rights, while the breast cancer laws attempt to further a patient's rights. Nonetheless, the language of the abortion laws could be used to challenge the breast cancer laws.

Are the Breast Cancer Consent Laws Useful Public Policy?

Two opposing arguments can be made. First, the laws are clearly useful public policy because they raise the consciousness of the health care professionals and result in provision of useful information to the patient. Second, they are not useful because they constitute an intrusion into the practice of medicine and hamper the physician from dealing with a particular patient. Further, they represent the camel's nose going under the tent. In other words, if the state is allowed to regulate consent for one particular type of treatment, what is to stop the state from regulating consent for all types of treatment and otherwise imposing on the physician-patient relationship?

Looking narrowly at the issue, the breast cancer laws can be seen as useful because of their desired result, but the slippery slope argument that the laws will be expanded into undesirable areas must be acknowledged.

Do the Laws Have Practical Problems?

There are several potential practical problems with the laws. Some of the problems have been noted above where each individual law is discussed. Additional problems include:

1. How can information be provided to patients who can't understand? Will physicians need to have consent auditors present?
2. In states requiring summaries, how will the booklets be updated? Who will be required to update them? How often should they be updated? If there is an advance in medical science not reflected in the booklets, clearly the health professional should provide the information to the patient even though this may be a technical violation of the state laws that require the booklet to be provided. Perhaps the physician could provide the booklet and then supplement with new information.
3. In states with booklet requirements, should the professional simply provide the information or should a preferred option be presented? Certainly a hallmark of professionalism is telling a patient or client what the available options are and then recommending what the professional feels is most appropriate for the patient. This is appropriate so long as all the information is first fairly presented in an accurate and unbiased way. The law should not be interpreted to diminish the ability of a professional to suggest appropriate options.
4. Will the laws make a difference? The mere existence of the laws has created a heightened awareness of breast cancer treatment issues, and so the laws have already made a difference. Whether that difference will continue in the long run cannot yet be determined, but it is likely that awareness will remain heightened.
5. What are the penalties for violation of the laws? Will the penalties be enforced? As noted, patients always have the ability to bring a civil suit based on lack of informed consent. These laws add two other possibilities.

   First is the possibility of a criminal misdemeanor for violation of the statute. It is hard to believe that the criminal law will come into effect unless a health care professional intentionally violates the law. A physician would have to publicly state that he or she intends to violate the law as a clear example of civil disobedience. Absent this type of intent, it is highly unlikely that the criminal law will be used as a sanction for violation of these laws.

   Second, some of the laws make specific reference to discipline by the licensing board for unprofessional conduct for violation of the laws. It is possible that repeated violations could be grounds for professional censure or reprimand. It is unlikely that unintentional violation of this type of law would be grounds for revoking a license. Perhaps the major penalty for violation would be public disclosure, which could result in loss of patients.

SUMMARY

Physicians must be certain to provide full information to their breast cancer patients of all medically appropriate treatment alternatives. They should make sure the patient understands and that the patient has made a reasoned choice prior to initiation of any therapy. The patient's choice should be documented as required by state law, and there should be a note in the patient's medical record.

The legislative approach of mandating a particular type of consent may be extended to other areas where society feels actual or potential abuse could occur. For example, the areas of electrocortical shock, psychosurgery, and unnecessary hysterectomy are likely areas for this type of law. These laws can be challenged as being improper interference with the practice of medicine, but if there is a societal consensus behind the laws, it is unlikely that a challenge will occur.

Medical societies may take heed of these developments and help develop a consistent approach for providing information to patients. To the extent that individual physicians and medical societies work toward establishing rapport with patients through provision of information, specific consent laws will be less necessary.

BIBLIOGRAPHY

1. Levine, RJ: *Ethics and Regulation of Clinical Research*. Urban and Schwarzenberg, 1986.
2. Rosoff, AJ: *Informed Consent: A Guide for Health Care Providers*. Aspen, 1981.
3. Rozovsky, FA: *Consent to Treatment: A Practical Guide*. Little, Brown & Company, 1984.
4. Specific state laws:
   a. California Health and Safety Code, Section 1704.5.
   b. Florida Statutes Annotated, 14A, Section 381.3812 (m) and 458.324.
   c. Kentucky Revised Statutes, 12, Section 311.935.
   d. Annotated Laws of Massachusetts, Chapter 111, Section 70E (h).
   e. Annotated Code of Maryland Health – General, Section 20-113.
   f. Michigan Compiled Laws Annotated, Sections 333.16221, 333.17013, and 333.17513.
   g. New Jersey Statutes Annotated, 45:9-22.2 and 45.9-22.3.
5. Laws of Pennsylvania, Act 1984 – 213; PL 10-68.
6. Virginia Code, Vol. 7A, Title 54-325.2:2.

6. *Epidemiology of Breast Cancer*

DAVID SCHOTTENFELD

Aside from nonmelanoma skin cancers, breast cancer is the most frequent cancer in Western European and North American women. In these countries, breast cancer accounts for about 4% of all deaths, 20% of all cancer deaths, and 25% of all cancer cases in women. Projections into the year 2000 anticipate between 1.1 and 1.4 million new cases of breast cancer per year throughout the world.

Incidence rates of female breast cancer exhibit substantial international variation (Table 1). The annual age-standardized incidence rates per 100,000 range from 85.6 among Hawaiian white women to 8.9 among Japanese women in Osaka. Countries at high risk include those in Northern and Western Europe and North America, while those at low risk include most countries of Africa, Latin America, and Asia. Countries of Eastern and Southern Europe exhibit rates that are intermediate.

In Western populations, age-adjusted mortality rates have been relatively stable over the past 30 years, whereas age-adjusted incidence rates have been increasing on an average of 1% to 2% per year. In a recent analysis of age-specific patterns of breast cancer mortality in the United States during 1950 to 1980, the rates under age 45 years have declined 10% to 15%, tended to increase, level off, then eventually decline at 45–59 years, and to have ultimately increased about 10% at ages 60 and older. Age-specific incidence rates between 1970 and 1980 have increased about 10% under 40 years, decreased 6% at 40–49 years, and increased 7% at 50–59 years and 10% to 20% at 60–69 years.[3]

The cross-sectional age-specific pattern in Western high-risk populations has revealed a bimodal curve, which has evoked speculation that breast cancer may be associated with two distinctive pathogenic mechanisms. Namely, age-specific incidence increases rapidly until approximately age 45 years, levels off transiently until age 50 years, and then increases again at a slower rate (Figure 1). In low-risk populations, such as in Japan, the incidence rises until the approximate age of onset of menopause, levels off, and then falls. The above pattern, which has been observed in cross-sectional data, has been cited as evidence that the pathogenesis of breast cancer has

Table 1. Age-Adjusted Breast Cancer (Female) Incidence* and Mortality† per 100,000 Population for Selected Countries

Country	Incidence	Mortality
North America		
United States		26.6
Connecticut	77.9	
Detroit		
White	71.3	
Black	62.5	
Los Angeles		
White	85.3	
Spanish	56.6	
Hawaii		
White	85.6	
Chinese	55.3	
Japanese	47.1	
Canada		28.1
Saskatchewan	62.6	
Ontario	64.6	
Europe		
Denmark	58.8	32.2
Hungary (Szabolcs)	20.6	25.0
Norway		22.1
Urban	55.0	
Rural	44.8	
Poland		17.4
Urban	36.5	
Rural	17.7	
Sweden	55.2	23.2
United Kingdom		34.3
Birmingham	56.4	
West Scotland	56.0	33.3
Yugoslavia (Slovenia)	34.2	14.9
Israel		27.7
Jews	59.9	
Non-Jews	11.0	
Japan		
Miyagi		
Urban	20.4	
Rural	14.1	
Osaka		
Urban	12.9	
Rural	8.9	

SOURCE: *Cancer Incidence in Five Continents, Volume IV (1982)
†World Health Statistics Annual, 1982–1984.

both premenopausal and postmenopausal components, and that the relative prominence of the postmenopausal component distinguishes patterns in high-risk countries from those in low-risk countries. It is of interest that after cohort analysis of data in low-risk countries, the shapes of the age-specific incidence curves are identical in Western and Asian populations. What is different is the magnitude of the rates during *both* the premenopausal and postmenopausal periods.[15]

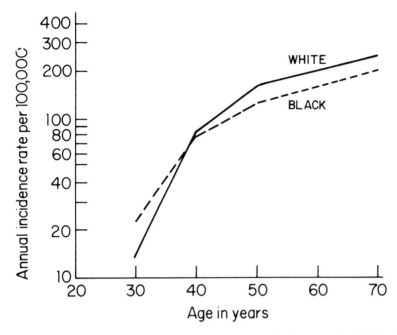

Figure 1. Breast cancer incidence rates in white and black women in the United States, 1969–1971. Data from the third National Cancer Survey.

Of interest is the view that the natural history of breast cancer may be influenced by two distinct temporal subsets of etiologic factors – breast cancer of premenopausal onset influenced significantly by genetic susceptibility and ovarian-pituitary dysfunction, and breast cancer of delayed onset or manifestation in the postmenopausal period, related more significantly to obesity, dietary factors, and endocrine interactions. The salient risk factors for breast cancer, delineated by epidemiologic studies (Table 2), have served to sharpen the focus of experimental research on reproductive endocrinology, endocrine factors controlling growth and development of mammary tissue, nutritional factors that promote tumorigenesis, and genetic mechanisms that regulate host susceptibility.

The natural history of neoplastic development evolves through stages of initiation, promotion, and autonomous progression. The clinical manifestations of a malignant neoplasm obscure recognition that symptomatic cancer is the phenotypic endpoint of a sequence of molecular and biochemical events occurring over an induction-latency period measured in years. In experimental systems, the length of the latency period varies with the type and dose of the initiating carcinogen and subsequent endogenous and exogenous growth-promoting factors, intrinsic susceptibility of target cells modulated by host immunogenetic characteristics, and tumor growth kinetics.

These concepts will be reviewed in the context of genetic, endocrine, and nutritional mechanisms of pathogenesis of human breast cancer.

Table 2.   Who is at Risk of Breast Cancer?

A. DEMOGRAPHIC

AGE   Incidence increases sharply after age 30, levels off around menopause (45–54 years), then rises thereafter, but not as steeply as before the premenopausal period.

SEX   One case of male breast cancer for 100 cases in women.

RACE   Incidence in North America and Western Europe 6-10 times higher than in Japan, most parts of Asia and Africa. American-born blacks with increasing incidence—black to U.S. white age-adjusted incidence ratio is 0.84, although rates tend to be higher in the blacks before age 40, and lower after age 40 (Fig.1).

SOCIO-ECONOMIC   Women of upper socioeconomic class have been at higher risk (50–100%) than women of lower, although this socioeconomic gradient in U.S. whites has diminished over time.

B. MARITAL STATUS AND PARITY

Beyond 40 years, incidence 50–100% higher in single women than in married women.

Nulliparous women at greater risk than women with first birth before 30 years.

Full-term pregnancy before age 18 associated with two-thirds reduction in risk, compared to nulliparous women.

Women with first live birth *after* age 35 have higher risk (about 50%) than nulliparous women.

High parity, in particular four or more births, confers independent protective effect, after adjusting for age at first birth.

Pregnancy outcome resulting in miscarriage, or of less than six months' duration, does not confer protection.

On the contrary, history of miscarriage(s) may be associated with increased risk.

C. MENSTRUATION

Slight trend of increasing risk with earlier age at menarche.

Onset of natural menopause at age 50 or older associated with twofold increase in risk when compared with women with natural onset before age 45.

Women who have had both ovaries removed before age 35, experience two-thirds reduction in risk when compared with women having a natural menopause.

D. FAMILY HISTORY

First-degree female relatives (paternal or maternal) of women with breast cancer—two- to threefold excess risk.

Both mother and sister, or two sisters, having history of breast cancer confers fivefold or greater excess risk in first-degree relatives.

Odds of history of breast cancer in mother or sister significantly higher when one or more first-degree relatives with diagnosis of breast cancer before onset of menopause, or bilateral breast cancer.

Familial cancer syndrome where autosomal dominant pattern of inheritance of premenopausal onset of breast and/or ovarian cancer, or Li-Fraumeni syndrome of early onset breast cancer, soft tissue sarcoma, brain tumors, leukemia, and adrenal and thyroid neoplasms within a pedigree.

E. OBESITY

Increase in body weight and body mass (weight/height^2) associated with about twofold increase in risk of postmenopausal diagnosis of breast cancer. Childhood obesity correlated with early age of menarche.

Table 2, continued

F. BENIGN BREAST DISEASE

Proliferative disease, such as ductal and lobular hyperplasia, with atypia is associated with more than eightfold increase in risk. This subgroup of benign breast disease accounts for approximately 5% of all categories of benign breast disease.

G. IONIZING RADIATION

Higher risk for each rad of exposure in younger women and in children.

Risk manifested after the age of 30 years, increasing with age, with minimal latency period of 10–15 years.

The age-specific pattern of radiation-induced breast cancer is superimposed upon the age-specific pattern of breast cancer in the general population.

The dose-response relationship generally interpreted to be linear.

H. SECOND PRIMARY CANCER—OVARY, ENDOMETRIUM, LARGE INTESTINE

In a patient with primary carcinoma of the ovary, the subsequent risk of breast cancer is increased three- to fourfold. In patients with endometrial carcinoma the risk of a subsequent breast cancer is increased 1.3–2.0 times the expectation in the general population. Similarly, the risk of breast cancer is almost twice that normally expected in women with previous colorectal cancer.

FAMILIAL HISTORY

The prevalence of breast cancer has been determined among the relatives of breast cancer patients and compared with general population statistics, or with the frequency among similar categories of family members of index persons without breast cancer. Early family studies provided evidence of a twofold to fourfold increased risk among parents, siblings, or offspring of breast cancer patients when compared with similar first-degree relatives of controls. Susceptibility to breast cancer apparently may be transmitted by male or female members, although expression of risk is highly selective for female members.

Familial clustering may be a consequence of relatives sharing common environmental exposures, such as dietary practices, rather than of inherited susceptibility. Earlier familial studies, however, did not seek to demonstrate heterogeneity in familial risk within pedigrees obtained from a representative sampling of breast cancer patients, or to search for genetic and environmental interactions.

Anderson[1] observed that familial risk among first-degree relatives of breast cancer patients varied in relation to age at diagnosis (premenopausal vs. postmenopausal) and laterality (unilateral vs. bilateral) in the index patients. Premenopausal onset of disease was associated with a threefold higher risk of breast cancer in first-degree relatives than in similarly aged controls, and bilateral breast cancer was associated with a fivefold increase in risk among relatives. In families selected initially on the basis of mother-daughter or sister-sister members with breast cancer, diagnosed in both instances prior to the onset of menopause and/or with bilateral breast cancer, the lifetime risk to other sisters and daughters approached 50%. In this highly selected group of families, this pattern was suggestive of autosomal dominant inheritance.

Family history also may have an important effect on the probability of developing a second primary cancer in the opposite breast. In premenopausal patients with breast cancer, in the presence of a family history in two first-degree relatives, the probability of developing breast cancer within 20 years was estimated to be 35%, or approximately twofold to threefold higher than in women with breast cancer without a family history. For a patient with postmenopausal breast cancer, the lifetime risk of developing cancer in the opposite breast varies from around 11% to 13% in patients without a family history, or with a family history limited to second-degree relatives, which is not different from the risk in the general population, to 20% to 25% in patients with a family history among first-degree relatives.[2]

There is substantial genetic heterogeneity in the risk of breast cancer among relatives within and among families. The assessment of risk when counseling family members will be guided by age at diagnosis, bilaterality and number of affected relatives, genetic relationship of unaffected relatives, and distribution of epidemiologic risk factors within the family. In most population-based studies, approximately 10% of breast cancer patients have family pedigrees with one or more first-degree relatives with breast cancer. Overall, perhaps 5% of families manifest genetically determined autosomal dominant susceptibility. The hereditary fraction, as determined by segregation analysis, would be about 10% for a population-based series of relatives of index patients with early onset (i.e., younger than 50 years) breast cancer.[16,17] Since breast cancer is a common disease, multiple cases or phenocopies may occur in families due to common cultural and environmental risk factors, without involving a genetic factor that may be controlling expression of susceptibility.

ENDOCRINE FACTORS

> . . . there is as yet no clear-cut pattern of abnormal hormone production or abnormal hormonal milieu found in women at increased risk for breast cancer.
>
> Kirschner (1977)[12]

In searching experimentally for endocrine factors in breast cancer, investigators have studied ovarian, pituitary, adrenal, and thyroid hormones that regulate mammary growth and function. Epidemiologic studies have described the relative protective effect of the first full-term pregnancy within 10 to 15 years after menarche, and that exposure of breast tissue to ionizing radiation before 20 years of age resulted in greater risk of cancer when compared with the effect of exposure in older age groups. These observations suggest that there is a period of increased risk for tumor initiation following the onset of puberty that is associated with endogenous hormonal stimulation of lobuloalveolar ductal proliferation and development. Reduction in risk because of early onset of menopause is also consistent with the inference that breast cancer is hormonally mediated, and that estrogens are essential factors in tumor expression. Studies to identify specific endogenous hormonal aberrations have consisted of comparisons of hormonal levels in blood and urine from breast cancer patients and controls, or in cross-sectional studies in groups of women at contrasting risk of breast cancer, and of prospective studies in which hormone levels in blood or urine from women who subsequently developed breast cancer were compared with levels in blood or urine from women who remained free of disease. The assays determined levels of various estrogens, androgens, progesterone, or prolactin. In general, these studies have failed to yield a clear understanding of the hormonal changes that promote the development of breast cancer.

Prolactin

Prolactin is a sustaining or promoting factor in the growth of mammary carcinoma in laboratory animals. Pituitary isografts, hypothalamic lesions, and drugs such as the phenothiazines, rauwolfia alkaloids, and methyldopa, which enhance prolactin secretion, increase the incidence of experimental mammary tumors when introduced *after* the administration of a carcinogen. This particular experimental model may be analogous to the epidemiologic observation that delayed first pregnancy, i.e., after age 35, was associated with an increased risk of breast cancer. Estrogens are potent stimulators of prolactin secretion in the rat and mouse, and both factors promote the growth of normal and neoplastic mammary tissue. Large doses of estrogen may inhibit mammary tumor growth by either blocking the binding of prolactin to tumor cell receptor sites or by interfering with the peripheral action of prolactin on mammary tumor cells. After the administration of a carcinogen and initiation of tumorigenesis, decreasing serum prolactin by hypophysectomy or by the use of such drugs as the ergot derivatives or pargyline, leads to decreased mammary tumor growth or tumor regression.[14]

The role of prolactin in human breast cancer is less certain. Significant prolactin stimulation occurs during pregnancy and lactation, and yet early pregnancy is protective, and cumulative months of breastfeeding are not correlated with the risk of breast cancer, and indeed may be protective in relation to premenopausal breast cancer. Blood prolactin bioactivity is not consistently aberrant in women with breast cancer, in high-risk family members, or in populations with high incidence rates when compared with those with low incidence rates.[8]

Table 3. Estrogen Receptors and Breast Cancer Risk Factors

Estrogen receptors have been detected in 50% to 70% of primary breast cancers.
Increasing proportion of estrogen receptor–positive breast cancer with increasing age, and among postmenopausal women.
Early age at menopause associated with higher proportion of estrogen receptor–positive breast cancer.
Higher proportion of estrogen receptor–negative breast cancers among blacks than among whites.
Poorly differentiated tumors are more often estrogen receptor–negative.
Receptor binding affinity significantly higher in familial than in nonfamilial breast cancer.
Higher proportion of estrogen receptor–negative breast cancers associated with prior long-term use of estrogen replacement therapy.
Higher proportion of estrogen receptor–positive breast cancers in obese postmenopausal women.

Estrogen Excess

Estrogens play a central role in augmenting initiation or promoting growth of human breast cancer. Mammary tissue responsive to estrogen stimulation contains intracellular receptor protein that binds specifically to the steroid molecule. The estrogen-binding proteins are located in the cytoplasm and nucleus of estrogen-responsive cells. Estrogen exerts its stimulatory effects on target cells through activation of gene transcription, resulting in induction of specific protein synthesis. Preliminary evidence suggests that receptor status varies in relation to established risk factors for breast cancer (Table 3).[24]

Estrogen administration has produced tumors in at least six species of mammalian animals, and in eight organ sites including breast, endometrium, and ovary. Critical factors in the experimental induction of mammary and reproductive organ tumors by exogenous estrogen are dosage, age at onset of exposure, and genetic susceptibility. Nulliparity and obesity are common risk factors in the epidemiology of reproductive organ and breast cancers occurring in postmenopausal women. Obesity increases levels of exposure to estrogen in the various target tissues, presumably by one or more of the following mechanisms: a) enhancing availability of androstenedione and the efficiency of its conversion to estrone (E_1) in peripheral tissues including fat cells, and b) decreasing sex hormone binding globulin (SHBG) and thus increasing the relative availability of "free" serum estrogen.[22]

The antiestrogenic effects of progestin on proliferating endometrium are believed to be mediated by decreasing estrogen receptor levels and by inducing enzymes that inactivate potent estrogen fractions such as estradiol. Implicit in both the "estrogen window" hypothesis and the "anovulatory–luteal insufficiency" hypothesis is the assumption that estrogen, unopposed by the modulating effect of progesterone, is a fundamental step in the pathogenesis of human breast cancer. It was suggested that anovulatory menstrual cycles were more frequent in women who subsequently develop breast cancer.[6,21] Korenman[13] viewed the intervals around the onset of menarche and before the onset of menopause as temporal "windows" of susceptibility because of the relative frequency of anovulatory menstrual cycles. It should be noted, however, that the concept that progesterone opposes the effect of estrogen is based on physiologic studies of endometrium and not breast. Indeed, both progestins and estrogens have been shown to be carcinogenic to the rodent breast.

Despite extensive research, uncertainty remains about the possible association between use of estrogen replacement therapy and the risk of breast cancer (Table 4). From the early 1960s, estrogen has been prescribed commonly for postmenopausal women in the United States, where in 1983, over two million prescriptions of noncontraceptive estrogens were issued. A major potential risk of such therapy is endometrial cancer, whereas the potential benefits of sustained treatment include reduced risks of osteoporosis and coronary heart disease. With respect to breast cancer, the majority of case-control studies have failed to show an association, or have failed to demonstrate a significant trend of increasing risk with increasing cumulative dose. In some instances, however, epidemiologic studies have shown 20% to 90% increases in overall risk, with demonstrably increasing risks in relationship to interval of follow-up, increasing dose, or in specific subsets of women. Ross et al.[20] reported that among women who have had a natural menopause, a total cumulative dose of conjugated estrogen of 1500 mg or more was associated with a relative risk of 2.5. In a retrospective cohort study by Hoover et al.,[11] the 1.8-fold increase in relative risk of breast cancer was evident in the women who were followed for at least 15 years. It would appear, therefore, that if a true increase in breast cancer risk does exist in noncontraceptive estrogen users, it is of lesser magnitude than that established for endometrial cancer, and may be of concern at higher doses or with protracted use.

The relationship between oral contraceptive use and the risk of breast cancer has been investigated in numerous epidemiologic studies. In general, the use of oral contraceptives has been shown neither to increase nor decrease risk. In the study of Rosenberg et al.,[19] the oral contraceptives did not further augment risk even within those subgroups of women with baseline risk factors, such as family history or benign breast disease, predisposing to breast cancer. Long-term use, about two years or longer, of combination oral contraceptives with relatively high progestogen content (i.e., formulations with the equivalent of 2.5 mg or more of norethindrone acetate) reduced the risk of benign breast disease about 50% to 60%.[23]

NUTRITION: INTERACTION WITH ENDOCRINE FACTORS

Female rats fed high-fat (20% to 25% by weight) diets and treated with a carcinogen, dimethylbenz(a)anthracene, develop a higher incidence of

Table 4. Risk of Breast Cancer in Postmenopausal Women Who Have Used Estrogen Replacement Therapy

FIRST AUTHOR (YEAR OF PUBLICATION)	CASES NUMBER	CASES SOURCE	CONTROLS NUMBER	CONTROLS SOURCE	RELATIVE RISK (95% CONFIDENCE INTERVAL)		
Ross (1980)[20]	131	retirement community	262	retirement community	Total study group ovaries removed	1.1 0.8	(0.8,1.9) (0.5,3.5)
Brinton (1981)*	881	breast cancer screenees	863	breast cancer screenees	Total study group ovaries removed natural menopause	1.2 1.5 1.2	(1.0,1.5) (0.9,2.8) (0.9,1.5)
Hoover (1981)[11]	324	Kaiser Foundation Health Plan	549	Kaiser Foundation Health Plan	Total study group ovaries removed natural menopause	1.4 1.5 1.3	(1.0,2.0) (0.3,6.6) (0.8,2.1)
Kelsey (1981)*	332	hospital	1353	hospital	ovaries removed natural menopause	0.9 0.9	(0.5,1.5) (0.6,1.2)
Kaufman (1984)*	925	hospital	1127	hospital	Total study group	0.9	(0.7,1.1)
Hiatt (1984)*	119	Kaiser Foundation Health Plan	119	Kaiser Foundation Health Plan	ovaries removed	0.7	(0.3,1.6)
La Vecchia (1986)*	1108	hospital	1281	hospital	Total study group	1.9	(1.4,2.8)
Wingo (1987)*	1369	population tumor registry	1645	community	Total study group ovaries removed natural menopause	1.0 1.3 0.8	(0.9,1.2) (0.9,1.9) (0.6,1.1)

*See Additional Readings.

mammary tumors than rats maintained on low-fat (0.5% to 5% by weight) diets. Polyunsaturated fats are somewhat more effective than saturated fats in promoting tumor development. The relationship of dietary fat and human breast cancer was suggested initially by correlation studies of per capita consumption of fats and oils in 24 countries with age-adjusted breast cancer incidence and mortality. Positive correlations within or among countries between average consumption levels and breast cancer rates were noted with total fat, total calories, animal fat, and animal protein. Correlational studies have not, however, shown a similar positive association with vegetable fat, which is primarily unsaturated.[4] Hems et al.[7] reported that temporal changes in breast cancer mortality in England and Wales were anticipated by prior shifts in consumption of fats, animal protein, and sugar.

Recent changes in breast cancer incidence and mortality within Japan and changing patterns of breast cancer in migrants from Japan to the United States are consistent with the effects of changing dietary practices. Hirayama[9] reported in a cohort study that frequency and amount of dietary consumption of meat, eggs, butter, and cheese by Japanese women was associated with an increased risk of dying of breast cancer. The study of patterns of cancer mortality in a migrant population and their offspring, when compared with those existing in the country of origin and the new host country, provides a unique opportunity to consider the etiological role of changing environmental factors. In Japanese migrants to California, the incidence of breast cancer in premenopausal women has now almost reached that of the United States white population. In general, first-generation migrants from low-risk to high-risk countries tend to develop breast cancer rates that are closer to the level in their country of origin. It is primarily in their descendants that the rates of breast cancer approach the increased levels manifested by women in the high-risk host country. These observations suggest that dietary intake early in life may be of particular etiologic importance.

The results of various cohort and case-control epidemiologic studies, however, have not consistently supported the association of increased consumption of dietary fat, meat, or dairy products, or of increased serum levels of cholesterol and lipoproteins, with the risk of breast cancer. For example, Graham et al.[5] did not observe any difference between cases and controls in their ingestion of total fat, or total animal or vegetable fat. In a study of Seventh-Day Adventists who generally follow a lacto-ovo-vegetarian diet, meat consumption was not associated with breast cancer risk.[18] Although Caucasian women have about a twofold greater risk of breast cancer than Japanese women in Hawaii, a recently conducted case-control study concluded that total fat or animal protein intake did not completely explain the differences in breast cancer risk between the two ethnic groups. Postmenopausal women, however, were found to have a significant trend of increasing risk with decreasing ingestion of Vitamin A.[10]

The correlation of breast cancer incidence and mortality trends with population dietary consumption patterns may be misleading. Population breast cancer trends may also be associated with changing temporal patterns of fertility, age at first birth, prescription of exogenous estrogens, and changing patterns of disease detection, diagnosis, and classification. In addition, the summary description of an average dietary pattern within a population may not reflect accurately the diets of those in that population who experience breast cancer. Although dietary fat has received the most attention, high intake of meat, animal fat, or other fats may be associated with lower intake of vegetables or other foods. Thus, dietary research with respect to breast cancer must consider the potential interactions of multiple components of the diet suspected of playing a role in the pathogenesis of human breast cancer.

Future research initiatives must attempt to resolve the current inconsistencies that confound interpretation and public policy implications of the role of dietary factors in human breast cancer. Food preferences are culturally interconnected and biochemically interactive. The almost single-minded focus on the putative role of excessive and maldistributed dietary fat has tended to ignore careful concomitant assessment of relative excesses or deficiencies of dietary sources of total calories, fat-soluble vitamins A and E, carotenoids, other antioxidants, and selenium. For each of these nutrient categories, there is experimental evidence that restriction of total calories or sufficiency of micronutrients may inhibit mammary tumorigenesis.

Dietary factors, broadly operating as either co-carcinogens or promoters in carcinogenesis, may be mediated through endocrine, immunological, or other biochemical mechanisms. For example, dietary fat may alter prolactin and estrogen bioactivity, and thereby directly affect mammary glandular growth and differentiation, and modulate prolactin and estrogen receptor content; induce phospholipid membrane abnormalities by changing composition or increasing peroxidation of membrane lipids; influence carcinogen metabolism or DNA repair processes; or any combination of the above. The endocrine effects of dietary fat in human breast cancer, and the relevance of obesity as a risk factor, may be expressed by enhancing responsiveness of target tissue.

REFERENCES

1. Anderson DE, Badzioch MD: Bilaterality in familial breast cancer patients. Cancer 56:2092, 1985.
2. Anderson DE, Badzioch MD: Risk of familial breast cancer. Cancer 56:383, 1985.
3. Blot WJ, Devesa SS, Fraumeni JF Jr: Declining breast cancer mortality among young American women. JNCI 78:451, 1987.

4. Carroll KK: Influence of diet on mammary cancer. Nutr Cancer 2:232, 1980.
5. Graham S, Marshall J, Mettlin C, et al.: Diet in the epidemiology of breast cancer. Am J Epidemiol 116:68, 1982.
6. Grattarola R: The premenstrual endometrial pattern of women with breast cancer: A study of progestational activity. Cancer 17:1119, 1964.
7. Hems G: The contribution of diet and childbearing to breast-cancer rates. Br J Cancer 37:974, 1978.
8. Henderson BE, Pike MC: Prolactin — An important hormone in breast neoplasia?, in Pike MC, Siiteri PK, Welsch CW (eds): *Hormones and Breast Cancer*, Banbury Report No. 8, Cold Spring Harbor Laboratory, 1981, p115.
9. Hirayama T: Epidemiology of breast cancer with special reference to the role of diet. Prev Med 7:173, 1978.
10. Hirohata T, Nomura AMY, Hankin JH, et al.: An epidemiologic study on the association between diet and breast cancer. JNCI 78:595, 1987.
11. Hoover R, Glass A, Finkle W, et al.: Conjugated estrogens and breast cancer risk in women. JNCI 67:815, 1981.
12. Kirschner MA: The role of hormones in the etiology of human breast cancer. Cancer 39:2716, 1977.
13. Korenman SG: Estrogen window hypothesis of the etiology of breast cancer. Lancet 1: 700, 1980.
14. Meites J: Relation of prolactin and estrogen to mammary tumorigenesis in the rat. JNCI 48: 1217, 1972.
15. Moolgavkar S, Day NE, Stevens RG: Two-stage model for carcinogenesis: Epidemiology of breast cancer in females. JNCI 65:559, 1980.
16. Ottman R, Pike MC, King MC, et al.: Practical guide for estimating risk for familial breast cancer. Lancet 2:556, 1983.
17. Ottman R, Pike MC, King MC, et al: Familial breast cancer in a population-based series. Am J Epidemiol 123:15, 1986.
18. Phillips RL, Snowdon DA: Association of meat and coffee use with cancers of the large bowel, breast and prostate among Seventh Day Adventists: preliminary results. Cancer Res 43:2403s, 1983.
19. Rosenberg L, Miller DR, Kaufman DW, et al.: Breast cancer and oral contraceptive use. Am J Epidemiol 119:167, 1984.
20. Ross RK, Paganini-Hill A, Gerkins VR: A case-control study of menopausal estrogen therapy and breast cancer. JAMA 243:1635, 1980.
21. Secreto G, Toniolo P, Berrino F, et al.: Increased androgenic activity and breast cancer risk in premenopausal women. Cancer Research 44:5902, 1984.
22. Siiteri PK, Hammond GL, Nisker JA: Increased availability of serum estrogens in breast cancer: A new hypothesis, in Pike MC, Siiteri PK, Welsch CW (eds): *Hormones and Breast Cancer*, Banbury Report No 8, Cold Spring Harbor Laboratory, 1981, p87.
23. Stadel BV, Schlesselman JJ: Oral contraceptive use and the risk of breast cancer in women with a "prior" history of benign breast disease. Am J Epidemiol 123:373, 1986.

24. Stanford JL, Szklo M, Brinton LA: Estrogen receptors and breast cancer. Epidemiol Rev 8:42, 1986.

ADDITIONAL READINGS

Brinton LA, Hoover RN, Szklo M, et al.: Menopausal estrogen use and risk of breast cancer. Cancer 47:2517, 1981.

Hiatt RA, Bawol R, Friedman GD, et al.: Exogenous estrogen and breast cancer after bilateral oophorectomy. Cancer 54:139, 1984.

Kaufman DW, Miller DR, Rosenberg L, et al.: Noncontraceptive estrogen use and the risk of breast cancer. JAMA 252:63, 1984.

Kelsey JL, Fischer DB, Holford TR, et al.: Exogenous estrogens and other factors in the epidemiology of breast cancer. JNCI 67:327, 1981.

Kelsey JL, Hildreth NG: *Breast and Gynecologic Cancer Epidemiology.* Boca Raton, CRC Press, Inc., 1983.

La Vecchia C, Decarli A, Parazzini F, et al.: Non-contraceptive oestrogens and the risk of breast cancer in women. Int J Cancer 38:853, 1986.

Wingo PA, Layde PM, Lee NC, et al.: The risk of breast cancer in postmenopausal women who have used estrogen replacement therapy. JAMA 257:209, 1987.

SECTION TWO

Issues in Diagnosis and Decision Making

7. Evaluation of Breast Masses

WILLIAM L. DONEGAN

A palpable mass continues to be the most frequent manifestation of primary breast cancer (Table 1). Most masses are found by patients themselves either accidentally or on breast self-examination, and most are benign, but because of its potential seriousness, a palpable mass in the breast requires prompt diagnosis. The size of a breast cancer at diagnosis is closely correlated with the prospects for cure. As discovery of a mass triggers a chain of time-consuming and often expensive diagnostic procedures, definition is important.

DEFINITION

A breast mass may be defined as a palpable density that a) has margins on all sides and b) is asymmetric with the opposite breast. In a multinodular breast it must be of a size or consistency that is different from the other tissues of the breast. Not to be mistaken for masses are certain normal formations. These include a prominent peripheral margin of firm breast tissue, the inner irregular edge of the doughnut of breast tissue that often surrounds the areola, vague aggregates in the upper outer quadrants, and the firm crescent of tissue often found near the inframammary fold. These are generally symmetric in the two breasts or lack a complete border.

It is useful to document the following characteristics of a mass: Mobility, Attachment to skin or deep tissues, Size in centimeters, Shape, Tenderness,

Table 1. Signs of 141 Consecutive Cancers 1982–86*

		No.	Percent
Palpable mass		91	65
Mammographic abnormality only		42	30
Calcifications	25		
Mass	9		
Calcifications and mass	8		
Nipple discharge only		5	3
Edema and redness ± mass		3	2

*Personal series

71

Location (centrally or in a particular quadrant), and Consistency. The first letters of these characteristics form an acronym, MASS and TLC; and will not be forgotten if every MASS is described with Tender Loving Care.

Masses discovered by physical examination may be visible as well as palpable because of size, skin retraction, or other changes in the overlying skin. After careful inspection, the most effective method for detection of a true mass is with the patient supine and the side to be examined slightly raised. The breast is flat and examination is performed with both hands compressing the flattened breast tissue against the chest wall with rotational movements of the fingers of both hands. Any mass that occurs within the bounds of the midline of the chest, the clavicle, the epigastrium, the midaxillary line, and the axilla may have origin in breast tissue. The best time to examine premenopausal women is seven days after the onset of the menstrual period when the breast is smallest.

LESIONS FREQUENTLY PRESENTING AS BREAST MASSES

The following are the most frequent lesions that present as breast masses. Many have distinctive characteristics.

1) Fibrocystic changes. Usually in premenopausal women. The mass may be irregular, mildly tender, rubbery, and in any quadrant of the breast.
2) Gross cysts. Occur in the breasts of premenopausal women or postmenopausal women on hormone replacement. They are generally spherical, vary from tender to nontender with soft or firm consistency, and are never associated with skin dimpling or deep attachment. Palpation is not reliable in distinguishing cysts from solid tumors.
3) Fibroadenoma. Characteristically found in the third or fourth decade of life. Typically spherical, nontender, highly mobile, firm, and without attachments to skin or deep tissues.
4) Carcinoma. Ordinarily occurs after age 30 with a frequency directly related to age. May be mildly tender or nontender, discrete or irregular, usually firm, and may dimple the skin and be attached to deep tissues. Likely when a mass is associated with axillary adenopathy.
5) Fat necrosis. Often preceded by a history of direct trauma with transient bruising; firm, irregular, nontender, and may produce skin retraction.
6) Mammary duct ectasia. Believed to have ductal ectasia as its origin; mildly tender or nontender, firm, irregular. Like fat necrosis, it can retract the skin and have all the gross features of carcinoma.
7) Lipoma. Located in the subcutaneous tissues, soft, and nontender, may be multiple and transilluminates.
8) Cystosarcoma phyllodes. Nontender, firm mass with discrete spherical shape that can achieve large size; when small they share the features of fibroadenomas but predominate in an older age group.

Masses are more common in the upper outer quadrant of the breast where most breast tissue is located. The probability of a mass representing cancer increases with age. Only mammary duct ectasia, fat necrosis, cancer, and a previous biopsy site with fibrosis can produce skin retraction.

Questionable or Uncertain Masses

If, on the basis of the physical examination, the presence of a mass is equivocal and a mammogram shows no definite abnormality, it is useful to reexamine the patient after a short interval. In premenopausal women, oral contraceptives should be discontinued and the reexamination timed for one week after the next menstrual period begins, when hormonal stimulation to the breast is at the lowest level. In postmenopausal women, replacement estrogens should be discontinued and the reexamination scheduled for one month. With withdrawal of hormonal stimulation, all suspicion may resolve or the presence of a mass may be more clearly evident.

Multiple Masses

Some patients present with multiple masses in one or both breasts. In these instances each mass must be evaluated individually. Not infrequently, patients present with bilateral simultaneous breast cancers. The occurrence of two individual cancers in the same breast is important to note since it would ordinarily make the patient ineligible for breast conserving therapy. When a mass is associated with an abnormal nipple discharge, it is often assumed that the mass is the cause of the discharge, but this may not be the case. If it is evident that the nipple discharge is arising from a different portion of the breast, the nature of both the mass and the discharge must be determined.

METHODS FOR DIAGNOSIS

Aspiration

When the presence of a mass is established, the first step is to determine whether it is solid or cystic. Aspiration is a highly useful method of determining this. It can be performed at the time of the physical examination. It requires only readily available equipment, i.e., a 21-gauge needle and a 10- to 30-cc syringe and is performed without local anesthesia. Its value is in a) quickly distinguishing simple cysts from solid tumors and b) providing cytologic material for diagnosis of solid tumors. Details of this technique are given in Chapter 9. Cysts are almost always benign. Intracystic carcinomas are rare, comprising less than 0.1% of all cysts and constituting less than one-half of 1% of all cancers. Simple cysts will contain fluid that varies from clear and straw-colored to turbid and dark green and will completely disappear after aspiration. Thirty percent will recur and require a second aspiration. Intracystic carcinomas will not be missed if they are suspected in the following circumstances: 1) the fluid is bloody or Hemoccult-positive; 2) the mass does not completely disappear; or 3) the cyst promptly refills and requires more than one additional aspiration. Routine cytologic examination of fluid from cyst aspirations is not necessary when these clinical signs are absent.

When no fluid is obtained on aspiration, the mass is likely not a cyst. In this event it is possible to retrieve material for cytologic preparation by passing the needle back and forth through the mass 2 to 3 times while suction is applied. Suction is released when withdrawing the needle, and a smear for cytology is prepared. If obtained properly, the material for cytology will be contained in the barrel of the needle rather than in the syringe. The needle is detached from the syringe, the syringe filled with air, and then reconnected to the needle. The contents of the needle are blown out on glass slides, quickly smeared, and the slides are dropped into 95% alcohol. Air drying is avoided to prevent artifacts. While the cytologic preparation will not always be sufficient to rule out cancer, a positive reading by an experienced pathologist is rarely in error, i.e., in no more than 0.2% of cases. The problems with fine needle aspiration cytology are 1) the occasional false positive and 2) it does not distinguish in situ from invasive cancer. While I do not consider a positive cytologic examination sufficiently accurate to initiate treatment, it does justify proceeding with a staging workup with the intent of obtaining histologic verification.

Ideally, mammograms are performed before rather than after aspiration so that edema or accidental hemorrhage does not obscure or complicate the mammographic findings. However, this is not convenient as it means a second trip to the physician's office, and a carefully performed aspiration will avoid these problems.

Ultrasound

The principal value of ultrasound (hand-held real time ultrasound) in evaluating palpable masses is in being able to distinguish noninvasively a cystic from a solid tumor. This determination can be made on mammographic masses and those too small to aspirate. In these cases, ultrasonically guided aspiration can be performed to confirm the cystic nature of a small deep-lying mass. Compared with aspiration, ultrasound is more expensive, less convenient, and not therapeutic. Its virtues are in being noninvasive, and in being able to evaluate masses detected on mammography that are too small to feel.

Table 2. Biopsy Results on Palpable Masses Compared with Mammographic Findings

Mammogram	Total No.	Cancer	Benign
Abnormal	127	63	64
Normal	103	13 (17%)	90
Not done	44	8	36
TOTAL	274	84	190

Mammograms

Bilateral mammography is an important adjunct for evaluating breast masses (or other breast complaints) in women over 30 years of age though some would move that age upward. It is best avoided for those younger because the breasts are dense and little useful information accrues from the examination; cancer is unusual in women under 25 years of age, and therefore an occult cancer is unlikely to be missed; and it is best to avoid irradiation of the young breast because it is more susceptible to carcinogenic effects.

Mammograms are important in the evaluation of breast masses for the following reasons: 1) They can confirm the likelihood of carcinoma, and the patient is prepared in advance for the likelihood of this diagnosis; 2) they can detect occult carcinoma in the same breast which may go undetected if the palpable mass is, in fact, benign; 3) they can detect occult carcinoma in the opposite breast and thereby avoid missing a case of bilateral breast cancer; 4) they may avoid a biopsy if the mammograms show the typical characteristics of a lipoma or a cyst (and the latter is further confirmed by ultrasound or aspiration).

A mammogram must be used in conjunction with a physical examination of the adult breast as neither alone is a sufficient examination. A number of cancers are not evident on mammograms.[1,3] In a review of patients with palpable breast masses who had mammography at the Medical College of Wisconsin, it was found that 17% of palpable masses ultimately diagnosed as cancer were not visualized on mammograms (Table 2). On the other hand, 7% of palpable masses ultimately diagnosed as benign were thought to be cancer on mammograms. It is evident that a normal mammogram does not rule out the presence of cancer, nor does a diagnosis of cancer on mammography guarantee its presence. Physical examination and mammography can independently provide indications for biopsy. The two examinations complement each other and must be used together for evaluation of the adult breast.

Mammographic abnormalities that may serve as indications for biopsy include: 1) a persistent mass; 2) fine clustered microcalcifications, i.e., five or more in a 1-cm square; 3) architectural distortion; 4) significant asymmetries of tissue.

CHANGING INDICATIONS FOR BREAST BIOPSY *

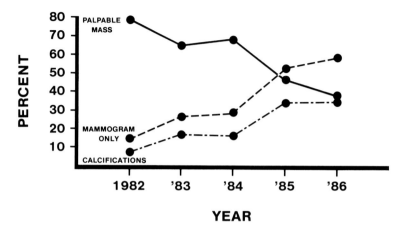

* Personal series - 506 consecutive biopsies

Figure 1. Progressively fewer breast cancers are presenting as masses; an increasing proportion is being found by mammography.

Thermography and Diaphanoscopy

Neither telethermography (the mapping of infrared radiation from the surface of the breast) or contact thermography using cholesterol crystals on a flexible film have an established place in the routine evaluation of breast masses. In a recent evaluation, both methods failed to detect five of eleven cancers.[7] In addition to limited sensitivity, especially for small cancers, thermographic changes in the breast are not specific, and false positives continue to pose a problem. Diaphanoscopy, or transillumination of the breast using a uniform wave length of light, helps to distinguish cysts from solid masses, but diffusion of light limits definition. It serves no purpose that is not better served by ultrasound.

Biopsy

Masses constitute the major indication for breast biopsies. In order of decreasing frequency, the indications are persistent mass, mammographic abnormalities, nipple discharge, and miscellaneous indications such as skin edema and axillary adenopathy. With recent emphasis on screening of asymptomatic women, however, mammographic abnormalities have become an increasingly frequent indication (Figure 1).

With rare exceptions breast biopsies are now performed as an outpatient procedure under local anesthesia. This approach has distinct advantages.[6] If cancer is diagnosed, treatment follows after an interval of several days, the

Table 3.   Indications for 506 Consecutive Breast Biopsies and Results

Indication	Total No.	(%)	Cancers No.	(%)
Palpable mass	272	(54)	93	(34)
Mammogram only	211	(42)	42	(20)
Calcifications	132		24	(18)
Mass	51		11	(22)
Calcification in mass	16		7	(44)
Asymmetry	10		0	(0)
Architectural distortion	2		0	(0)
Nipple discharge only	16	(3)	3	(19)
Edema ± erythema	3	(0.6)	1	(33)
Chronic fistula	3	(0.6)	0	(0)
Abscess	1	(0.2)	0	(0)
TOTAL	506		139	(28)

so-called two-step procedure.[4] The advantages of the two-step procedure are: 1) since most biopsies reveal benign lesions, unnecessary hospitalizations are avoided, and there is less time commitment and expense to patients; 2) diagnosis is established on a firm basis with time for study of permanent sections and pathologic consultation if necessary; 3) an interval is provided during which treatment can be discussed with the patient on the basis of a definite diagnosis, treatment alternatives discussed, and an agreement reached between patient and physician. Staging procedures will be limited to those who definitely require them, with a resultant saving of time and expense. An interval of up to two weeks between biopsy and treatment has been attended with no obvious detrimental effect on prognosis.[2]

Two techniques of biopsy are employed for histologic diagnosis. The first, core needle biopsy, is an office procedure and is suitable for large tumors that are easy targets. While false negatives are frequent, false positive diagnoses are an extreme rarity. In studies of Tru-Cut needle biopsies 67% to 90% of cancers are diagnosed and no false positives are recorded.[5] For smaller lesions an open surgical biopsy is performed with excision of small masses and incisional biopsy of large ones. Sufficient tissue is removed to obtain estrogen receptor and progesterone receptor protein determinations on fresh tumor. Electrosurgical dissection is avoided in order to ensure the viability of receptors. In a series of 506 breast biopsies at the Medical College of Wisconsin, 34% of masses proved to be carcinomas (Table 3). The probability of carcinoma increased with age from 2% in 20 to 30 year olds progressively up to 100% in women 80 years of age or older.

AN ALGORITHM FOR MANAGEMENT OF BREAST MASSES

The algorithm shown in Figure 2 provides a basis for evaluating breast masses using physical examination, fine needle aspiration, mammography,

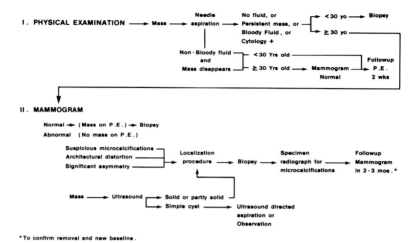

Figure 2. An algorithm for management of breast masses. Suggested course of action for evaluation of breast masses and abnormal findings on mammography. With permission of W. B. Saunders Co., Philadelphia.

and biopsy. It is axiomatic that masses in the breast require a diagnosis. Tumor size is directly correlated with the probability of histologic involvement of axillary lymph nodes, and both are the most important determinant of stage.

These biologic features have a far more important influence on prognosis than variations in local, regional, or systemic adjuvant therapy, hence prompt diagnosis of breast masses is encouraged.

REFERENCES

1. Cahill CJ, Boulter PS, Gibbs NM, et al.: Features of mammographically negative breast tumours. Br J Surg 68:882–884, 1981.
2. Fisher ER, Sass R, Fisher B: Biologic considerations regarding the one and two step procedures in the management of patients with invasive carcinoma of the breast. Surg Gynecol Obstet 161:245–249, 1985.
3. Mann BD, Giuliano AE, Bassett LW, et al.: Delayed diagnosis of breast cancer as a result of normal mammograms. Arch Surg 118:23–24, 1983.
4. Margolese RG: Response: The case for the two-step biopsy procedure for breast cancer. CA 32:51–57,1982.
5. Minkowitz S, Moskowitz R, Khafif RA, et al.: Tru-Cut needle biopsy of the breast. An analysis of its specificity and sensitivity. Cancer 57:320–323, 1986.
6. Saltzstein EC, Mann RW, Chua TY, et al.: Outpatient breast biopsy. Arch Surg 109:287–290, 1974.
7. Sterns E E, Curtis A C, Miller, S, et al.: Thermography in breast diagnosis. Cancer 50:323–325, 1982.

8. Mammography: Changing Role and Concepts

DAVID R. PENNES
DORIT D. ADLER

Although mammography was performed as early as 1927,[15] it was not until 1969 that a dedicated mammography unit was commercially produced.[11] Technical advances since the 1970s have improved mammographic image quality, while decreasing radiation dose by more than a factor of 10.[18]

SCREENING MAMMOGRAPHY

The first randomized trial to assess the potential benefits of screening mammography was conducted by the Health Insurance Plan of New York (HIP) between 1963 and 1970.[24,25] This project demonstrated a 40% reduction in breast cancer mortality in screenees over the age of 50, compared to the control population. In women under age 50, the HIP trial was unable to demonstrate reduced mortality from breast cancer, a finding that is likely related to the less sophisticated mammographic technique employed during the 1960s, compounded by the difficulty obtaining diagnostic images of dense breasts in young women.[6] Because breast cancer is often an indolent neoplasm, the screening benefit to women under age 50 may become apparent only on long-term follow-up, and there is some evidence that late follow-up may demonstrate this benefit in younger women who participated in the HIP trial.[23]

The Breast Cancer Detection Demonstration Project (BCDDP) was a large-scale screening endeavor between 1973 and 1981, conceived by the American Cancer Society and funded by the National Cancer Institute.[3] In large part because of improvements in film technique, as well as greater interpretive expertise, the breast cancer detection rates for similar populations were approximately double those of the HIP trial for similar populations on the initial screening examination. In addition, the size of the detected cancers was smaller, with in situ carcinomas, and invasive carcinomas less than 1 cm in size, constituting 36% of cancers detected in the BCDDP, as opposed to only 8% in the HIP study. Unlike the HIP study, the BCDDP did not randomize patients into screened and nonscreened groups, and there was no proven benefit to screening women under age 50. Nevertheless, inferential analysis of the BCDDP data suggests a randomized trial would demonstrate a mortality reduction of at least 50% in women aged 40 years and older.[6]

The initial results from two randomized screening trials begun in 1977 in Sweden[31] have demonstrated a 40% reduction in deaths from breast cancer in women aged 50 to 74 years, although there was an insufficient number of women aged 40-49 with breast cancer to unequivocally prove screening benefit of mammography in that age group. Nevertheless, the finding of fewer cases of advanced breast cancer among younger women who had undergone screening as compared to the nonscreened population suggests that a mortality reduction may be demonstrated on long-term follow-up in the 40-49 year age group.[6]

The incidence of radiation-induced breast cancer is well known from studies of survivors of the atomic bombings in Hiroshima and Nagasaki,[33] sanatorium patients from Massachusetts and Canada who underwent repeated chest fluoroscopic procedures during treatment for tuberculosis,[5,14] and patients who underwent radiation therapy for postpartum mastitis,[26] or other benign breast diseases,[4] and in radium watch face painters.[1] It is generally accepted that doses of 100 rads or more lead to increases in breast cancer, with a latency period of approximately 10 years, and that the increased risk of breast cancer persists throughout the individual's lifetime. With current techniques, the radiation dose from a mammogram is in the range of 0.1 rad and represents a tenfold reduction in radiation exposure since the 1960s, with an immeasurable improvement in image quality. With regard to the risk/benefit ratio of screening mammography, Feig states:

> The existence of low dose radiation risk has neither been proven nor disproven. If there is a risk from the low doses used in current mammographic techniques, it is immeasurably small, especially when compared with the overwhelmingly large incidence of naturally occurring breast cancers, many of which could be detected by mammography at an early curable stage. This risk, if it does exist, would be lowest among women exposed over 30 years of age, a fortunate circumstance since this group would benefit most from mammography.[7]

Given the current knowledge of radiation risk, as well as the remarkable decrease in radiation dose, controversy over the risk/benefit ratio of screening mammography that raged in the 1970s should no longer be an issue in women of screening age. As a result of the studies of women exposed to large doses of radiation, as well as the results of the HIP and BCDDP studies, the American Cancer Society formulated recommendations for screening mammography in 1982,[21] which were later modified in 1983 to include periodic screening of women aged 40-49[22] (Table 1). These recom-

Table 1. Mammography Screening Recommendations of the American Cancer Society for Asymptomatic Women[21,22]

Age	Recommended Screening Interval
35–39	Baseline mammogram
40–49	Mammograms every 1–2 years
≥50	Annual mammograms

mendations are in general accordance with those of other organizations, including the American College of Radiology, the American College of Physicians, the National Cancer Institute, the American College of Obstetrics and Gynecology, and the American Academy of Family Physicians. Currently only a small percentage of American women follow these guidelines.[10] The reasons for poor compliance are multiple, and include physician referral and the cost of the examination. Although patient and physician education are encouraged, it is clear that full implementation of the American Cancer Society recommendations would result in a demand that is greatly beyond the current capabilities of radiologic facilities and manpower.[10] In consideration of the increased number of surgical biopsies and follow-up that would result from such an effort, the true magnitude of the effects of mass screening become apparent.

DIAGNOSIS

In contradistinction to screening mammography, which is performed on asymptomatic women, a diagnostic mammogram is warranted in women above the age of 35 who present with a palpable mass. A tailored examination may be performed in younger women. In addition to demonstrating the characteristics of the mass, the mammogram aids in identifying other abnormalities in the same and contralateral breast. Such findings may be important in future management decisions.

TECHNIQUE

Breast radiography is currently performed using two techniques: film/screen mammography and xeroradiography. Film/screen mammography is comparable to other plain radiographic examinations in diagnostic radiology, resulting in images that are viewed using light boxes. Xeroradiography is a radiographic technique developed by the Xerox Corporation in 1971, employing an electrostatically charged selenium plate and fine particles of an electrically charged blue powder. Images are recorded on paper and viewed using reflected rather than transmitted light. Radiologists in the United States are divided approximately equally between film/screen, and xeroradiographic mammography, although in recent years, film/screen mammography has gained popularity. While we prefer film/screen mammography, each technique has its strengths and limitations. State-of-the-art dedicated film/screen and xeroradiographic units both provide diagnostic mammograms at acceptably low radiation doses, and the decision to use one or the other imaging technique is primarily based on training and experience. The essential feature is that the highest quality examination be performed.

Although single-view mammograms have been advocated for mass screening,[20] in general, a screening or diagnostic mammogram consists of two or three views of each breast, performed on a dedicated mammographic unit. The views are obtained with firm compression of the breast in the craniocaudal, mediolateral, and oblique projections. Additional views, including special projections or magnification views, are employed to clarify suspicious abnormalities and constitute a "tailored" mammographic examination. Correlation with the breast physical examination and the results of cytologic examination (see below) will result in the lowest possible false negative rate. It is essential to remember that there is approximately an 8% to 10% false negative rate for mammography. A report of a "normal" mammogram should not dissuade the referring clinician from proceeding with other examinations such as a surgical biopsy for a clinically suspicious finding. Because of the inherently higher costs, the tailored mammographic approach is not practical in low-cost mass screening programs.[30]

MAMMOGRAPHIC FEATURES OF BREAST DISEASE

The main radiographic findings indicating malignancy are mass, retraction, calcification, and breast edema. With few exceptions, such as a densely calcified adenofibroma (Figure 1), or radiolucent masses representing lipomas (Figure 2), it is rarely possible to state with absolute certainty that a mass demonstrated on a mammogram is unequivocally benign. Nevertheless, there are radiographic features that can be used to predict with a high degree of accuracy, the nature of a given mass. Most important are density and marginal characteristics of a mass. The presence of a dense, spiculated mass (Figure 3) is essentially diagnostic of malignancy in the absence of previous biopsy. In contrast, a low-density, smoothly marginated mass (Figure 4) favors a benign lesion, such as a cyst or adenofibroma. Benign lesions frequently are surrounded by a thin radiolucent halo. It is usually impossible to differentiate a cyst from an adenofibroma mammographically, although such differentiation may be readily achieved using ultrasound or aspiration.

Approximately 40% of breast carcinomas contain mammographically visible microcalcifications,[12] and the presence of microcalcifications is

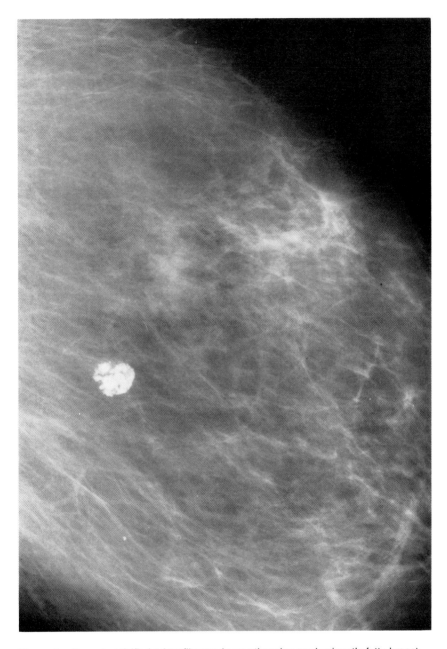

Figure 1. Densely calcified adenofibroma in an otherwise predominantly fatty breast.

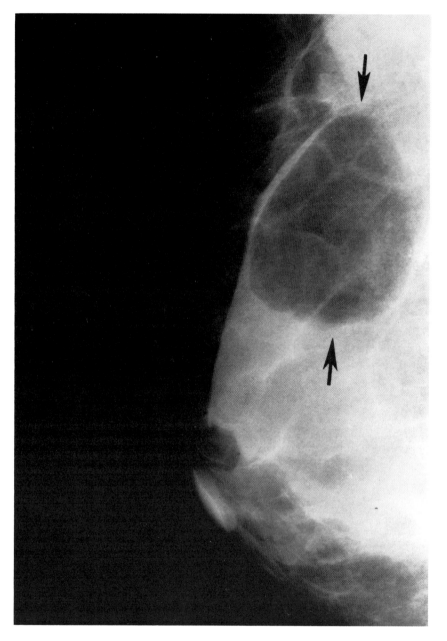

Figure 2. Lipoma (arrows) is apparent by virtue of the localized lucent (fatty) composition surrounded by glandular breast parenchyma.

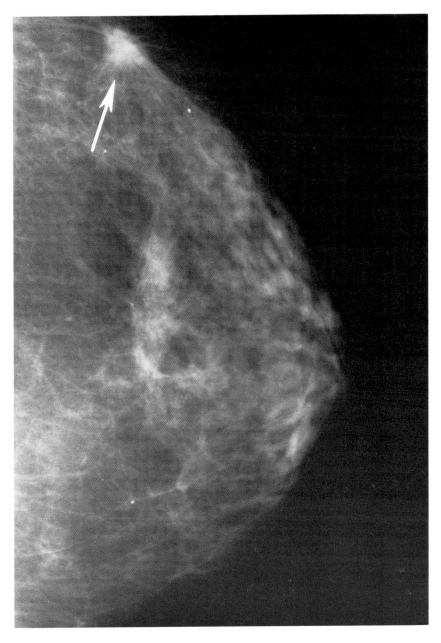

Figure 3. Lateral view demonstrates a small dense spiculated cancer (arrow) in the cranial portion of the breast.

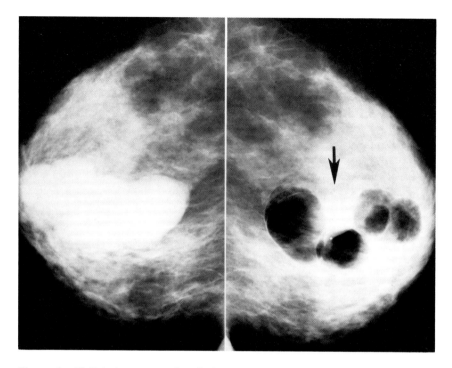

Figure 4. Multiple large, smooth-walled masses (left) were aspirated, yielding typical straw-colored cyst fluid. Pneumocystogram (right) demonstrates no intracystic masses. One cyst (arrow) was not punctured.

sometimes the sole radiographic indicator of nonpalpable cancers.[27] In view of this fact, the detection and evaluation of breast calcifications assumes utmost importance.

Microcalcifications occurring in a cluster are suspicious for malignancy, particularly if the calcifications vary in size and shape and are arranged in a linear configuration (Figure 5). Benign conditions such as sclerosing adenosis can produce clustered microcalcifications indistinguishable from those of a cancer, and generally account for the benign biopsies performed for such calcifications. In instances where the calcifications are homogeneous in size and form, the probability of malignancy is diminished. Such findings may be followed with more frequent periodic mammograms to assess for interval change, which is generally an indication for surgical biopsy. Occasionally, dermal calcifications (Figure 6) can simulate breast calcifications, although the former often have a characteristic appearance and location. Secretory disease (mammary duct ectasia) is a benign condition resulting in multiple homogeneous needlelike calcifications, clearly distinguishable from malignant calcifications (Figure 7).

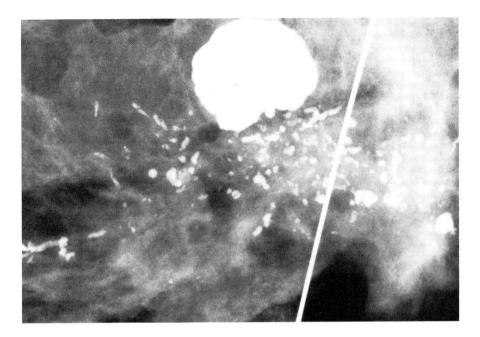

Figure 5.   Coned down view of a specimen radiograph (part of localization wire visualized) demonstrates focal malignant calcifications, varying in size and shape, in a linear and branched configuration. A heavily calcified adenofibroma is adjacent to the malignant calcifications.

In addition to the presence of masses or calcifications, there are indirect, nonspecific mammographic signs of malignancy. Such features include a developing density on the mammogram, not associated with a discrete mass or calcifications. Prominent ducts, architectural distortion, and breast edema are additional nonspecific signs that can be seen in conjunction with malignancy or a variety of benign conditions.

SPECIAL PROCEDURES

Magnification Radiography

In 1977, mammographic units capable of performing magnification views first became commercially available. Such capability has proved extremely useful in the evaluation of microcalcifications and the marginal characteristics of masses. Magnification views have become an important component of the tailored approach to mammography.[28]

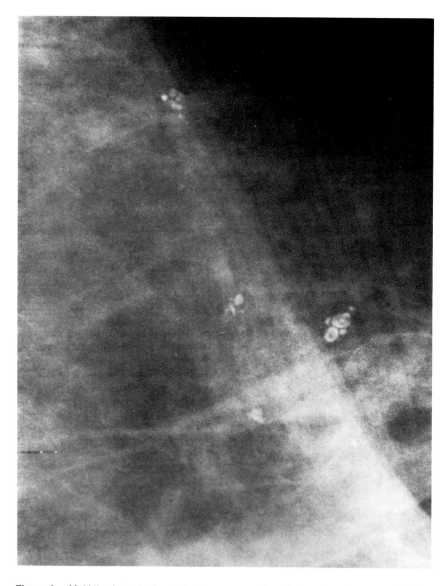

Figure 6. Multiple clusters of calcifications, many with radiolucent centers, are typical for dermal calcifications. Additional tangential projections confirmed that these calcifications were cutaneous in origin.

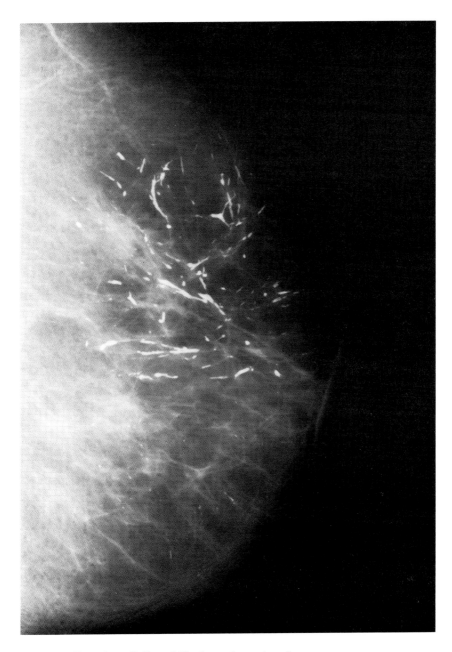

Figure 7. Typical needlelike calcifications of secretory disease.

Ductography

Spontaneous bloody or blood-tinged serous nipple discharges usually result from benign intraductal papillomas, although occasionally intraductal carcinomas can present in this manner. Such discharges must be differentiated from the common and innocent blue, green, or milky breast discharges resulting from fibrocystic disease.

The evaluation of a patient with a nipple discharge may include cytologic evaluation of the discharge. In addition, a duct injection can identify the involved duct or ducts as well as direct the surgeon to a particular quadrant in the breast. The performance of a ductogram requires that the discharge be present at the time of the examination, and entails the insertion of a blunt-tipped 30-gauge needle into the affected duct. After cannulation of the duct, a small volume of water-soluble contrast medium is injected, and orthogonal views are obtained. Filling defects (Figure 8), representing intraductal papillomas, are usually multiple and are radiographically indistinguishable from intraductal carcinomas.

Pneumocystography

Following aspiration of a cyst, the introduction of an equivalent volume of air (Figure 4) allows identification of the occasional intracystic papilloma or carcinoma (Figure 9). In addition, the introduction of air into a cyst may prevent cyst recurrence.[32]

Fine Needle Aspiration Biopsy

Fine needle aspiration biopsy (FNAB) can be performed for both palpable[9] and nonpalpable breast abnormalities. The introduction of coordinate, or perforated, compression plates for use in conjunction with dedicated mammography units allows accurate positioning of needles into nonpalpable masses or clustered calcifications for the purpose of obtaining cellular material for cytologic analysis. With experience on the part of the radiologist performing the procedure, as well as the pathologist interpreting the specimens, FNAB has proved to be a highly accurate and cost-effective procedure.[19] Although the specimens are subject to sampling error, particularly in the case of very small lesions, the use of FNAB provides additional information regarding the benign nature of lesions with a low suspicion for malignancy, especially if a lesion is to be followed with mammographic follow-up rather than excisional biopsy. A positive cytologic result may facilitate "one-stage" breast surgery.

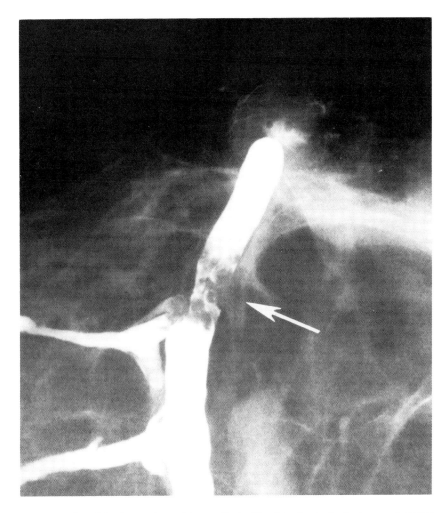

Figure 8. Duct injection performed in a patient with a bloody nipple discharge. A dilated duct containing a multilobular filling defect (arrow) is demonstrated. The finding at surgery represented a benign ductal papilloma.

Localization of Nonpalpable Abnormalities

Nonpalpable lesions can be easily localized by the radiologist for surgical excision. Several types of hook-wires are commercially available that can be accurately positioned adjacent to a radiographically suspicious abnormality (Figure 10).[13,16] In all instances of excision of a nonpalpable breast abnormality, specimen radiography (Figure 11) is essential to assure that the abnormality is contained in the resected specimen and to establish the completeness of the excision.

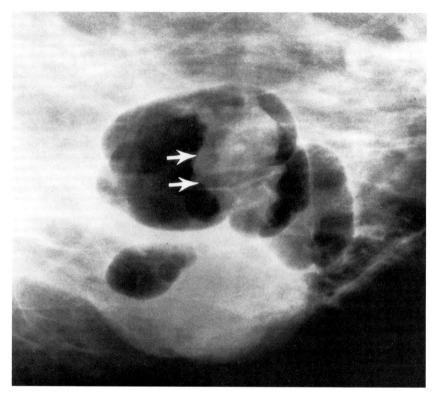

Figure 9. Aspiration of a cyst yielded bloody fluid, and the pneumocystogram demonstrated an intraluminal filling defect (arrows). Excision demonstrated a benign intracystic papilloma.

OTHER BREAST IMAGING MODALITIES

As indicated above, mammography has its limitations, particularly in women with dense breasts. Multiple attempts have been made to find a non-ionizing imaging technique as good as, or superior to, mammography for breast cancer screening and diagnosis. Unfortunately, thus far all such attempts have failed, and mammography remains the "gold standard." To a limited extent, however, ultrasound can play an important role in special settings.

Ultrasound is excellent in determining whether a mass is cystic or solid, and a 1984 statement by the American College of Radiology indicated that the main role of ultrasound should be restricted to this purpose.[2] Sonography should not be used for breast cancer screening. Breast ultrasound can be accomplished using either a dedicated automated water-path scanner or a high-frequency real-time hand-held probe. Due to the relative ease of

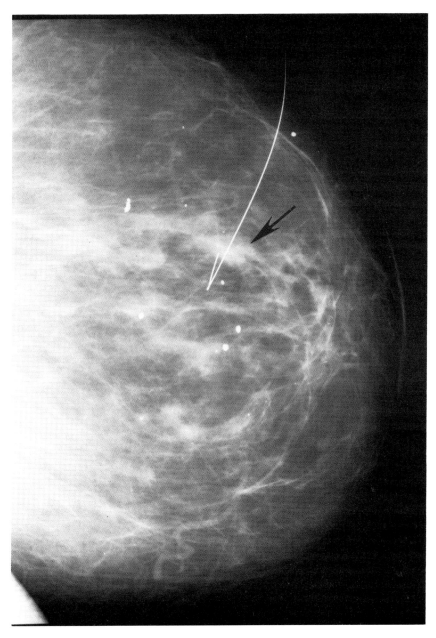

Figure 10. Hook-wire is in position, adjacent to a small nonpalpable cancer (arrow). Several coarse benign calcifications are scattered in the breast.

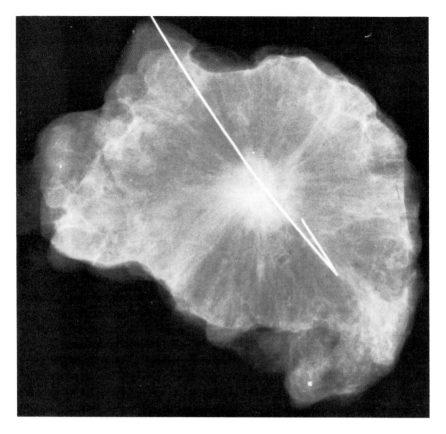

Figure 11.   Specimen radiograph of cancer shown in Figure 3 confirms surgical excision of this nonpalpable tumor.

use and availability, the latter alternative is currently more frequently employed. Accuracy rates for sonographic differentiation of cystic from solid masses ranges from 96% to 100%.[8,29] Unfortunately, however, ultrasound suffers from the inability to detect microcalcifications, difficulty in consistently demonstrating small masses, and the overlap of sonographic features for benign and malignant solid masses.[17] Generally, we favor aspiration of both palpable and nonpalpable masses in lieu of ultrasound examinations due to the simplicity of performing the procedure, the ability to obtain samples for cytologic analysis in the case of solid masses, and the therapeutic benefit of cyst aspiration.

In addition to mammography and ultrasound, other breast imaging techniques have been used or are currently undergoing evaluation. Thermography, which came into wide use in the 1970s, resulted in sensitivity and specificity too low to be considered clinically useful and was eliminated from the BCDDP screening program. The American College of Radiology currently regards thermography as an experimental technique with no established clinical indications. Diaphanography (light scanning) of the breast is a technique that has been in existence since the 1920s, with recent technical refinements using far red and near-infrared light. Currently, diaphanography should be regarded as an experimental technique with unproven benefit, although evaluation and technical improvements are ongoing. Other techniques including digital subtraction angiography of breast masses, magnetic resonance imaging, and dual energy mammography are also currently undergoing evaluation and must be considered experimental at this time.

SUMMARY

In the past decade, improved mammographic technique, at a fraction of the radiation dose, has improved the ability to detect nonpalpable, early breast cancers and has resulted in a reduction in mortality and morbidity from breast cancer. The use of specialized techniques, including magnification radiography and fine needle aspiration biopsy of nonpalpable lesions, frequently allows a preoperative diagnosis of malignancy with a high degree of certainty. Widespread availability of low-cost, high-quality screening mammography has yet to be achieved.

REFERENCES

1. Adams EE, Brues AM: Breast cancer in female radium dial workers first employed before 1930. J Occup Med 22:583–587, 1980.
2. American College of Radiology, Policy Statement on Sonography for the Detection and Diagnosis of Breast Disease. Prepared by the Committee on Breast Imaging of the Commission on Diagnostic Radiology, 1984.
3. Baker LH: The Breast Cancer Detection Demonstration Project: 5 year summary report. Cancer 32:194–225, 1982.
4. Baral E, Larrson LE, Mattson B: Breast cancer following irradiation of the breast. Cancer 40:2905–2910, 1977.
5. Boice JD, Monson RB: Breast cancer following repeated fluoroscopic examinations of the chest. JNCI 59:823–832, 1977.
6. Feig SA: Screening mammography: benefits and risks, in Moskowitz M (ed): *Diagnostic Categorical Course in Breast Imaging*. Chicago, Radiological Society of North America, 1986, pp. 75–84.
7. Feig SA: Assessment of the hypothetical risk from mammography and evaluation of the potential benefit. Radiol Clin North Am 21:173–191, 1983.
8. Fleischer AC, Muhletaler CA, Reynolds VH, et al: Palpable breast

masses: Evaluation by high frequency, hand-held real-time sonography and xeromammography. Radiology 148:813–817, 1983.

9. Frable WJ: Needle aspiration of the breast. Cancer 53:671–676, 1984.
10. Hall FM: Screening mammography—potential problems on the horizon. N Engl J Med 314:53–55, 1986.
11. Haus AG: Physical principles and radiation dose in mammography. Med Radiogr Photogr 58:70–80, 1982.
12. Hoeffken W, Lanyi M: *Mammography.* Philadelphia, WB Saunders Company, 1977, p 162.
13. Homer MJ: Nonpalpable breast lesion localizer using a curved-end retractable wire. Radiology 157:259–260, 1985.
14. Howe GR: Epidemiology of radiogenic breast cancer, in Boice JD Jr, Fraumeni JF Jr (eds.): *Radiation Carcinogenesis: Epidemiology and Biological Significance.* New York, Raven, 119–129, 1984.
15. Kleinschmidt O: In Zweifel-Payr (ed.): Klinik der bosartigen Geschwulste, Vol IV, Leipzig, Hirzel, 1927.
16. Kopans DB, Meyer JE: Versatile spring hookwire breast lesion localizer. AJR 138:586–587, 1982.
17. Kopans DB, Meyer JE, Lindfors KK: Whole breast US imaging: Four year follow-up. Radiology 157:505–507, 1985.
18. Kopans DB, Meyer JE, Sadowsky N: Breast imaging. N Engl J Med 310:960–967, 1984.
19. Lannin DR, Silverman JF, Pories WJ, et al.: Cost effectiveness of fine needle biopsy of the breast. Ann Surg 203:474–479, 1986.
20. Lundgren B, Jakobsson S: Single view mammography: A simple and efficient approach to breast cancer screening. Cancer 38:1124–1129, 1976.
21. Mammography: A statement of the American Cancer Society. CA 32:226–230, 1982.
22. Mammography guidelines 1983: Background statement and update of cancer-related checkup guidelines for breast cancer detection in asymptomatic women age 40–49. CA 33:255, 1983.
23. Moskowitz M: Minimal breast cancer redux. Radiol Clin North Am 21:93–113, 1983.
24. Shapiro S: Evidence of screening for breast cancer from a randomized trial. Cancer 39:2772–2782, 1977.
25. Shapiro S, Venet W, Strax P, et al.: Ten-to-fourteen year effect of screening on breast cancer mortality. JNCI 69:349–355, 1982.
26. Shore RE, Hempelmann LH, Kowaluk E, et al.: Breast neoplasms in women treated with x-rays for acute post-partum mastitis. JNCI 59:813–822, 1977.
27. Sickles EA: Mammographic features of 300 consecutive non-palpable breast cancers. AJR 146:661–663, 1986.
28. Sickles EA: Microfocal spot magnification mammography using xeroradiographic and film-screen recording systems. Radiology 131:599–607, 1979.
29. Sickles EA, Filly RA, Callen PW: Benign breast lesions: Ultrasound detection and diagnosis. Radiology 151:467–470, 1984.

30. Sickles EA, Weber WN, Galvin HB, et al.: Mammography screening: How to operate successfully at low cost. Radiology 160:95–97, 1986.
31. Tabar L, Fagerberg CJG, Gad A, et al.: Reduction in mortality from breast cancer after mass screening with mammography: Randomized trial from the Breast Cancer Screening Working Group of the Swedish National Board of Health and Welfare. Lancet 1:829–832, 1985.
32. Tabar L, Pentek Z, Dean PB: The diagnostic and therapeutic value of breast cyst puncture and pneumocystography. Radiology 141:659–663, 1981.
33. Tokunaga M, Norman JE Jr, Asano M, et al.: Malignant breast neoplasms among atomic bomb survivors, Hiroshima and Nagasaki, 1950–1974. JNCI 62:1347–1359, 1979.

9. *Fine Needle Aspiration: The New Diagnostic Technique?*

BERNARD NAYLOR

Fine needle aspiration has finally "arrived" as a diagnostic technique in North America. The impetus to its development began with the seminal publications of Papanicolaou and Traut who, in the early 1940s, described the finding of cancer cells in cellular samples from the female genital tract, an event which ushered in the beginnings of cytopathology as we know it today. These two publications and the numerous subsequent publications authored by Papanicolaou stimulated clinicians and pathologists to apply the cytologic method to the diagnosis of cancer in the other systems of the body. Thus developed the era of cytopathology where the cells to be examined were either spontaneously exfoliated or were obtained by scraping the area to be investigated.

The next broad development has been to obtain cells by aspirating them from superficially or deeply situated organs: fine needle aspiration (FNA) cytology. Although the diagnosis of neoplasms by FNA was practiced in the United States more than 50 years ago it, never enjoyed widespread use.[2] Only in about the last five years has its use become widespread and accepted. It was the wide use and advocacy of the method in Sweden that attracted the attention of a small number of pathologists in North America who went abroad, familiarized themselves with the method, and brought it back to these shores. At The University of Michigan we benefited from the Swedish experience when, in 1983, a visiting radiologist from Sweden began to aspirate routinely lesions of the breast at our Breast Cancer Detection Center. Prior to his arrival, FNA cytology of the breast was virtually not practiced in our institution.

From the point of view of the pathologists who have examined the specimens, our experience with FNA cytology of the breast since we began it three years ago has been extremely satisfying: the specimens have been abundant, the preparations excellent, the challenge stimulating, and the results gratifying. Furthermore, working closely with the radiologists and

99

the clinicians attached to our Breast Care Center has enabled us to be kept aware of the impact of our diagnostic endeavors.

As an outcome of our experience over the last three years, I shall address four aspects of FNA cytology of the breast: 1) procuring the specimen, 2) types of breast lesions that can be diagnosed by FNA, 3) our method of reporting, and 4) results.

PROCURING THE SPECIMEN

The method described below could not be simpler. It will enable you to make smears that can be stained by the Papanicolaou method, which is used routinely in cytopathology laboratories in North America.

What Is Needed to Perform a Fine Needle Aspiration?

The equipment required is simple and inexpensive (see Appendix).

1. Disposable 20-ml plastic syringe with Luer-Lok tip.
2. Syringe holder. It is entirely possible to aspirate lesions *without* a syringe holder; however, most prefer to use one since it allows one hand to fix or secure the lesion and the other hand to control the movement of the syringe and apply suction.
3. Disposable 22-gauge needles, preferably with *clear* plastic hubs. This simple feature enables the aspirator to see the first drop of material leaving the shaft of the needle and entering the hub. The importance of this is explained below.
4. Glass slides with one end frosted for writing on the identification of the patient with *lead pencil*.

How is the Fine Needle Aspiration Done?

Before beginning the procedure, inform the patient that you are going to "suck out" (not "aspirate") some cells with a needle. The procedure is as follows:

1. Anesthesia is rarely needed.
2. Fix the mass with your fingers.
3. Cleanse the skin with an alcohol swab. Before you insert the needle, dry the area with a piece of gauze. If you do this, it is less likely to sting when the needle is inserted.
4. Carefully poise the needle, just touching the point of insertion. Introduce the needle through the skin and advance it into the mass.
5. When the needle has entered the mass, apply suction.
6. Move the needle back and forth in the mass while applying the suction.
7. The moment any aspirated material is seen in the clear plastic hub, *release*

the suction and withdraw the needle. (If the needle hub were opaque more blood might be aspirated, thereby diluting the cellularity of the specimen.)

8. If after about 10 to 15 seconds no material is seen in the plastic hub, *release the suction* and withdraw the needle.

How Should the Specimen Be Handled?

1. Remove the needle from the syringe, suck air into the syringe, reattach the needle. Do all of this quickly, before any clotting takes place.
2. Express a drop of fluid about 2 to 3 mm in diameter onto the center of the glass slide.
3. With the beveled edge of the needle facing down, spread the cellular sample in a longitudinal and criss-cross manner, taking about 5 to 6 seconds, and then spray-fix the smear *before the slightest trace of drying occurs.* (Hold the nozzle of the spray fixative about 10″ from the smear.)

   Make 1 to 3 smears from each insertion. Flush out the syringe and needle in saline. Send this cell suspension to the laboratory in addition to the smears.

   Repeat the procedure twice for a total of three insertions.
4. Send the spray-fixed smears and the saline suspension of cells to the laboratory.

TYPES OF LESIONS THAT CAN BE DIAGNOSED BY FNA

Certain types of lesions can be diagnosed with certainty or, in correlation with the clinical and mammographic findings, their presence may be strongly suggested. In some situations the cytologic findings may be said to be "consistent with" a certain type of lesion.

1. *Carcinoma of the breast.* This is the malignant neoplasm of the breast most frequently diagnosed by FNA cytology (Figure 1). With an adequate specimen, the pathologist should be able not only to diagnose cancer, but also to specify what type it is, e.g., adenocarcinoma. We are not able to determine by FNA whether the carcinoma is only intraductal or invasive, nor do we specify as to whether it is a ductal or a lobular carcinoma.
2. *Other malignant neoplasms.* Other primary malignant neoplasms of the breast are uncommon; we have diagnosed only two over the three-year period, one a malignant lymphoma (Figure 2), the other a sarcoma of unknown type. Metastatic malignant neoplasms are also uncommon; we have diagnosed three: one metastatic malignant melanoma and two metastatic adenocarcinomas. Since some neoplasms metastatic to the breast closely resemble primary breast carcinomas, it is important that the person sending the specimen to the laboratory provides any history of previous neoplasm.
3. *Fibroadenoma.* Fibroadenoma may give an unequivocal cytologic picture (Figure 3). On the other hand, the cytologic picture may be only suggestive of or consistent with the diagnosis of fibroadenoma. Whatever the cytologic picture is, it should be possible to state that the cells in the preparation are

benign, even though it may not be possible to conclude with certainty that they are derived from a fibroadenoma.

4. *Fibrocystic "disease."* The only unequivocal evidence of fibrocystic changes that can be discerned in a fine needle aspirate is the presence of so-called apocrine metaplastic cells (Figure 4). These cells are the manifestation of a metaplastic change that commonly takes place in the epithelial lining of the cystic component of this condition. The other components, essentially a manifestation of lobular or ductal epithelial hyperplasia, cannot be discerned as such. Cells from such areas appear as fragments of benign mammary epithelium with no other distinctive features except, possibly, for some papillary formation.

5. *Intramammary lymph node.* The aspirate from an intramammary lymph node consists of numerous benign-appearing lymphoid cells (Figure 5); frequently, no other type of cell is present in the aspirate. This finding, combined with the clinical findings (if any) and the characteristic mammographic appearance, is strong presumptive evidence that the nodule aspirated is an intramammary lymph node.

6. *Fat necrosis.* We suggest the presence of fat necrosis when we find globules of what is presumably lipid released from damaged fat cells engulfed by macrophages (Figure 6).

7. *Subareolar papillomatosis.* An aspirate from a focus of subareolar papillomatosis gives a profusely cellular specimen composed of large cohesive sheets of

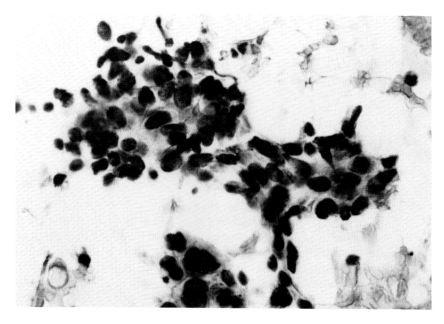

Figure 1.   Adenocarcinoma. This irregularly shaped fragment composed of loosely cohesive cells with hyperchromatic nuclei of various shapes and sizes is unequivocally malignant.

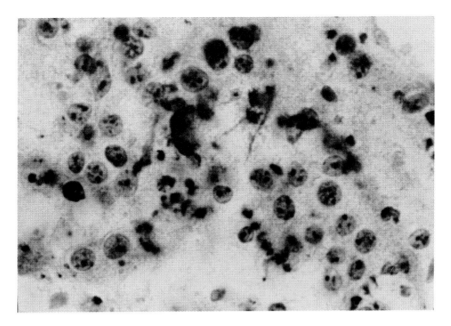

Figure 2. Malignant lymphoma. This field of noncohesive cells dominated by fairly uniform, round nuclei that contain large nucleoli is diagnostic of malignant lymphoma.

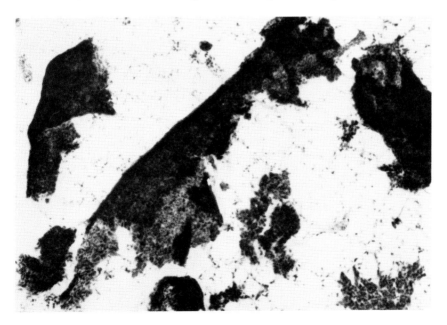

Figure 3. Fibroadenoma. These large fragments of mammary epithelium composed of small, uniform cells interspersed by numerous small, bare nuclei, is diagnostic of fibroadenoma.

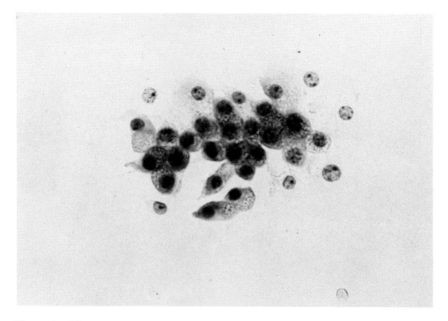

Figure 4. Fibrocystic disease. This flat sheet of large cells with finely granular cytoplasm and neatly round, relatively small nuclei containing prominent nucleoli is an example of apocrine metaplasia, a manifestation of fibrocystic disease.

benign-appearing mammary epithelial cells, many with a papillary configuration (Figure 7).

8. *Chronic subareolar abscess.* This specific clinicopathologic entity, believed to be the result of chronic inflammation of a lactiferous duct that has become dilated and undergone squamous metaplasia, gives a characteristic cytologic picture consisting of inflammatory cells and keratinizing and nonkeratinizing squamous epithelial cells (Figure 8).

REPORTING OF CYTOLOGIC SPECIMENS

Reports should be brief, accurate, and as specific as possible. However, as mentioned above, in certain benign conditions it may be possible to state that the cellular findings are only "consistent with" a specific lesion. Even so, a useful service may be provided by reporting that any mammary epithelial cells in the aspirate look benign.

When cells of malignant neoplasms are aspirated, we state that neoplastic cells are present and what type they are, in most cases adenocarcinoma. Reports expressing only various degrees of suspicion for the presence of cancer cannot be avoided although we are reluctant to issue such equivocal but alarming reports. We strive to avoid them.

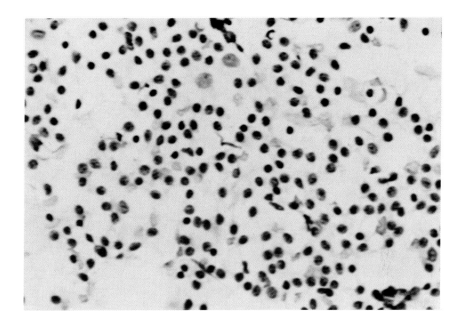

Figure 5. Intramammary lymph node. This field, composed almost exclusively of numerous benign appearing lymphocytes, is characteristic of an aspirate of an intramammary lymph node.

Certain benign lesions may be diagnosed and reported with specificity or with at least a strong suggestion as to the nature of the lesion. Even though the type of lesion may not be unequivocally diagnosed, one should be able to state that there is no cytologic evidence of malignancy.

Many aspirates contain only nonspecific cellular findings, such as blood, adipose tissue, and fragments of benign-appearing mammary epithelium. In such situations, the mammary epithelium may be derived from the clinically or radiographically detected abnormality in the breast; on the other hand, it may have been aspirated from normal breast tissue at the periphery of a lesion. In such cases we merely list our cytologic findings and do not specify as to whether neoplasm is or is not present.

We do not report specimens as being unsatisfactory, even when they contain no cells or very few cells. We describe what we see — or do not see. Some lesions, for example an area of fibrosis, may yield few or no cells on aspiration. To label such an aspirate "unsatisfactory" is unjustified; in fact, the person who carried out the aspiration may be very satisfied with the *non*-finding of cells since this could corroborate a clinical impression that the lesion consists essentially of fibrous connective tissue.

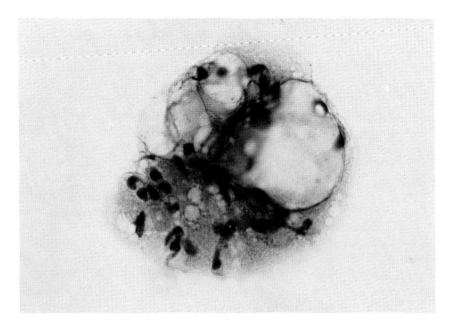

Figure 6.   Fat necrosis. This droplet of aspirate is composed of numerous globules, presumably released lipid. The nuclei in this droplet are those of macrophages, an inflammatory response to the lipid.

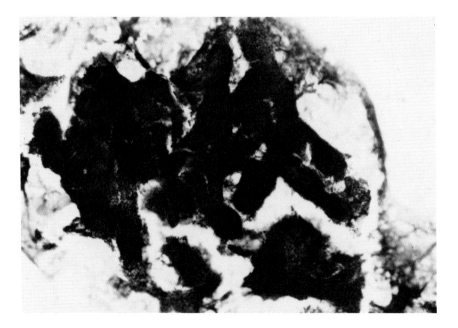

Figure 7.   Subareolar papillomatosis. This smear contains many large coalescent papillary fragments of mammary epithelium, typical of subareolar papillomatosis.

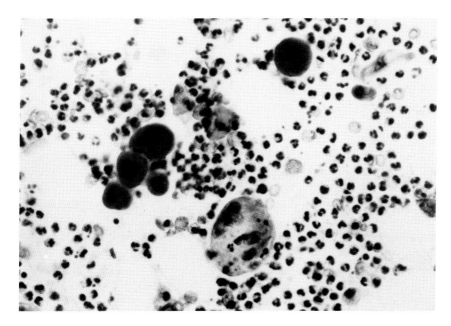

Figure 8.   Chronic subareolar abscess. This field illustrates numerous neutrophilic leuko-
cytes, a large multinucleated macrophage, several dark, round squamous epithelial cells, and numerous polygonal "empty" spaces that contain very lightly
stained anucleate flakes of keratin derived from metaplastic squamous epithelium. This picture is characteristic of chronic subareolar abscess.

RESULTS

Our series of 1200 aspirates included 161 cases of clinically palpable,
histologically confirmed breast cancer. One hundred thirty-one of these
neoplasms were unequivocally diagnosed as cancer by FNA, giving a sensitivity of 81.3%. Our reports contain one false suspicious report and six
reports in which we had commented on a degree of cytologic atypia, which
induced the clinicians to perform biopsy but where no malignant lesion was
found. With increasing experience, the frequency of such reports has
sharply diminished.

Differences between the rate of positives in studies of FNA of breast
cancer are related to many factors: differences in the clinical presentation of
the lesions, different techniques of aspiration, and variation in the pathologist's interpretation of the aspirated material. However, as a recent study
has shown, the most significant variable in the accuracy of FNA cytology of
the breast is the size of the lesion and the proficiency of the individual
performing the procedure.[1] With a skilled and experienced physician, positive aspiration results should be obtained in over 80% of breast cancers.
Failure to achieve 70% positive results in confirmed cases of breast cancer

indicates that something is wrong, either in the procurement or the interpretation of the specimens.

In our Breast Care Center several different persons perform the aspirations, often the radiologists performing mammography. Some of these radiologists have acquired a large experience in aspirating breast lesions, while their junior colleagues and the occasional surgeon aspirator have had much less experience. It is entirely possible that if all the breast aspirations were performed only by those radiologists who have a large experience with the technique, the sensitivity of the method would increase.

It is a controversial matter as to whether a biopsy should always be performed after a negative FNA result. In our experience, and as has been previously reported, the meaning of a negative aspiration result varies greatly with the proficiency of the physician performing the procedure.[1] The guidelines for biopsy confirmation must be influenced by the clinical risk factors, the characteristics of the lesion (particularly tissue texture), and the mammographic appearance of the lesion.

In all areas of breast disease it is extremely important that effective lines of communications exist between the persons performing the aspirations and the pathologists interpreting them. This viewpoint was pithily summarized by Stewart in 1933: "Diagnosis by aspiration is as reliable as the combined intelligence of the clinician and pathologist make it."[3]

APPENDIX

1. Disposable plastic syringes: standard hospital equipment.
2. Syringe holder.
   A. Cameco Syringe Pistol. Made of aluminum and stainless steel. Sterilizeable. Cost $165.00 plus $4.50 shipping (UPS). Obtain from Precision Dynamics Corporation, 13880 Del Sur Street, San Fernando, CA 91340, (818-897-1111). Remember to state the size of the syringe the holder should take: 20 ml.
   B. Aspir-Gun. Made of plastic. Non-sterilizeable. Holds only a 20 ml syringe. Cost $45.00 if payment made with order. Obtain from Everest Company, 5 Sherman Street, Linden, NJ 07036 (201-925-2012).
3. Disposable needles with clear plastic hubs. We use Monoject℗ needles. The most useful is the 22 gauge × 1 1/2" needle.

REFERENCES

1. Barrows GH, Anderson TJ, Lamb JL, et al.: Fine-needle aspiration of breast cancer. Relationship of clinical factors to cytology results in 689 primary malignancies. Cancer 58:1493-1498, 1986.
2. Frable WJ: *Thin-Needle Aspiration Biopsy.* Philadelphia, W.B. Saunders Co., 1983.
3. Stewart FW: The diagnosis of tumors by aspiration. Am J Pathol 9:801-812, 1933.

10. Technique of Segmental Mastectomy: The National Surgical Adjuvant Breast Project (NSABP) Experience

RICHARD G. MARGOLESE

Recent surveys of surgical practices have shown that the use of segmental mastectomy for the treatment of primary breast cancer is increasing.[1,2] The initial results of the National Surgical Adjuvant Breast Project (NSABP) Protocol B-06 have indicated that segmental mastectomy and axillary dissection with postoperative breast radiation is comparable to modified radical mastectomy in terms of disease-free survival and overall survival.[3]

A review of the NSABP experience has revealed some common technical errors in the performance of segmental mastectomy. While the primary goal is complete local control and removal of all tumor, it is important to keep in mind the ancillary goal of cosmetic outcome. It has become clear that certain technical definitions and recommendations will help ensure the proper performance of this procedure.

In order to meet the criterion of complete removal, pathological verification of the status of resection margins must be obtained. This requires thoughtful planning of the operation and careful collaboration with the pathologist (Figure 1).

BASIC TECHNIQUE

The ideal setting for a partial mastectomy is a small tumor in a field with no previous biopsy. The biopsy is the segmental mastectomy. This avoids the problems of segmental mastectomy as a second procedure, where hematoma and ecchymosis surrounding a cavity cause a confusing environment for the surgeon. It is much easier to approach a tumor that is well-defined and clearly palpable.

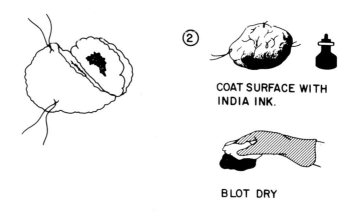

COAT SURFACE WITH
INDIA INK.

BLOT DRY

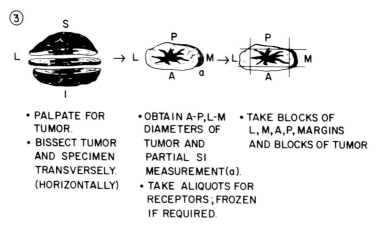

- PALPATE FOR
  TUMOR.
- BISSECT TUMOR
  AND SPECIMEN
  TRANSVERSELY.
  (HORIZONTALLY)

- OBTAIN A-P,L-M
  DIAMETERS OF
  TUMOR AND
  PARTIAL SI
  MEASUREMENT(a).
- TAKE ALIQUOTS FOR
  RECEPTORS; FROZEN
  IF REQUIRED.

- TAKE BLOCKS OF
  L, M, A, P, MARGINS
  AND BLOCKS OF TUMOR

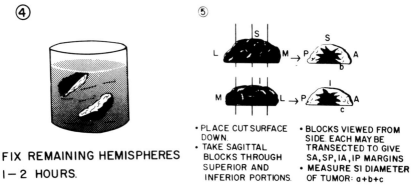

FIX REMAINING HEMISPHERES
1-2 HOURS.

- PLACE CUT SURFACE
  DOWN.
- TAKE SAGITTAL
  BLOCKS THROUGH
  SUPERIOR AND
  INFERIOR PORTIONS.

- BLOCKS VIEWED FROM
  SIDE. EACH MAY BE
  TRANSECTED TO GIVE
  SA, SP, IA, IP MARGINS
- MEASURE SI DIAMETER
  OF TUMOR: a+b+c

Figure 1. Recommended NSABP procedure for pathological preparation of segmental mastectomy specimens.

A small ellipse of skin can be left over the center of the tumor mass to orient the pathologist, but this is not necessary. The incisions are deepened in either direction away from the incision, but true flaps are not made. The tumor is outlined by continued palpation, and as the lateral walls are deepened, the tumor mass with the surrounding cuff of about 1 cm of normal tissue can be grasped and the remainder of the contours of the excision defined by continued palpation and the specimen removed. Although fascia on pectoralis major may be removed, this is not necessary either.

The most important aspect of the operation is control of the resection margins. Marking sutures are placed at 12 o'clock superiorly and 3 or 9 o'clock laterally in order to orient the specimen for the pathologist (Figure 1). If skin was not taken, a suture should also be placed at the superficial aspect. If there is any doubt grossly about limits of resection, frozen sections can be taken from the biopsy cavity corresponding to tissue opposite the doubtful area. Immediate assessment of adequacy of margins allows for resection of more tissue if indicated.

Incision Placement

Frequently, the placement of an incision for a benign tumor will be very different than for a carcinoma at the same site. For example, if an indeterminate periareolar mass is found on fine needle aspiration cytology to be benign, a cosmetic circumareolar incision would be indicated. However, if the cytologic diagnosis is suspicious or diagnostic for cancer, an incision over the mass would be better.

Use of Two Incisions

In general, an incision should not be extended to encompass the axillary dissection. Although one incision may suffice for lesions which are indeed high in the tail of the breast, the tendency to combine these incisions is generally overdone, resulting in avoidable poor cosmesis (Figure 2). For a tumor situated in the upper outer quadrant, stretching a radial incision up into the axilla results in a long suture line crossing the lines of tension, and the most common result is contraction and flattening of the scar. A transverse or circumferential incision for the segmental mastectomy and a separate axillary incision for the dissection are always better even when the two incisions are only 2 or 3 cm apart. The single-incision option should only be used when the tumor is so high that it falls within the axillary incision without any extension of that incision. When in doubt, use two incisions.

When it is remembered that the axillary phase of the operation is more for staging than for therapy, and that patients with lesions in the other three quadrants of the breast always have a two-incision procedure, it can be seen that there is no merit in stretching the axillary incision to encompass the tumor when there is even the slightest chance of avoidable cosmetic problems. The so-called en bloc resection is not a consideration.

Lesions in the lower half of the breast should not have skin sacrificed. If a transverse incision is used and a segment of skin is removed, the distance from the areola to the inframammary fold is shortened and the breast will be distorted unnecessarily, with loss of volume and collapse inferiorly (Figure 3).

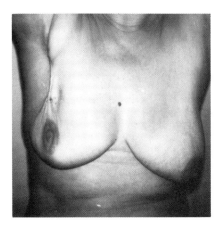 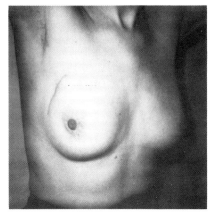

Figure 2.   a) A radial excision extended to the axilla causing flattening and scarring, which is avoidable. b) The use of two incisions for an upper outer quadrant tumor: improved cosmetic outcome with equivalent control of tumor and axillary node dissection.

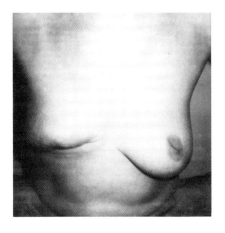 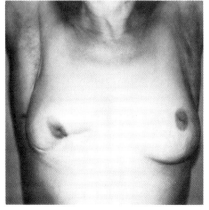

Figure 3.   Excessive removal of skin in the lower part of the breast causes collapse and distortion, which is avoidable.

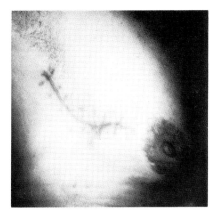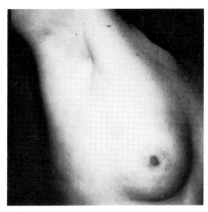

Figure 4.   a) Improper skin closure with tightly tied mattress sutures causes scarring and cross-hatching. b) Another patient with a similarly situated tumor shows better healing with appropriate surgical technique.

Parenchymal Reconstruction

In general, reconstruction should be specifically avoided. Cosmetic results are always superior if the spaces are allowed to fill with fibrin and organize. This gives a cosmetic contour and consistency that is close to normal and always superior to the condition caused by approximating breast tissue with large sutures. For this reason drains should never be used in the segmental mastectomy incision. Meticulous hemostasis should be obtained, however, because a hematoma may heal by fibrosis and give the consistency of a hard mass.

Skin Closure

Cosmetic principles of skin closure should be used and a subcuticular fine (5-0) Dexon is recommended. Alternatively, skin clips may be used and should be removed on the third or fourth day with Steri-strip support continuing. Interrupted nylon or silk sutures, especially mattress sutures, can often cause cross-hatching and should be avoided (Figure 4). The skin over the breast is soft, thin, and well vascularized and heals similarly to a thyroidectomy incision. If proper technique is followed, most such scars will be thin and flat.

Volume of Tissue Resected

The total volume resected depends on the size of the tumor, and the ratio of the tumor size to breast size will dictate which patients may not be suitable for this procedure. The goal is clear margins; therefore, a zone approximately 10 mm thick grossly should be included. If these margins are clear, there seems to be little point in excising more tissue. If doubt exists, frozen section of one or more areas can provide definitive information.

SUMMARY

Simultaneous consideration of both principles (complete resection and cosmetic preservation) provides a rational approach to priorities. Careful attention to the other details will result in the best cosmesis.

REFERENCES

1. Fisher B, Bauer M, Margolese R, et al: Five-year results of a randomized clinical trial comparing total mastectomy and segmental mastectomy with or without radiation in the treatment of breast cancer. N Engl J Med 312:665–673, 1985.
2. Nemoto T, Vana J, Bedwani RN, et al: Management and survival of female breast cancer: Results of a national survey by the American College of Surgeons. Cancer 45:2917–2924, 1980.
3. Wilson R, Donegan WL, Mettlin C, et al: The 1982 national survey of carcinoma of the breast in the United States by The American College of Surgeons. Surg Gynecol Obstet 159:309–318, 1984.

11. Changing Role of the Pathologist in the Diagnosis of Breast Lesions

HAROLD A. OBERMAN

The management of breast lesions has changed dramatically in the past 15 years, and this has occasioned equal modification of the pathologist's handling of breast specimens. For example, a major symposium held in 1969, The Pathology of Breast Lesions, contained no mention of screening mammography, fine needle aspiration cytology, primary radiation therapy, or "lumpectomy," and failed to recognize such current problems as assessment of margins of lumpectomy specimens, significance and diagnosis of the nonpalpable breast lesion or hormonal receptor determinations.[1] In addition, diagnosis of breast lesions at that time was primarily centered on intraoperative frozen section diagnosis followed by definitive treatment, with the patient being aware of the diagnosis only at the conclusion of the procedure.

INITIAL PROCESSING OF THE BREAST BIOPSY

Today the pathologist is usually asked to assess a breast biopsy obtained in an ambulatory care setting rather than from an anesthetized patient in the operating room. This allows for a less hurried approach to diagnosis and the opportunity for thorough assessment of the specimen before decisions are made about the definitive management of the patient.

Rather than being presented with a grossly defined breast mass, the pathologist is often confronted by a lesion that has been identified initially by mammographic evaluation of the breast, with notation of abnormal microcalcifications. Therefore, the pathologist must examine a specimen with no grossly discernible abnormality. In such instances, there is absolute necessity that the area of abnormality detected by the radiologist be visualized under the examining microscope. In order to accomplish such evalua-

115

tion, it is necessary that the excised specimen first be subjected to specimen mammography to ensure that the abnormal area has been removed. Localization of the areas of microcalcification in the specimen for microscopic examination may necessitate multiple sections of the specimen, on occasion assisted by radiographic examination of the paraffin blocks.

In many instances, initial diagnosis of a breast lesion is accomplished by fine needle aspiration cytology or by core biopsy using such techniques as the Tru-Cut needle. In these instances, the pathologist is required to diagnose a specimen using criteria that differ from those customarily employed when examining an entire lesion.[3]

FROZEN SECTION DIAGNOSIS

Given the aforementioned changes in the evaluation of a breast abnormality, what is the role of frozen section diagnosis? Frozen section techniques came to be routinely practiced when intraoperative diagnosis was mandatory. While frozen section diagnosis of a grossly defined lesion is remarkably accurate, there seems little reason to require such haste in diagnosis, as well as added expense, especially in light of the occasional falsely positive diagnosis, in this era of outpatient biopsy. In addition, frozen section diagnosis may result in distortion of the specimen for subsequent permanent section evaluation. This is a particularly important consideration when dealing with very small lesions or with papillary lesions. In both of these instances, performance of a frozen section may distort the specimen and interfere with diagnosis.

On occasion, frozen section diagnosis of a biopsy obtained in the outpatient clinic may be appropriate so that the overly anxious patient can be given provisional information about the character of the excised lesion. The technique also may find use in surgical management of the lesion that has been diagnosed as carcinoma solely on the basis of fine needle aspiration cytology. Intraoperative tissue confirmation of the diagnosis by frozen section is advisable before definitive treatment in this situation.

DETERMINATION OF HORMONAL RECEPTORS

A sample of grossly evident neoplasm should be obtained from the biopsy and submitted for determination of estrogen and progesterone receptors. Such tissue should be frozen, preferably in liquid nitrogen, within no more than 30 minutes after its excision. In those instances where initial diagnosis has been made on the basis of fine needle aspiration cytology, tissue for hormonal receptors is obtained at the time of subsequent wide local excision or modified radical mastectomy. When performing a mastectomy, it is important to obtain the sample for hormonal receptor determinations before the mastectomy has been completed to ensure that it is frozen within 30 minutes of loss of its blood supply. This can be accomplished by removing the neoplasm before performing the mastectomy.

Hormonal receptor assays are performed only on grossly evident neoplasm since at least 1 gm (approximately 1 cm³) of neoplasm is necessary for the evaluation. Frozen section diagnosis is not necessary to determine whether such assays should be performed. We freeze any grossly suspicious lesion and retain it for subsequent evaluation. Actual performance of the assays depends upon the results of permanent sections at a later date. It must be emphasized that the first responsibility of the pathologist in assessment of a breast biopsy specimen is diagnosis, and not performance of hormonal receptor assays. Therefore, there is no need to be concerned with such assays in the evaluation of the nonpalpable breast lesion. In that situation, even if carcinoma is present, the amount of neoplasm is usually so small that assays performed on the excised material may prove to be falsely negative.

While immunocytochemical techniques are available for determination of both estrogen and progesterone receptors, they are expensive, and there is concern about the correlation of the results with cytosol techniques. In contrast to results of the cytosol technique, which can be quantitated, interpretation of the immunocytochemical procedure is qualitative and is subject to variability of observer assessment of depth of nuclear staining. Current techniques require use of frozen sections of fresh material, so that this assay would not be applicable for paraffin-embedded specimens. It is unlikely that this procedure will allow the determination of hormonal receptors in intraductal, or very small invasive, carcinomas because one would be reluctant to risk tissue distortion of such specimens from freezing. It seems probable that this technique may find earliest applicability for fine needle aspiration cytology specimens. However, ultimately it should replace cytosol methodology.

MICROSCOPIC DIAGNOSIS OF CARCINOMA

Biopsies of minute abnormalities seen on screening mammography often result in the need for the pathologist to recognize malignant change in a less well developed setting. The most common diagnostic problem to be presented to consultant pathologists is the distinction of intraductal carcinoma from intraductal hyperplasia. All breast carcinoma begins within the duct system. Neoplastic change is characterized by proliferation of intraductal epithelial cells, resulting in a homogeneous growth pattern. The neoplastic cells grow into the duct lumen, and may present as solid, fenestrated, cribriform, or micropapillary growth patterns (Figure 1). In each instance, there

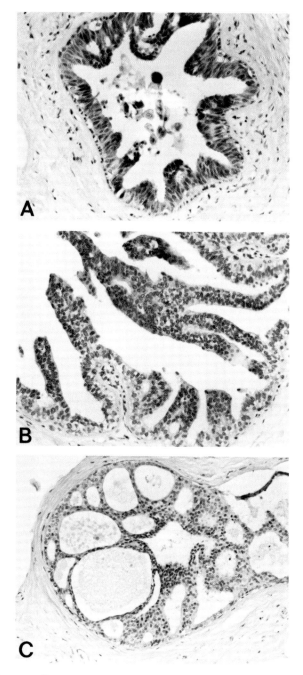

Figure 1. Patterns of intraductal carcinoma. *(a)* Involvement of duct circumference without necrosis or occlusion; *(b)* micropapillary growth; *(c)* cribriform proliferation
of neoplastic cells.

are benign counterparts of these growth patterns which must be distinguished. In approximately one-third of cases, the intraductal malignancy is
multifocal, involving multiple ducts in the excised segment of breast. On
occasion, only a small aggregate of ducts are involved. Are these apparent
early expressions of breast disease truly cancer? Follow-up studies of
patients whose lesions were underdiagnosed, resulting only in excisional
biopsy, have been used to resolve this issue. Subsequent carcinoma of the
ipsilateral breast developed in ten of fifteen of these patients treated at
Memorial Sloan-Kettering Cancer Center, and eight of these ten neoplasms
proved to be invasive.[18] No subsequent neoplasm developed in the contralateral breast in these patients after a mean follow-up interval of approximately ten years. This high incidence of subsequent invasive neoplasm in
the ipsilateral breast of such patients, often at the biopsy site, leaves little
doubt of the malignant character of these lesions.

FURTHER ASSESSMENT OF THE LESION

While the prognosis of patients who have neoplasm confined to the mammary duct system (intraductal carcinoma) is excellent after appropriate
treatment, stromal invasion of neoplastic cells significantly worsens the
prognosis. This requires careful sampling of the specimen, as the invasive
component may be of minimal extent in the biopsy specimen. It is important that the pathologist distinguish stromal invasion of neoplasm from
extension of neoplasm into lobular ducts.[5] The latter may simulate invasion
(Figure 2).

Once the pathologist has defined the presence of invasion, it is necessary
to assess the specimen for the presence of neoplastic invasion of lymphatics.
Recent studies have shown that this has significance comparable to that of
lymph nodal involvement.[10] This is especially true for those patients with T1
tumors (tumors measuring up to 2.0 cm in greatest dimension). In these
patients who lacked axillary lymph nodal involvement, the recurrence rate
of neoplasm was approximately ten times greater when lymphatic invasion
was present than when it was absent.

Regardless of whether the patient is to have a mastectomy or is to be
treated by lumpectomy followed by radiation therapy, axillary lymph nodal
excision is performed. This provides for staging of the neoplasm and planning for adjuvant treatment, and also removes involved lymph nodes that
subsequently might result in large axillary masses that would be difficult to
manage. The surgeon should tag the apex of the axillary dissection so that
the pathologist can assess the extent of lymph nodal involvement. When the
axillary contents are removed *in toto*, lymph nodes adjacent to the chest
wall below the pectoralis minor muscle should be segregated from those
beneath the muscle and those above it. This allows for improved assessment

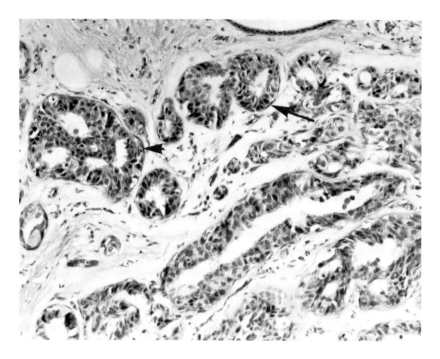

Figure 2. Extension of intraductal carcinoma into lobular ducts simulating stromal invasion. Presence of myoepithelial cells around lobular ducts (arrows) distinguishes this from invasive carcinoma.

of extent of involvement by neoplasm. While the pathologist must determine the number of lymph nodes involved, we have found little value in
defining such factors as sinus histiocytosis or nodal follicular hyperplasia.
In our experience, less than 1% of patients diagnosed as having intraductal
carcinoma are found to have simultaneous metastatic neoplasm in axillary
lymph nodes. When such metastases are encountered, it is a reflection of
the difficulty of recognizing small foci of stromal invasion with the usual
sampling techniques. Even though the pathologist may take multiple samples of a biopsy specimen containing multifocal intraductal carcinoma,
small foci of invasion can be undetected.

The pathologist must assess the adequacy of excision of neoplasms
treated by wide local excision ("lumpectomy"). This requires close cooperation between surgeon and pathologist. The surgeon must orient the lumpectomy specimen for the pathologist by placing sutures at the superior and
lateral aspects of the specimen. The specimen then is coated with dye, such
as India ink, and blotted dry, permitting microscopic recognition of margins of excision. The specimen should be bisected during the operation to
allow the pathologist to assess gross adequacy of margins, and to allow the

surgeon to reexcise the biopsy cavity. Permanent sections then are taken from the various surgical margins. Frozen section assessment of these margins should not be necessary.

The pathologist must evaluate the lumpectomy specimen for the presence of multifocal intraductal carcinoma because this is the best predictor of subsequent recurrence. A recent report noted that patients with extensive intraductal involvement had a 22% incidence of local recurrence five years following radiation therapy, but other patients a 1% incidence.[9]

We do not attempt to perform nuclear grading of neoplasms. This criterion has not proven useful in anticipating recurrence;[9] moreover, the degree of interobserver variability in interpretation of this criterion invalidates its usefulness in the usual surgical pathology laboratory.[7]

SIGNIFICANCE OF "SMALL" CANCERS

The concept of minimal carcinoma of the breast refers to a form of carcinoma wherein the prognosis does not differ significantly from that of intraductal carcinoma. When initially defined, minimal carcinoma implied the presence of an invasive carcinoma whose greatest diameter was no greater than 0.5 cm, or of an intraductal or lobular carcinoma in situ, unassociated with *clinically* abnormal axillary lymph nodes.[6] The concept since has been refined to include invasive neoplasms less than 1.0 cm, unassociated with microscopic evidence of metastatic carcinoma in the axillary lymph nodes.[2] One form of invasive carcinoma, usually detected by the mammographer, which is associated with an excellent prognosis, is tubular carcinoma. Such neoplasms average less than 1.0 cm in diameter, and in our experience, rarely exceed 2.0 cm.[14] The neoplasms are characterized by a haphazard infiltration of mammary stroma by well-formed, angulated ducts (Figure 3). This apparently represents an early expression of stromal invasion. It is important that this growth pattern be distinguished from sclerosing adenosis, as well as from other newly recognized forms of adenosis, by the pathologist.[13]

The term "early carcinoma" is a misnomer. When one considers the doubling time of carcinomas of breast, it is likely that the earliest lesion that can be detected by palpation must have been present for at least two to three years, and perhaps as long as eight to ten years.[16] Some have questioned the clinical significance of carcinomas detected solely by screening mammography. In studies conducted in the early and middle 1970s, over half of such neoplasms manifested stromal invasion when initially detected.[15] Moreover, minute primary breast neoplasms may be associated with massive axillary involvement, as in the instance of the so-called occult carcinoma of the breast.[17] Therefore, there seems little reason to deny the clinical significance of such lesions.

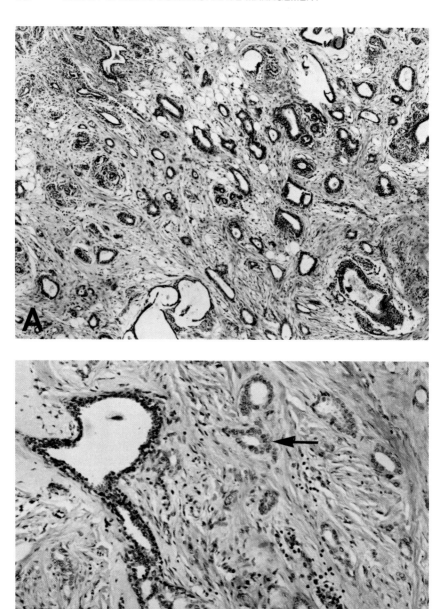

Figure 3. Invasive tubular carcinoma. *(a)* Haphazard infiltration of stroma by angulated ducts of uniform size; *(b)* absence of myoepithelial cells around invasive ducts (arrow) (compare with Figure 2).

LOBULAR CARCINOMA IN SITU

A unique form of carcinoma of the breast, initially recognized in 1941, is lobular carcinoma in situ. In this lesion, lobular ducts are distended by a uniform population of relatively bland, poorly cohesive cells (Figure 4). The lesion is characterized by multicentricity and a propensity for involvement of both breasts. Depending upon the extent of contralateral breast evaluation, and the thoroughness of assessment of the biopsy, 30% to 50% of patients have simultaneous bilateral neoplasm. In most instances, lobular carcinoma in situ is detected by chance, in the course of examination of a biopsy performed for cysts or for microcalcifications related to sclerosing adenosis.

There is debate whether this represents a variant form of noninvasive carcinoma or is a marker lesion defining a high risk for subsequent invasive neoplasm. In addition, long-term follow-up studies of patients with this lesion who have not been subjected to mastectomy have resulted in some divergence of opinion regarding their management.[8,19] The study from Memorial Sloan-Kettering Cancer Center indicated that 22% of patients developed ipsilateral cancer after a mean follow-up interval of 24 years, while a like number developed contralateral carcinoma over the same inter-

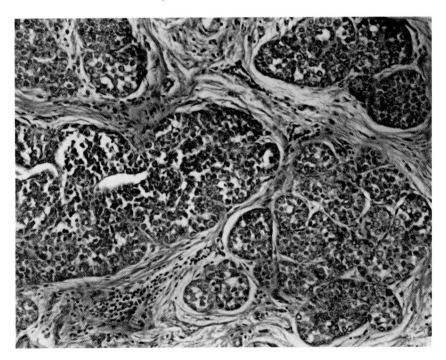

Figure 4.   Lobular carcinoma in situ. All lobular ducts are distended by uniformly sized cells lacking atypism.

val, although the latter group of patients also include some with lobular carcinoma in situ in the contralateral breast. The Columbia University study resulted in a lower incidence of subsequent ipsilateral and contralateral carcinoma, but the mean follow-up interval was eight years shorter.

While some advocate aggressive treatment of such lesions, others who consider this a marker lesion for subsequent malignancy believe that a course of careful clinical observation will suffice, especially for those patients beyond their sixth decade of life. The extent of disease cannot be defined in a small biopsy specimen in this condition because of the common presence of multifocal involvement. Therefore, lumpectomy would seem to play little role in the management of patients with this diagnosis. The current alternative lies between mastectomy and careful clinical observation. We believe that it is appropriate to individualize to some extent in the management of such patients. This implies that other risk factors, as well as the patient's age and willingness to engage in a seemingly experimental program of clinical observation, are taken into consideration.

At the time of diagnosis of lobular carcinoma in situ, the contralateral breast must be biopsied before a treatment program can be defined. This implies that a rather generous biopsy of the upper outer quadrant of the breast be obtained, especially from the segment within a radius of 5 cm from the nipple since this area contains relatively more mammary parenchyma than other quadrants.

SUMMARY

While the assessment of breast specimens by the pathologist has changed greatly in the past decade, with new radiologic screening expertise and the advent of primary radiation therapy for breast carcinoma, we may anticipate additional changes in the near future. Better assessment of growth rate of neoplasms through such techniques as DNA quantitation and nuclear cytometry may provide improved prognostic information.[4,11,12] Similarly, as previously noted, it is likely that the current cytosol method for assessment of hormonal receptors will be replaced by immunocytochemical techniques, which will allow assessment of much smaller lesions. Nevertheless, for the foreseeable future, the diagnosis of carcinoma will continue to rest upon the light microscopic interpretation of the breast biopsy by the well-trained pathologist.

REFERENCES

1. Ackerman LV: Lesions of the mammary gland. American Society of Clinical Pathologists, Chicago, 1969.
2. Ackerman LV, Katzenstein AL: The concept of minimal breast cancer

and pathologist's role in the diagnosis of early carcinoma. Cancer 39:2755, 1977.

3. Bauermeister DE: The role and limitations of frozen section and needle aspiration biopsy in breast cancer diagnosis. Cancer 46:947–949, 1980.
4. Beak JPA: The relative prognostic significance of nucleolar morphometry in invasive ductal breast cancer. Histopathology 9:437–444, 1985.
5. Fisher ER, Sass R, Fisher B, et al.: Pathologic findings from the national surgical adjuvant breast project (protocol 6) I. Intraductal carcinoma (DCIS). Cancer 56:197–208, 1986.
6. Gallager HW, Martin JE: Early phases in the development of breast cancer. Cancer 24:1170–1178, 1969.
7. Gilchrist KW, Kalish L, Gould VE, et al.: Interobserver reproducibility of histopathological features in stage II breast cancer. Breast Cancer Res Treat 5:3–10, 1985.
8. Haagensen CD, Lane N, Lattes R, et al.: Lobular neoplasia (so-called lobular carcinoma in situ) of the breast. Cancer 42:737–769, 1978.
9. Harris JR, Recht A, Schnitt S, et al.: Current status of conservative surgery and radiotherapy as primary local treatment for early carcinoma of the breast. Breast Cancer Res Treat 5:245–255, 1985.
10. Lee AKC, DeLellis RA, Silverman ML, et al.: Lymphatic and blood vessel invasion in breast carcinoma. Hum Pathol 17:984–987, 1986.
11. McDivitt RW, Stone KR, Craig RB, et al.: A comparison of human breast cancer cell kinetics measured by flow cytometry and thymidine labeling. Lab Invest 52:287–291, 1985.
12. Meyer JS: Cell kinetic measurements of human tumors. Hum Pathol 13:874–877, 1982.
13. Oberman HA: Benign breast lesions confused with carcinoma. In McDivitt RW, Oberman HA, Ozzello L, and Kaufman N (eds.): *The Breast*. Baltimore, Williams & Wilkins, 1984, pp. 1–33.
14. Oberman HA, Fidler WJ: Tubular carcinoma of the breast. Am J Surg Pathol 3:387–395, 1979.
15. Patchefsky AS, Shaber GS, Schwartz GF, et al.: The pathology of breast cancer detected by mass population screening. Cancer 40:1659–1670, 1977.
16. Pearlman AW: Breast cancer—influence of growth rate on prognosis and treatment evaluation. Cancer 38:1826–1833, 1976.
17. Rosen PP: Axillary lymph node metastases in patients with occult non-invasive breast carcinoma. Cancer 46:1298–1306, 1980.
18. Rosen PP, Braun DW, Kinne DE: The clinical significance of pre-invasive breast carcinoma. Cancer 46:919–925, 1980.
19. Rosen PP, Lieberman PH, Braun DW, et al.: Lobular carcinoma in situ of the breast. Am J Surg Pathol 2:225–251, 1978.

SECTION THREE

Issues in the Management of the Patient with Breast Cancer

12. The Surgeon's Role in the Management of the Patient with Breast Cancer

WILLIAM W. COON

Although many physicians may become involved in the diagnosis and management of the patient with breast cancer, the surgeon usually plays a principal role in this process. As a surgeon who has been involved with the treatment of this disease for more than 35 years, I have been asked to make some comments regarding my personal philosophy and current attitudes regarding diagnosis and therapy; these opinions do not necessarily represent the approach of all of my many colleagues who share in the management of breast cancer at the University of Michigan Medical Center. The more one peruses the thousands of papers published on this topic, the less dogmatic he becomes concerning what represents the optimal approach to diagnosis and treatment. The following comments represent some of my current opinions, which may well change in the future as more definitive data become available.

DIAGNOSIS OF BREAST CANCER

With very few exceptions, the woman who consults her physician because of a palpable lump in the breast is apprehensive and anxious and is seeking a prompt answer to whether the lump could represent a breast cancer. Good patient care, which includes concern for the individual's psychologic well-being, necessitates that the patient be seen and evaluated promptly. If, after examining the lump, there is any concern about a possible cancer, every woman age 30 or over should have bilateral mammograms performed; in younger women, mammography may be considered if the mass is particularly worrisome but with the realization that differentiation of cancer from benign masses is less accurate because of the greater density of breast tissue. Even in the patient with clinically obvious breast cancer, mammography can be helpful in defining whether multicentric or bilateral lesions are present;

129

foreknowledge of these conditions aids greatly in planning operative management.

Needle aspiration cytology of palpable or mammographically demonstrable lesions has been helpful in eliminating the discomfort of open biopsy in the group of patients in whom aspiration biopsy is positive for carcinoma. An aspiration interpreted as benign or acellular has little relevance since the area of concern may have been missed. A negative aspiration cytology should be followed by open biopsy if there is sufficient concern after physical exam or mammography that the lesion might be malignant. In this litigious age, a valid argument can be made that any lesion suspicious enough to require aspiration cytology should be biopsied if negative. However, with the availability of pathologists highly skilled in interpreting aspiration specimens, I am performing this procedure in many patients whom I would have previously followed with frequent examinations. On this basis, if the patient is followed with frequent exams and is informed of the uncertain character of the lesion and is comfortable with a period of follow-up rather than immediate biopsy, this process in selected patients would appear to be more cost-effective and eliminate some of the multiple biopsies some women undergo during their lifetimes.[7]

Similarly, the cost-effectiveness of sending all fluid aspirated from breast cysts for cytologic examination is debatable. If cyst fluid contains any evidence of blood, pathologic examination is imperative. If the cyst recurs after aspiration, biopsy is indicated. Pneumocystography has been helpful in ruling out an intracystic carcinoma.

Every breast biopsy should be approached with the assumption that the lesion may be malignant. This concept is important in planning the incision so that "lumpectomy" will be complete and the biopsy scar will not interfere with the most cosmetic incision for mastectomy. The incision should be placed directly over the lump and should usually extend transversely, as I feel that transverse mastectomy incisions provide optimal cosmesis and are most satisfactory for subsequent breast reconstruction. Partial circumareolar incisions are only suitable for small subareolar lesions. Each specimen is sent without preservative for determination, if positive for cancer, of estrogen and progesterone receptor activity.

Approximately 99% of our breast biopsies are performed under local anesthesia, including needle localization procedures. The rare exceptions involve deep-lying lesions in women with very large breasts and operations in patients who are uncooperative or who refuse local anesthesia. Concomitant biopsy and mastectomy under general anesthesia is outmoded. The opportunity for the woman to learn the definitive diagnosis after biopsy and then, if cancer is diagnosed, to consider alternative methods of treatment is essential to the current management of this condition. Whether immediate examination by frozen section of gross lesions removed at biopsy should be routine has been debated with our pathologists. Although this represents an additional cost, most women are so anxious concerning the diagnosis that they welcome the assurance that they will be told the result of the frozen section examination before they leave the biopsy suite; it is explained to every patient, however, that a "benign" diagnosis on frozen section is not definitive and that, in several percent of instances, permanent sections will demonstrate a cancer undetected by the limited immediate exam. No needle localization biopsies are submitted to frozen section in order to preserve all tissue for more definitive studies.

The biopsy technique required to define whether the lesion has been completely excised will be discussed by Dr. Margolese. This consideration is of importance for women who are potential candidates for "lumpectomy." A major problem is women who are referred to us for a second opinion regarding lumpectomy who have had a breast biopsy elsewhere; it is often impossible to determine from the operative note and prepared slides whether the primary lesion has been completely excised. If reexcision of the biopsy site is contemplated because of concern regarding residual neoplasm, the reaction associated with the first operation often makes determination of adequacy of the reexcision extremely difficult and adds to the deformity of the segment of breast. Marriyo et al. have recently reported a 27% incidence of residual disease at the biopsy site in needle-localized mammographically detected cancers.[8]

DISCUSSION WITH THE PATIENT OF ALTERNATIVE TREATMENTS

While a number of states have now mandated that the several methods for treatment of breast cancer be discussed with each patient, it is important that the surgeon interpret for the patient the advantages and disadvantages of each method and the appropriateness of each therapeutic approach for that particular patient. The problem that every well-read physician encounters in attempting to present an honest and valid assessment of various therapies is that one can find studies to support or denigrate each modality of treatment. In many instances, one can say that at the present time we do not know that one treatment is better than another. The validity of many reports of a specific treatment is confused by selection and time biases and inadequate duration of follow-up.

"Lumpectomy," Axillary Dissection, and Radiotherapy

Many patients present to our breast care clinic seeking this alternative to mastectomy. Several studies that have indicated that this is a satisfactory therapy have been limited to women with solitary lesions 2 cm in size or smaller; other reports have included lesions up to 4 cm.[2] The patient should be told that local recurrence (or evolution of a new multicentric cancer) will occur at an estimated rate of 1% to 2% per year, that more frequent long-term follow-up is required to detect this potential recurrence, and that not all (probably only 1/2) of recurrences will be "curable" by subsequent mastectomy. Perhaps larger lesions in women with large breasts can also be managed by this approach, but the patient should be told that, in this instance, the treatment is "experimental" in the sense that no definitive data are available to prove this postulate; in fact, the recently reported results of the National Surgical Adjuvant Breast Project (NSABP) Protocol B-06 indicate the recurrence is higher in lesions greater than or equal to 2.0 cm, those with high histologic and nuclear grades, or intralymphatic extension.[3] Evidence of possible multifocality by biopsy or mammogram (other clusters of calcifications, etc.) is another contraindication to this procedure. Lumpectomy without added radiotherapy is unacceptable in view of the much higher recurrence rates reported in the NSABP trial.[2]

Occasionally, in elderly patients with small lesions and severe associated disease that increases the risk of general anesthesia, we have recommended lumpectomy and radiotherapy without axillary dissection.

Radical Mastectomy

The evolution of the modified radical mastectomy over the past 20 to 30 years has resulted in considerable improvement in the cosmetic appearance of the chest wall and the ease of breast reconstruction. Only in the rare case of deep-lying lesions invading the pectoral fascia is conventional radical mastectomy indicated. Although a few additional level III lymph nodes may be removed with the standard (Halsted) mastectomy, no convincing data are available to demonstrate a significant increase in survival.[1] Extended radical mastectomy has not been practiced at our institution for several decades; although Urban has reported a somewhat improved survival in patients with large medial lesions, it is doubtful whether this more extensive and morbid procedure will achieve any better results than with the addition of adjuvant chemotherapy to modified or Halsted radical mastectomy. A prospective randomized trial of Halsted mastectomy versus extended radical mastectomy has shown no difference in survival at ten years.[1]

At the time of discussion of mastectomy with the patient, the possibility of breast reconstruction is also discussed. Our plastic surgeons feel that better results are obtained if the reconstruction is delayed approximately six months. This permits the prior administration of adjuvant chemotherapy to women with involved axillary nodes and allows the patient to make a more reasoned decision concerning breast reconstruction when some of the apprehension and emotional upset following the initial diagnosis of cancer has lessened; many patients who are initially in favor of breast reconstruction change their minds about a further operative procedure after later consideration and discussion with their families.

Very extensive and "inflammatory" breast cancers are now managed initially with chemotherapy, radiation, or a combination of both. The patient's cancer is monitored for response to treatment; if sufficient regression of the cancer is achieved, palliative mastectomy is performed in an effort to prevent the development of neoplastic ulceration over the chest wall.

TECHNICAL CONSIDERATIONS

My preferred incision is transverse or slightly oblique, since this approach provides the optimal cosmesis for women who elect to have subsequent breast reconstruction. Unless the cancer is extensive and invading through the capsule of the breast into the subcutaneous tissues, development of thin skin flaps is not only illogical but predisposes to skin necrosis.[6] In modified radical mastectomy, the pectoralis minor muscle is not divided, since Moosman's excellent anatomic studies have demonstrated that division of this muscle will frequently result in division of the lateral pectoral nerve and denervation of the lower third of the pectoralis major with subsequent atrophy.[9] No consistent attempt is made to remove the interpectoral nodes since prior studies have shown that isolated involvement of these nodes seldom occurs, and that when these nodes contain cancer, there is usually extensive axillary nodal involvement as well, obviating the likelihood of operative "cure" of the lesion.[12]

Regardless of the amount of drainage from the axillary drain postoperatively, the drain is removed by the fifth or sixth postoperative day, since leaving the drain in place for a longer period is linked to a high frequency of drain tract infection. Fluid rarely reaccumulates after drain removal, but if it does, it is aspirated with needle and syringe.

OTHER ISSUES IN MANAGEMENT OF BREAST CANCER

Random Contralateral Biopsy

In the absence of any significant mammographic abnormality in the opposite breast, biopsies are routinely performed only in patients with lobular carcinoma (invasive or in situ).

Atypical Ductal and Lobular Hyperplasia

The extensive studies by Page et al.[10] have demonstrated that this diagnosis (which requires the opinion of a skilled pathologist) is linked to a greater than fourfold increase in risk for subsequent development of carcinoma. When this diagnosis is made in a woman who relates a family history of breast carcinoma in a primary relative, the risk increases to eight- to tenfold. These patients are placed in our "high risk" group and followed with every-three-month physical examination and annual mammography.

Carcinoma in Situ

This issue has engendered a great deal of controversy regarding proper management. The statistical data and alternatives in treatment are discussed at length with the patient. I have several patients whose breast biopsies have shown a single focus in one high-powered field of ductal or lobular carcinoma and who have elected to be followed closely; as long as the patient appreciates the risks, as best we can define them, this seems to be a reasonable approach. However, if the in situ change is more extensive, further treatment would appear to be preferable. Whether further segmental resection of breast tissue, total mastectomy, radiotherapy, or modified radical mastectomy is a satisfactory or optimal treatment has not been defined. A major concern is whether the patient may harbor a focus of invasive carcinoma elsewhere in that breast.[11]

In patients with lobular carcinoma in situ, the comparably increased risk of development of invasive carcinoma in the opposite breast is discussed; frequent follow-up of the opposite breast is recommended unless contralateral biopsy shows similar changes. "Prophylactic" removal of the other breast is not recommended unless the patient requests such a procedure for psychologic reasons.

Recent studies of in situ intraductal carcinomas have shown a very high frequency of multifocality in the same breast;[4,5] these findings lead one more to consider mastectomy in these individuals.

Follow-up

Each physician has his or her own program for following patients with breast cancer. I examine all patients every three months for three years and continue this interval for patients treated by lumpectomy and radiotherapy. The intervals between exams are gradually lengthened for mastectomy patients. Mammograms of the opposite breast are performed at least annually, sometimes more frequently in lumpectomy patients who are followed with our radiotherapists at joint visits.

SUMMARY

In summary, we should recognize the many aspects of breast cancer concerning which we have no definitive answers at present. The surgeon should be selective in management of individual patients and honest in discussions with respect to what we do not know. He or she should respect the autonomy of the patient, her right to share in decisions regarding therapy once she is adequately informed. However, it is obligatory that the patient be counselled if, in her particular case, a given form of therapy is less desirable or if a relatively new treatment is being proposed, the long-term results of which are not yet known.

REFERENCES

1. Donegan WL, Sugarbaker ED, Handley RS, et al.: The management of primary operable breast cancer; a comparison of time and mortality factors after standard, extended, and modified radical mastectomy. Proceedings of the Sixth National Cancer Conference, pp 135–143, Philadelphia, J. B. Lippincott, 1970.
2. Fisher B, Bauer M, Margolese R et al.: Five-year results of a randomized clinical trial comparing total mastectomy and segmental mastectomy with or without radiation in the treatment of breast cancer. N Engl J Med 312:665–673, 1985.
3. Fisher ER, Sass R, Fisher B, et al.: Pathologic findings from the National Surgical Adjuvant Breast Project (Protocol 6). II. Relation of local breast recurrence to multicentricity. Cancer 57:1717–1724, 1986.
4. Gump FE, Habif DV, Logerfo P, et al.: The extent and distribution of cancer in breasts with palpable primary tumors. Ann Surg 204:384–390, 1986.
5. Holland R, Veling SH, Mravunac M, et al.: Histologic multifocality of Tis, T1–2 breast carcinomas. Cancer 56:979–990, 1985.
6. Krohn IT, Cooper DR, Bassett JG: Radical mastectomy: Thick vs. thin skin flaps. Arch Surg 117:760–763, 1982.
7. Lannin DR, Silverman JF, Walker C, et al.: Cost-effectiveness of fine needle biopsy of the breast. Ann Surg 203:474–480, 1986.
8. Marriyo G, Jolly PC, Hall MH: Non-palpable breast cancer: Needle localized biopsy for diagnosis and considerations for treatment. Am J Surg 151:599–602, 1986.
9. Moosman DH: Anatomy of the pectoral nerves and their preservation in modified mastectomy. Am J Surg 137:883–886, 1980.
10. Page DL, Dupont WD, Rogers LW, et al.: Atypical hyperplastic lesions of the female breast. Cancer 55:2698–2708, 1985.
11. Rosen PP, Sinie R, Schottenfeld D, et al.: Noninvasive breast carcinoma. Frequency of unsuspected invasion and implications for treatment. Ann Surg 189:377–382, 1979.
12. Veronesi U, Volagussa P: Inefficacy of internal mammary node dissection in breast cancer surgery. Cancer 47:171–175, 1981.

13. The Treatment of Breast Cancer with Excision Followed by Radiation Therapy

ALLEN S. LICHTER

Breast cancer was formerly thought to be a disease that progressed in a predictable manner. The breast itself was affected first; then after a time, the disease progressed to the lymph nodes, where it remained in place. After another delay, the disease disseminated to distant organs. In fact, in the late 1800s when the surgical therapy for breast cancer was being codified, the concept of bloodborne metastases was given little credence. Halsted and other surgeons of the time felt that breast cancer spread to other organs in direct continuity with the primary breast cancer. Halsted once wrote, "Although it undoubtedly occurs, I am not sure that I have observed from breast cancer metastases which seem definitely to have been conveyed by way of the blood vessels."[17] Rather, he felt that breast cancer spreads with a "quite uninterrupted connection between the original focus and all the outlying deposits of cancer."[17]

When one believes that breast cancer spreads in a logical stepwise progression, then one may be encouraged to perform greater and greater amounts of local dissection in an attempt to completely excise and cure the disease. Thus Halsted, Handley, and other surgeons of the time described extensive radical surgical procedures to remove the cancerous breast and adjacent lymph node–bearing regions.[18,19] In the late 1800s, breast cancer presented as advanced disease more often than not. It was likely true that local control was increased when these locally advanced tumors were treated with operations that removed substantial amounts of tissue, thus eliminating occult surgical transection of tumor masses. However, it is still doubtful that these radical operations changed the cure rate of breast cancer compared to lesser surgical procedures.[4]

It is worth noting that in the 1920s and 1930s several small series of patients treated with breast tumor excision plus breast irradiation were reported within larger series of postoperative radiation patients.[1,13,31] While the results in these small groups of patients were encouraging, the observation was never followed up in this country. To large measure, the radiation machines in the early 1900s produced very low energy X-rays that gave a high surface dose. In order to get sufficient amounts of radiation deep into the breast, the surface structures had to be given enough radiation such that fibrosis, telangiectasia, and other adverse cosmetic consequences resulted. Therefore, the treatment of breast cancer was left almost entirely in the hands of the surgeon, who was armed with a radical operation. It was in this setting that change began to occur.

EARLY EXPERIENCES WITH PRIMARY RADIOTHERAPY

The first physician to raise a strong case against mastectomy and in favor of excision followed by radiation was a British surgeon, Mr. Geoffrey Keynes from St. Bartholomew's Hospital in London. The brother of the famous British economist, John Maynard Keynes, Sir Geoffrey was a Renaissance man with deep interest and major accomplishments in both medicine and the arts. He was the first surgeon to advocate and show the effectiveness of thymectomy for myasthenia gravis.[23] He turned his attention to breast cancer in the 1920s, a time when no surgeon was advocating treatment of breast cancer with other than a radical mastectomy. He would excise the cancerous breast mass, and then, to avert the deleterious skin changes produced by low-energy X-rays, he would implant the breast with a series of radium needles. In 1937, Keynes published the survival rates from his treatment, comparing these with the results of patients treated in a nearby hospital with surgical therapy only.[24] The results are seen in Table 1, and the comparability of the data is remarkable. It should be further noted that the patients whose disease was confined to the breast were only clinically staged by Keynes, but were surgically staged with the mastectomy treatment. Because many patients whose clinical exam of the axilla is negative do, in reality, have positive lymph nodes, the results are even more impressive. Attention was beginning to be paid to Keynes' results. However, the Second World War interrupted the research. Not only was Keynes assigned to the Royal Air Force, thus interrupting his general surgical practice, but the bombing of London became imminent. Since radium has a half-life of 1620 years and produces lethal colorless, odorless radon gas, it was felt prudent to remove the supply of radium from London. When he returned from the war, Keynes could not reestablish the follow-up of patients he had previously treated with excision plus radiation, and he went on to investigate other areas of medicine.[23]

Other physicians began to experiment with nonmastectomy treatment. Cheatle, in London, suggested that a combination of external radiation followed by interstitial radium implant might be a useful treatment for

Table 1. Results of Excision Plus Radium by Keynes

	5 Year Survival	
Extent of Disease	Excision Plus Radium	Mastectomy
Confined to breast	71.4%	69.1%
Positive axilla	29.3	30.5
Inoperable	23.6	—

primary breast cancer.[8] In France, Baclesse used a protracted course of external radiation to avoid deleterious skin changes.[3] His results treating locally advanced breast cancers were encouraging. In Finland, Mustakallio reported worthwhile treatment results in operable cancer treated with lumpectomy and relatively low dose radiation to the breast.[28]

In North America, the thread of interest in nonmastectomy treatment was taken up by Dr. Vera Peters at the Princess Margaret Hospital in Toronto.[30] She began to treat patients in the late 1940s with excision plus radiation, usually confined to patients who refused mastectomy. By the 1970s she had accumulated a large series of patients and reported her results using a matched pair analysis. In this analysis, each excision-plus-radiation patient was compared to three mastectomy-plus-radiation patients who were matched for age, tumor size, and year of admission into the Princess Margaret Hospital. The results from this analysis, actuarially plotted to 30 years, indicate that her treatment was successful in curing patients of breast cancer without the need to surgically remove the entire breast.[30]

THE ERA OF HIGH-ENERGY RADIATION COMBINED WITH INTERSTITIAL IMPLANT IN THE TREATMENT OF BREAST CANCER

Over the last 10 to 15 years, a variety of institutions in Europe and the United States have gained a great deal of experience with treatment of breast cancer using excision followed by radiation. Three French institutions, Institute Curie,[7] Cretiel,[32] and Marseilles,[2] have the greatest experience with this technique. Their results are summarized in Table 2 and show excellent long-term survival. Some of their local control data are difficult to interpret since many larger tumors were not excised due to the fear of distorting the breast. This meant that some patients were actually treated with preoperative irradiation with the full expectation that they would need to have mastectomy to provide local control. Another area in which the French data are not easily comparable to the United States data involves the use of axillary dissection. Many of the French patients were treated without axillary dissection, a treatment philosophy that has not been widely practiced in the United States.

Table 2.   Results of Nonmastectomy Treatment—French Data

Institution	Stage	No. Patients	Survival	
			5 Year	10 Year
Curie[7]	$T_1T_2N_0$	321	—	71%
	T_2N_1	89	—	42
Creteil[32]	T_1	99	99%	65
	T_2	235	82	69
Marseilles[2]	$T_1T_2N_1$	568	87	76
	$T_1T_2N_1$	212	77	67

In the United States, a number of centers have published long-term results (Table 3). The senior institution in this regard is the Joint Center for Radiation Therapy (JCRT) at Harvard Medical School in Boston.[20] Under the direction of Dr. Samuel Hellman, the JCRT actively began to recruit patients for treatment with excision plus radiation in the early 1970s. They have the largest experience of any institution in the United States and their local control and survival results are comparable to any surgical series ever reported. They are currently treating over 400 patients each year with this technique.

THE RISE OF INTEREST IN NONMASTECTOMY TREATMENT

Several reasons can be cited to explain the rapid increase in the use of nonmastectomy treatment for primary breast cancer. Over the past 30 years, medical science has developed a new understanding of the biology of breast cancer. As summarized by Dr. Bernard Fisher[15] (Table 4), it is no longer believed that Halstedian concepts of breast cancer spread are valid. Breast cancer frequently spreads through bloodborne routes and is often disseminated by the time the patient comes to the attention of her physician. Variations in cure rate attributable to the type of local treatment given to the breast tumor are unlikely to be seen, provided the local treatments are effective in eradicating the local tumor. Since local recurrence rates average between 5% and 10% following excision plus radiation, a figure that is actually slightly lower than the overall chest wall recurrence following mas-

Table 3.   Results of Nonmastectomy Treatment—American Data

Institution	No. Patients	Disease-Free 5 Year Survival	
		Stage I	Stage II
JCRT[20]	265	93%	84%
Yale[33]	179	88	66
U. Penn[11]	196	86	69
M.D. Anderson[27]	291	85	78

Table 4.   Changes in the Biologic Concepts Regarding Breast Cancer

Halsted	Modern
Lymph nodes are perfect barriers to tumor passage	Tumor cells often bypass regional lymph nodes
Lymph nodes are the instigators of further spread	Lymph nodes are indicators of potential spread
Bloodborne metastases are of little importance	Bloodborne metastases are critical
Breast cancer is primarily a local-regional disease	Breast cancer is frequently a systemic disease
The extent of the surgical operation is the major determinant of survival	Variations in local-regional treatment are unlikely to affect survival

From Fisher[15]

tectomy, it is not surprising that survival rates are comparable to treatment with mastectomy.

The Two-Stage Approach to Treatment of Breast Cancer

Another important development that has allowed nonmastectomy therapy to flourish is the use of the outpatient biopsy. For decades, breast cancer was treated differently from any other cancer in the body. A patient with a lump in the breast was taken to the operating room and had a biopsy under general anesthesia. The biopsy was diagnosed immediately using a frozen section, and if positive, the patient immediately underwent mastectomy. This obviously left little or no opportunity for discussion of alternative therapies, as the mastectomy was done before the patient was actually aware of the diagnosis. How the treatment of breast cancer got started down this path at a time it was considered safe to perform a biopsy of any other cancer in any other body site before initiating treatment is difficult to reconstruct. However, this so-called one-stage procedure still has advocates despite the inability to substantiate an advantage of this procedure over a two-stage approach.[40] It has now been established beyond doubt that a biopsy that is separated by days to weeks from primary breast cancer treatment is not deleterious, and this two-stage approach is now the standard of care in most hospitals in the United States.[6,12,26,36] A further advance has been the use of fine needle aspiration cytology to make a diagnosis of breast cancer even before biopsy.[29,43] It is now possible to see a patient with a newly diagnosed breast mass, obtain an immediate mammogram and fine needle aspiration, confirm a diagnosis of breast cancer, and begin to discuss treatment options within a few hours of seeing the patient for the first time. Today, women have the opportunity to participate in the decision as to which type of breast cancer treatment they will have, rather than our former approach to patients where patient input into treatment was nearly impossible.

It would be a mistake to ignore the contribution that the women's movement has made in popularizing nonmastectomy treatment of breast cancer. In many respects, this was not a therapy that was developed through laboratory and clinical research and then announced in the medical literature. Rather, it was a technique that scratched and clawed its way into recognition, propelled in part by the interest of women in their own health care needs. Articles in women's magazines frequently discussed breast cancer and made women aware of this emerging alternative.

RANDOMIZED TRIALS IN NONMASTECTOMY TREATMENT OF BREAST CANCER

Four modern trials have addressed in a prospectively randomized fashion the efficacy of nonmastectomy treatment for breast cancer.[14,16,35,41] The results of these four studies are summarized in Table 5. While the entry criteria have differed in each of these four studies, and the radiation and surgical techniques have differed slightly, the conclusions from all four studies are remarkably similar. That is, there is no statistical difference between the survival rate of patients treated with mastectomy versus patients treated with excision plus radiation at five years, or out to ten years in the case of the Milan study.

The National Surgical Adjuvant Breast Project (NSABP) trial is especially interesting to analyze. Instead of simply comparing mastectomy to excision plus radiation, the NSABP utilized a third arm that involved wide excision with pathologically free margins and no further radiation. Cure rates in these patients were identical in all groups. With a mean follow-up of three years, they have observed an approximately 30% rate of local recurrence in those patients treated with wide local excision alone compared to 8% in patients treated with the same operation followed by local radiation. In node-positive patients where chemotherapy was added, the local recurrence rate was less than 3%. Since women who failed wide local excision are customarily treated with mastectomy at the time of failure, the maximum chance at breast preservation clearly comes through the use of a combination of surgical excision along with carefully applied radiation therapy.

Table 5. 5 Year Survivals in Randomized Trials of Nonmastectomy Treatment

	No. Pts.	Excision Plus Radiation	Mastectomy
Milan[41,42]	701	85%	85.5%
Gustave-Roussey[35]	179	95	91
NSABP[16]	1843	84	76
NCI[14]	197	No Difference*	

*13 mastectomy failures; 12 radiation failures

THE TECHNIQUE OF TREATMENT WITH EXCISION PLUS RADIATION

The radiation dose required to sterilize microscopic disease is considerably less than the dose required to sterilize a gross tumor mass. Therefore, a basic concept in the successful treatment of breast cancer without mastectomy involves the careful surgical removal of the tumor. Remaining behind are small amounts of microscopic cancer that can be controlled by doses of radiation that leave the breast in a cosmetically acceptable state. The technique of surgical tumor removal has been discussed elsewhere in this volume and will not be pursued in detail here. One should point out, however, the importance of surgical clips being left to demarcate the tumor bed. One of the most difficult problems in radiotherapeutic treatment of breast cancer is deciding exactly where the tumor was, especially since many of these masses are excised for diagnostic purposes prior to the radiotherapist becoming involved in the case. When surgical clips are placed to define the tumor bed, the ability to accurately localize the boost dose of radiation becomes much easier (Figure 1). The other major aspect of surgical therapy in the nonmastectomy treatment of breast cancer involves the axillary dissection. This aspect of the treatment is discussed elsewhere in this volume and will not be discussed in detail here except to say that most centers favor a more formal axillary dissection of at least levels one and two of the axillary lymph nodes.[21] This is in contradistinction to an operation known as "axillary sampling" in which a variable number of lymph nodes at ill-defined levels of the axilla are removed. There is little reason to suppose that more or less axillary lymph node tissue should be removed for mastectomy therapy than for nonmastectomy therapy. All the major randomized clinical trials involving nonmastectomy therapy have utilized formal axillary dissection. The operation can be successfully performed and recovers the same amount of lymph nodal tissue as an axillary dissection associated with a full mastectomy.[10]

Following the excision plus axillary dissection, usually 10 to 14 days is allowed to elapse before the start of radiation therapy. This is necessary, in large part, to allow for adequate recovery of arm motion so that the patient's arm can be held up and away from the body during radiation (Figure 2). The breast is irradiated through tangentially directed fields that treat the breast and a small amount of underlying lung (Figure 3). Forty-five hundred to 5000 rad are delivered in five to five and one-half weeks. The treatment is tolerated well with few, if any, immediate side effects. Most of our patients who are working continue to work at least part-time during their therapy, and many continue to work full-time.

If the lymph nodes in the axilla are positive, we recommended systemic therapy in the form of hormone therapy, cytotoxic chemotherapy, or both. If chemotherapy is chosen, we generally deliver the first two cycles of

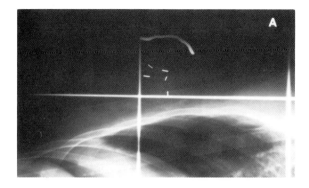

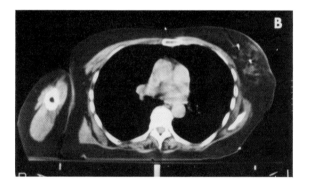

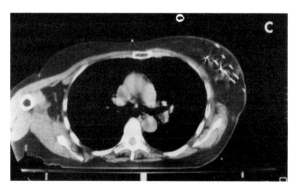

Figure 1. *(a)* A tangential X-ray of the breast following tumor excision. The heavy wire marks the excision scar and surgical clips delineate the excision bed. *(b)* On CT scans, the location of the clips are well seen. *(c)* The breast boost with iridium seeds can be tailored to encompass the clips at the deep surgical margins.

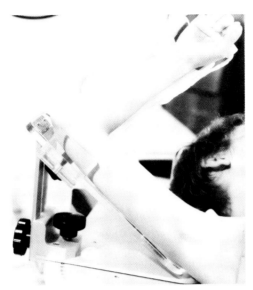

Figure 2. The treatment position for radiation therapy of breast cancer. The arm is held up and away from the body to avoid delivering unnecessary radiation to this structure. A special calibrated arm board is used to aid positioning.

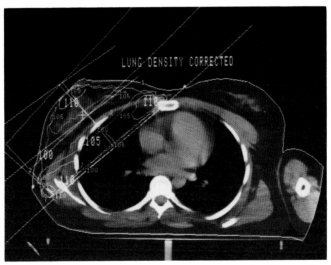

Figure 3. A breast treatment plan superimposed on the CT scan. Two tangential fields treat the breast and a rim of underlying lung. The plan is corrected to account for the reduced density of lung tissue compared to soft tissue.

chemotherapy before starting radiation. This means that radiation begins about six weeks postoperatively (Figure 4).

After whole breast irradiation is completed, a boost dose of radiation is given to the tumor bed. Having clips placed in the tumor bed facilitates this boost. The boost can be done with either an iridium needle implant or with an electron beam (Figure 5). It should be pointed out that the NSABP trial employed no boost treatment in addition to the 4500 rad delivered to the entire breast. Their local recurrence rate of 7.7% compares favorably to local recurrence rate in other published series. However, patients in the NSABP trial were required to have pathologically confirmed clear margins at the time of excision. Furthermore, these pathologically free margins had to be obtained at the first excision, and any patient whose tumor margins were positive was required to have mastectomy rather than having a re-excision.

Chemotherapy in the NSABP trial further decreased the incidence of local failure. In general, most patients seen for radiation treatment today do not have a clean excision with pathologically free margins performed on the first biopsy. In an attempt to preserve a cosmetically acceptable breast, re-excisions, when required, are designed to take out the minimum amount of tissue consistent with good surgical oncology practice. Until the need for boost radiation is further defined, we continue to employ a boost dose to all

SCHEDULE FOR RADIATION PLUS
CHEMOTHERAPY IN NODE-POSITIVE PATIENTS

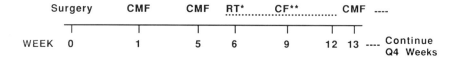

*   5 Weeks Whole Breast Radiation, Then
Boost With Iridium or Electron Beam

**   Methotrexate Held During Radiation

Figure 4.   The treatment sequence for treating breast cancer with excision plus radiation.

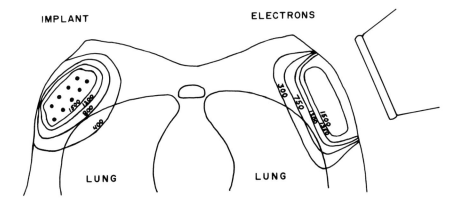

Figure 5. The contrast between electron beam and implant boosts to the tumor bed. Both dose the tumor bed adequately. With electrons, more of the dose is delivered to the skin.

patients. It is likely, however, that patients who have extremely wide local excision, patients who have well-circumscribed pure invasive carcinoma without an intraductal component, and patients who are to receive adjuvant chemotherapy will be the first group of patients to be regularly treated without the necessity of radiation boost fields.

COMPLICATIONS OF TREATMENT

The major complications associated with nonmastectomy treatment of breast cancer are listed in Table 6. The most serious complication is radiation pneumonitis, which can, on occasion, lead to marked symptoms. Thankfully, this complication is also the rarest complication of all those listed. At The University of Michigan, there has been a single case of cough and infiltrate on chest X-ray that symptomatically lasted for about one month and has left no sequela. This experience relates to more than 200 patients treated, and therefore we believe the incidence of this complication is less then 1%. Soreness in the breast is universal following radiation therapy. Usually this soreness is intermittent and manifests itself with a twinge of pain lasting one or two seconds every several weeks or several months. However, some patients will have more soreness in the chest wall or breast, which will frequently respond to a course of anti-inflammatory therapy. Rib fractures occur in approximately 5% of the patients treated. These are self-limiting in that they heal in a relatively short period of time, as other rib fractures do.

LOCAL RECURRENCE AND ITS MANAGEMENT

Local recurrence appears in approximately 5% to 10% of patients. It is likely that some of these patients have a true local recurrence, that is, the regrowth of tumor cells that were present at the time of the initial breast tumor. Such recurrences are located within the initial tumor quadrant. Some patients, however, have a regrowth of a new tumor that was not present at the time of initial treatment and represents a *de novo* appearance of a new clone of malignant cells. These recurrences often manifest themselves in quadrants not originally involved with tumor, but it is frequently impossible to differentiate between these two events. Once a local recurrence appears, treatment is mastectomy.

The pathophysiology of a local breast recurrence is considerably different from the pathophysiology of a chest wall recurrence following a mastectomy. In the latter event, virtually all patients manifest systemic disease over time, and almost all will succumb to metastatic breast cancer.[5] The outlook for patients who fail locally in the intact breast is considerably brighter. Several studies have shown that somewhat over half of these patients are controlled with mastectomy.[9,22,34] In the Toronto experience,[9] if the lesion is detected early and the disease has not gone on to involve residual axillary lymph nodes, the survival of patients who have had a breast recurrence virtually superimposes on the survival of those patients who have remained recurrence free. This underscores the importance of careful follow-up with physical exam and mammography in order to detect local recurrence at its earliest stages. Application of mastectomy can then be highly successful in curing the disease.

At least one institution has reported performing a second conservative treatment on women who have a local failure in the intact breast.[25] Such a therapeutic approach would appear, on the surface, to be rather risky. However, further follow-up of these patients may define a subset of patients who can have a second nonmastectomy approach. We currently treat all patients who have local failure with total mastectomy.

Table 6.   Complications of Nonmastectomy Therapy

Rib fracture	5%
Pneumonitis	<1
Chest wall pain	10–20
Arm edema	5
Poor cosmesis	5

CANDIDATES FOR TREATMENT WITH EXCISION, AXILLARY DISSECTION, AND FULL COURSE RADIATION

The criteria for inclusion into a treatment protocol involving lumpectomy postradiation are outlined in Table 7. Not listed is the most important criterion, the woman's desire to preserve her breast. While it is true that most women have this objective, one should not assume that all women regard this as a major goal of breast cancer treatment. For those patients who, for one reason or another, sincerely express no concern over breast preservation, mastectomy is recommended because of its proved effectiveness and the rapidity of treatment. Most women are in and out of the hospital within five days, and mastectomy (without reconstruction) can probably be delivered at lower cost than nonmastectomy treatment. For those women who wish to preserve their breast, the following criteria should be satisfied:

Patient Age

In general, most clinics do not regard patient age as a relative indication or contraindication for nonmastectomy treatment. We have treated women from age 20 through age 90. It is true that younger women, who have a longer remaining life span, are at risk for any late sequelae of radiation treatment for a long period of time. However, it is often younger women who are very motivated towards breast preservation. Issues concerning possible long-term side effects, although unknown, must be frankly aired with these young women. Once they are fully informed, we routinely offer nonmastectomy treatment to women in their twenties and thirties. To date, we have not been disappointed with this philosophy.

Tumor Size and Location

A great deal of confusion surrounds the criteria of tumor size and location for nonmastectomy therapy. While the Milan study used 2 cm as a cutoff point, and the NSABP used 4 cm, it should be emphasized that these were arbitrary size dimensions for study purposes. Most investigators believe that there is no absolute size criterion that can be applied uniformly. The overriding concern is the size of the mass in relation to the size of the breast. Women with large breasts and relatively centrally located lesions can have 5- or 6-cm tumors removed with cosmetically acceptable results and satisfactory surgi-

Table 7.   Criteria for Treatment with Nonmastectomy Therapy

Age	Any age
Tumor size	Any tumor that can be cosmetically excised
Location	Any; central tumors may require excision of nipple-areola complex
Breast size	Any size
Histology	Invasive or intraductal; extensive intraductal change requires wide excision
Mammography	All suspicious califications removed

cal margins. On the other hand, patients with small breasts can be difficult to treat even if their tumors are 2 or 3 cm in size, depending on the location of the tumor. For each patient that we evaluate, we individualize whether the mass can be removed completely and leave a cosmetically acceptable outcome. If this can be accomplished, the patient is, in general, a candidate for nonmastectomy therapy.

Location of the tumor within the breast is another relative rather than absolute factor. For example, a large tumor in the inferior part of the breast can often be removed in a more cosmetically acceptable fashion than a similarly sized tumor in the superior part of the breast, because in normal upright position the inferior aspect of the breast is frequently not visible. A significant deformity in the inferior part of the breast can be more easily concealed than the same type of surgical defect located in the upper aspect of the mammary gland. Subareolar tumors, or even Paget's disease of the breast, should also be considered for radiation treatment. In the past, some surgeons and radiotherapists have felt that subareolar tumors should not be treated with breast-sparing therapy because the nipple, areola, or both may have to be removed. However, a cosmetically intact breast without a nipple/areola is still superior in appearance to virtually all plastic surgical reconstructions. Therefore, we routinely offer nonmastectomy therapy even to women whose nipple/areola might have to be partially or completely excised in order to completely remove the tumor. The results have been very satisfactory in our eyes as well as in the opinion of our patients.

Breast Size

Breast size is another area where absolute criteria should not be set. In general, women with small breasts have more cosmetically superior outcomes than women who are large breasted, because a change in breast size is often less apparent in small-breasted women. It is not true, however, that women with large breasts cannot be treated with radiation. Cosmetically acceptable results can be produced when care and attention are given to radiation treatment planning. In some patients, a slightly higher energy X-ray beam should be used.

It should also be remembered that very full-breasted women have great difficulties with mastectomy. The size of the remaining breast can often be a severe impediment when it is not counterbalanced by an equal mass of tissue on the contralateral chest wall. Full-breasted women have the most difficulty having breast reconstruction, often having to undergo reduction mammoplasty of the contralateral breast.

Following radiation, women with full breasts can be more difficult to follow because finding small masses on palpation can be difficult, and the density of the mammogram postradiation can make it hard to recognize subtle changes. However, we have yet to turn a patient away from nonmastectomy treatment solely on the basis of breast size.

Histologic Subtype

Knowing that 5% to 10% of women treated with nonmastectomy therapy fail treatment and require subsequent mastectomy, researchers in Boston retrospectively analyzed histologic subtypes in an attempt to discover whether failure patterns could be predicted. Their results are extremely important.[38,39] They have found that women with pure invasive carcinoma have a failure rate that is less than 2%. In contrast, women who have an intraductal tumor extending outside the boundaries of the main tumor mass have local failure rates of up to 25%. There is no proved explanation for this observation. Most likely, women who have extensive amounts of intraductal carcinoma beyond the area of invasive neoplasm have had large amounts of unsuspected tumor left behind following excisional biopsy. The volume of tumor may have been too great to have been controlled with local radiation. In addition, the boost fields for these patients may not have encompassed all of the cancerous tissue. Based on these findings, it is clear that women with an intraductal component to their tumor are the patients that should have careful reexcision of their primary tumor mass. One should attempt to achieve clear margins on this reexcision. When we find extensive amounts of intraductal carcinoma infiltrating in all areas of the reexcision specimen, then we are hesitant to claim that we have cleared all the tumor from the patient's breast. We seriously consider performing primary mastectomy in these women. For those women whose reexcision shows no identifiable residual tumor or shows small scattered foci of intraductal carcinoma with clear margins, we feel confident in treating with full course radiation. It should be emphasized that no survival decrement has been seen in women who have had extensive intraductal carcinoma with recurrence postradiation. Therefore, we still treat women who might be at high risk for tumor recurrence because of extensive intraductal carcinoma in the reexcision specimen, as long as they understand the advantages and disadvantages of this approach. Subsequent mastectomy for a local failure can still be performed.

Mammographic Appearance

It is critical to perform bilateral mammography on every patient who is being considered for nonmastectomy treatment. The ipsilateral breast must be cleared of all suspicious microcalcifications before treatment begins. Since the mammogram will be one of the major methods for follow-up of each patient, having an excellent baseline mammogram is very important and having a mammogram that is free of suspicious microcalcifications is also critical. When suspicious microcalcifications are left behind, follow-up mammograms always become difficult to interpret and one is always uncertain whether there is a persistence or recurrence of tumor. Occasionally a patient will present with widespread suspicious calcification throughout the breast. These are patients in whom we do not perform nonmastectomy treatment.

FOLLOW-UP OF PATIENTS TREATED WITH NONMASTECTOMY THERAPY

We routinely follow our patients at three-month intervals for the first two years, four-month intervals for the next two years, and then six-month intervals thereafter. Chest X-ray and liver function studies are obtained yearly. The first ipsilateral mammogram is obtained six months following treatment. By that time, the acute effects of radiation have subsided, and one gets a clear look at how the breast appears following treatment. A bilateral mammogram is obtained at 12 months following treatment and every year thereafter. Other studies, such as bone scan, are employed as symptoms or physical findings warrant.

There is always some difficulty with physical examination in a patient who has been treated with nonmastectomy therapy. Frequently there is induration in the region of the tumor bed caused by surgical excision and radiation. In general, this induration is two-dimensional. That is, it has a width and a length but only a vague and ill-defined thickness. We believe that this two-dimensional thickening is due to fibrosis and watch the region carefully. Detailed drawings at the time of each follow-up examination greatly facilitate this process. Any lesion that has a three-dimensional aspect needs to be sampled, either with fine needle aspiration or with incisional biopsy. All new microcalcifications suggestive of malignant disease also must be carefully explored. While many of these regions represent calcifications within areas of fat necrosis following radiation, there is no obvious way to tell on mammography or physical examination whether spiculated microcalcification represents a benign or malignant process.

IS NONMASTECTOMY TREATMENT ACTUALLY SUPERIOR TO MASTECTOMY?

In the past, the onus was on nonmastectomy treatment to prove that it was equivalent to mastectomy, since mastectomy was the "gold standard" of breast cancer care. All modern studies and single-institution reports indicate that this equivalence exists. However, some interesting data are emerging that allow one to speculate that nonmastectomy treatment may turn out to be superior. These issues are explored below.

There is little question today that the psychosocial impact of nonmastectomy treatment is considerably less than that of mastectomy treatment. In a tightly controlled, randomized prospective trial, Schain et al. at the National Cancer Institute (NCI) have shown that virtually every psychological parameter measured is significantly less disturbed in nonmastectomy-treated patients compared with their mastectomy counterparts.[37] This extends beyond questions of body image and body perception to include such areas as general anxiety, feelings of being in control, sadness, and guilt. These issues are discussed in more detail elsewhere in this volume.

It should also be pointed out that three modern studies that have randomized nonmastectomy treatment all show an advantage in survival for nonmastectomy patients. The NCI study (data unpublished) continues to show a nonsignificant advantage for the lumpectomy patients. The NSABP shows a survival advantage at the P = 0.07 level.[16] The Milan study shows that there is a nonsignificant advantage to nonmastectomy therapy overall (P = 0.13), and when node-positive patients are analyzed separately, the nonmastectomy group has an overall survival advantage (P = 0.08).[42] All these studies bear further watching. It is conceivable that nonmastectomy therapy, for reasons that we can only speculate upon at this point, may turn out to have survival advantages for patients so treated.

SUMMARY

In experienced surgical and radiotherapeutic hands, and with meticulous attention to detail, nonmastectomy treatment of breast cancer can now be considered a legitimate and acceptable alternative for most patients with operable breast cancer. The mammogram should indicate a mass that can be surgically cleared, leaving the breast with no suspicious microcalcifications. Tumor size and location should be balanced against the overall size of the breast so that proper cosmesis can be assured following local tumor excision. Axillary dissection should remove lymph nodes at least at levels one and two, using an incision that is separate from the one for excision of the primary neoplasm. The pathologic specimen must be evaluated carefully for areas of intraductal carcinoma outside the primary tumor mass. In women who have this particular histologic finding, a reexcision of the tumor bed should be performed. Careful follow-up with breast self-examination, physician examination, and mammography are critical to the overall success of this treatment approach.

REFERENCES

1. Adair F E: The role of surgery and irradiation in cancer of the breast. JAMA 121:553–559, 1943.
2. Amalric R, Santamaria F, Robert F, et al: Conservative therapy of operable breast cancer—Results at five, ten, and fifteen years in 2216 consecutive cases, Harris JR, Hellman S, Silen W (Eds): *Conservative Management of Breast Cancer. New Surgical and Radiotherapeutic Techniques.* Philadelphia, Lippincott, 1983, pp 15–21.
3. Baclesse F: Roentgen therapy as the sole method of treatment of cancer of the breast. Am J Roentgen Rad Ther 62:311–319, 1949.

4. Baum M, Edwards MH: Management of early carcinoma of the breast. Lancet 2:85, 1972.

5. Bedwinek JM, Lee J, Fineberg B, et al: Prognostic indicators in patients with isolated local-regional recurrence of breast cancer. Cancer 47:2232–2235, 1981.

6. Bertario L, Reduzzi D, Piromalli, D, et al: Outpatient biopsy of breast cancer — Influence on survival. Ann Surg 201:64–67, 1985.

7. Calle R, Vilcoq JR, Pilleron JP, et al: Conservative treatment of operable breast carcinoma by irradiation with or without limited surgery — 10 year results, in Harris JR, Hellman S, Silen W (Eds): *Conservative Management of Breast Cancer. New Surgical and Radiotherapeutic Techniques.* Philadelphia, Lippincott, 1983, pp 3–9.

8. Cheatle L: A lecture on treatment of mammary carcinoma by radiation. Br Med J 1:807–811, 1930.

9. Clark RM: Alternatives to mastectomy — The Princess Margaret Hospital experience, in Harris JR, Hellman S, Silen W (Eds): *Conservative Management of Breast Cancer. New Surgical and Radiotherapeutic Techniques.* Philadelphia, Lippincott, 1983, pp 35–46.

10. Danforth DN, Findlay PA, McDonald HD, et al: Complete axillary node dissection for stage I-II carcinoma of the breast. J Clin Oncol 4:655–662, 1986.

11. Danoff BF, Goodman RL: Excisional biopsy, axillary node dissection and definitive radiotherapy for stage I and II breast cancer. (Abstract) Int J Radiat Oncol Biol Phys 9:113–114, 1983.

12. Donegan WL: Diagnosis, in Donegan WL, Spratt JS, (Eds): *Cancer of the Breast: Major Problems in Clinical Surgery.* 2nd edition, Philadelphia, W.B. Saunders, 5:78, 1979.

13. Evans WA, Levcutia T: Deep roentgen-ray therapy of mammary carcinoma. Am J Roentgenol 42:866–882, 1939.

14. Findlay PA, Lippman ME, Danforth Jr D et al: Mastectomy vs. radiotherapy as treatment for stage I-II breast cancer: A prospective randomized trial at the National Cancer Institute. World J Surg 9:671–675, 1985.

15. Fisher B, Redmond C, Fisher ER: The contribution of recent NSABP clinical trials of primary breast cancer therapy to an understanding of tumor biology — An overview of findings. Cancer 46:1009–1025, 1980.

16. Fisher B, Bauer M, Margolese R, et al: Five year results of a randomized clinical trial comparing total mastectomy and segmental mastectomy with or without radiation in the treatment of breast cancer. N Engl J Med 312:665–673, 1985.

17. Halsted WS: The results of radical operations for the cure of carcinoma of the breast. Ann Surg 46:1–19, 1907.

18. Halsted WS: The results of operations for the care of cancer of the breast performed at the Johns Hopkins Hospital from June, 1889 to January, 1894. Ann Surg 200:497,1984.

19. Handley WS: Cancer of the Breast. John Murry, London, 1906.

20. Harris JR, Hellman S: The results of primary radiation therapy for early breast cancer at the Joint Center for Radiation Therapy, in Harris

JR, Hellman S, Silen W (Eds): *Conservative Management of Breast Cancer. New Surgical and Radiotherapeutic Techniques.* Philadelphia, Lippincott,1983, pp 47-52.

21. Harris JR, Hellman S, Kinne DW: Limited surgery and radiotherapy for early breast cancer. N Engl J Med 313:1365-1368, 1985.

22. Harris JR, Recht A, Amalric R, et al: Time course and prognosis of local recurrence following primary radiation therapy for early breast cancer. J Clin Oncol 2:37-41, 1984.

23. Keynes G: *The Gates of Memory.* Oxford, Clarendon Press, 1981.

24. Keynes G: Conservative treatment of cancer of the breast. Br Med J pp 643-647, 1937.

25. Kurtz J M, Amalric R, Brandone H, et al: A second chance to preserve the breast: Results of wide excision for breast recurrence after lumpectomy and irradiation (abstr). Int J Radiat Oncol Biol Phys 11(Suppl. 1):103, 1985.

26. Margolese RG: The case for two-step biopsy procedure for breast cancer. Cancer 32:51-57, 1982.

27. Montague ED: Conservative surgery and radiation therapy in the treatment of operable breast cancer. Cancer 53:700-704, 1984.

28. Mustakallio S: Conservative treatment of breast carcinoma — Review of 25 years of follow-up. Clin Radiol 23:110-116, 1972.

29. Norton LW, Davis JR, Wiens JL, et al: Accuracy of aspiration cytology in detecting breast cancer. Surgery 96:806-814, 1984.

30. Peters MV: Wedge resection with or without radiation in early breast cancer. Int J Radiat Oncol Biol Phys 2:1151-1156, 1977.

31. Pfahler GE: Results of radiation therapy in 1,022 private cases of carcinoma of the breast from 1902-1928. Am J Roentgenol 27:497-508, 1932.

32. Pierquin B: Conservative treatment for carcinoma of the breast: Experience of Creteil—Ten year results, in Harris JR, Hellman S, Silen W (Eds): *Conservative Management of Breast Cancer. New Surgical and Radiotherapeutic Techniques.* Philadelphia, Lippincott, 1983, pp 11-14.

33. Prosnitz LR, Goldenberg IS, Weshler Z, et al: Radiotherapy instead of mastectomy for breast cancer—The Yale experience, in Harris JR, Hellman S, Silen W (Eds): *Conservative Management of Breast Cancer. New Surgical and Radiotherapeutic Techniques.* Philadelphia, Lippincott, 1983, pp 61-70.

34. Recht A, Silver B, Schnitt S, et al: Breast relapse following primary radiation therapy for early breast cancer. I. Classification, frequency, and salvage. Int J Radiat Oncol Biol Phys 11:1271-1276, 1985.

35. Sarrazin D, Le M, Rouesse J, et al: Conservative treatment versus mastectomy in breast cancer tumors with macroscopic diameter of 20 millimeters or less. Cancer 53:1209-1213, 1984.

36. Scanlon EF: The case for and against two-step procedure for the surgical treatment of breast cancer. Cancer 53:677-680, 1984.

37. Schain W, Findley P, d'Angelo T, et al: A prospective psychosocial assessment of breast cancer patients receiving mastectomy or radiation

therapy in a randomized clinical trial (abstr). Proc Am Soc Clin Oncol 4:248, 1985.

38. Schnitt SJ, Connolly JL, Recht A, et al: Breast relapse following primary radiation therapy for early breast cancer. II. Detection, pathologic features, and prognostic significance. Int J Radiat Oncol Biol Phys 11:1277–1284, 1985.

39. Schnitt SJ, Connolly JL, Harris JR, et al: Pathologic prediction of early local recurrence in stage I and II breast cancer treated by primary radiation therapy. Cancer 53:1049–1057, 1984.

40. Urban JA: The case against delayed operation for breast cancer. CA 21:132–133, 1971.

41. Veronesi U, DelVecchio M, Greco M, et al: Results of quadrantectomy, axillary dissection, and radiotherapy (QUART) in T1N0 patients, in Harris JR, Hellman S, Silen W (Eds): *Conservative Management of Breast Cancer. New Surgical and Radiotherapeutic Techniques.* Philadelphia, Lippincott, 1983, pp 91–99.

42. Veronesi U, Banfic A, DelVecchio M, et al: Comparison of Halsted mastectomy with quadrantectomy, axillary dissection, and radiotherapy in early breast cancer: Long-term results. Eur J Cancer Clin Oncol 22:1085–1090, 1986.

43. Wanebo HJ, Feldman PS, Wilhelm MC, et al: Fine needle aspiration cytology in lieu of open biopsy in management of primary breast cancer. Ann Surg 199:569–579, 1984.

14. Contemporary Chemotherapy

ROBERT L. CODY
MAX S. WICHA

The rational use of chemotherapy and hormonal manipulation in the treatment of patients with breast cancer demands thorough pretreatment evaluation and staging as well as a complete understanding of the natural history of breast cancer. The realistic goal for patients with locoregional breast cancer should be complete eradication of cancer (cure) with fewest long-term side effects. Studies in the treatment of women with locally advanced breast cancer hold promise for cure, but unfortunately, metastatic breast cancer remains incurable and the goals of therapy are palliative. We will review, by stage, the treatment management of women with localized, locally advanced, and metastatic breast cancer.

LOCAL-REGIONAL DISEASE (STAGE I, II)

The concepts of adjuvant chemotherapy are based on hypotheses formulated in the laboratory study of animal models of cancer, which were then applied to the treatment of cancer in humans. In animal models, it was shown that chemotherapy is more effective after the tumor burden is reduced substantially by surgical resection, and that there is an inverse relationship between body tumor burden and probability of a complete eradication of transplantable tumors.[26] Confirmation of these hypotheses developed in the laboratory has been difficult in spontaneous human malignancies, but Fisher's study[15] shows the inverse relationship between the size of a breast cancer primary and the patient's survival. Timing of adjuvant chemotherapy has demonstrated importance in eradication of experimental metastases in animal models, after resection of the primary.[20] However, none of these hypotheses can be directly tested in human subjects.

The demonstration that postoperative adjuvant chemotherapy was useful in breast cancer began with the studies initiated by the National Surgical Adjuvant Breast and Bowel Project (NSABP) in 1958 and with the Milan Cancer Institute studies beginning in 1973. These two series of studies have had major impact on therapy for breast cancer in the United States (Table 1).

The first NSABP trial (B-01) began in 1958. Eight hundred twenty-six patients were randomized to treatment with thiotepa or placebo given in the perioperative period in an attempt to eliminate circulating tumor cells.[17] After a ten-year follow-up, a significant survival advantage was noted in premenopausal women with four or more positive nodes treated with thiotepa compared with the placebo group.

In 1972, the NSABP B-05 protocol was begun; 370 patients with Stage II breast cancer were randomized to receive L-phenylalanine mustard (L-PAM) or placebo for two years. The initial[16] and subsequent follow-up reports[63] continue to show an advantage in disease-free survival for the L-PAM treated group. Further examination of the data shows that the primary benefits of this therapy are seen in women less than or equal to 49 years of age with one to three positive axillary lymph nodes.

The NSABP B-07[18] and B-08[63] trials were an extension of the B-05 protocol. In B-07, the single agent L-PAM was randomized against L-PAM plus 5-FU (5-fluorouracil) (P + F). The combination of P + F showed an advantage over prednisone alone in women more than 49 years old and with more than or equal to four positive lymph nodes, but the disease-free survival (DFS) and overall survival (OS) advantage disappeared after the eighth year of analysis. Protocol B-08[63] randomized treatment with PF or PF plus methotrexate (PF + M). This study failed to show an advantage for the three-drug treatment even when analyzed in subgroups according to age and node status.

In 1973, the Milan Cancer Institute initiated a study comparing cyclophosphamide, methotrexate, and 5-FU (CMF) vs placebo.[6] In this study, women with Stage II breast cancer were randomized to 12 monthly cycles of combination chemotherapy or no treatment. The initial publication in 1976[6] reported a highly significant reduction in relapse rate in all subgroups treated with chemotherapy. When this data was reanalyzed at three[62] and subsequently at ten[7] years, the relapse-free survival (RFS) advantage and overall survival (OS) persisted only for the premenopausal patients. With the promising early results from the 1973 Milan trial, that group next addressed the issue of duration of chemotherapy. In the 1975 study, patients were randomized to either 6 or 12 monthly cycles of CMF. At five-year follow-up no differences were seen in the two groups in RFS, OS, or treatment-related complications, while both groups maintained RFS (63%) and OS (75%) similar to the original Milan study. No differences were seen when patients were examined according to menopausal status or estrogen receptor content of the tumor, but in both groups outcome was related to the number of axillary nodes involved.[56]

The Southwest Oncology Group conducted a randomized trial of one year of adjuvant CMFVP (cyclophosphamide, methotrexate, 5-FU, vincris-

Table 1. Randomized Trials of Adjuvant Chemotherapy in Stage II Breast Cancer

Study	Reference	No. Patients Studied	Duration	Treatment Arms	Results
NSABP B0-1	(17)	826	5 doses	thiotepa vs placebo	10 yr survival advantage[a] in thiotepa group
NSABP B0-5	(16)	370	2 yr	L-PAM vs placebo	10 yr survival advantage[b] for L-PAM group
NSABP B-07	(18)	741	2 yr	L-PAM vs L-PAM + 5-FU	8 yr DFS and OS in PF[c]
NSABP B-08	(63)	737	2 yr	PF vs P + methotrexate + 5-FU	No advantage to PMF vs PF[d]
Milan 1973	(6)	386	12 cycles	CMF vs control	10 yr RFS and OS advantages for premenopausal patients[e]
Milan 1975	(56)	459	CMF 6 cycles vs CMF 12 cycles		5 yr results no difference in RFS or OS between groups[f]
SWOG 1975	(25,43)	366		CMFVP vs 2 yrs L-PAM	8 yr RFS and OS advantage for combination therapy[g]
CALGB 1975	(20)	330	1 yr	CMFVP vs CMF	No advantage for 5 drugs[h]
Ludwig I (1978)	(37)	241	12 cycles	CMF vs CMF + P	4 yr DFS no Δ or OS Δ[i]

[a]Restricted to < 49 year women with ≥ 4 + nodes
[b]Restricted to < 49; 1–3 + nodes
[c]Restricted to > 49 ≥ 4 + nodes, beyond 8 yr followup no change between P vs PF
[d]Age and nodal subgroups showed no advantage in DFS
[e]No benefits in postmenopausal patients
[f]Subset analysis showed no difference in 6 vs 12 cycles RFS + OS similar to treatment group from 1973 study
[g]Benefit to postmenopausal patients, greatest benefit to premenopausal > 4 nodes (18)
[h]In contrast to SWOG study (16) no advantage in postmenopausal women
[i]The prednisone group able to receive increased doses of CMF with prednisone, no change in outcome

tine, and prednisone) given for one year vs L-PAM (L-phenylalanine mustard) given for two years. In 1982, at 42-month follow-up, the results of this trial were reported.[25] Disease-free survival was significantly longer for CMFVP-treated patients compared with the L-PAM group. This DFS advantage extended through the major subgroups: premenopausal, postmenopausal, one to three positive nodes, and four or more positive nodes. The investigators noted no correlation between the interval from mastectomy to institution of chemotherapy (range one to six weeks) and DFS and OS. At the eight-year follow-up,[43] CMFVP treatment continues to show an advantage in DFS and OS for the entire group and all the subgroups; however, the differences in the postmenopausal patients are not statistically significant in either DFS or OS.

The Cancer and Acute Leukemia Group B compared cyclophosphamide, methotrexate, 5-FU, vincristine, and prednisone (schedule different from that used by Southwest Oncology Group) to cyclophosphamide, methotrexate, 5-FU (identical to the Milan study).[25] The long-term analysis of that study shows no advantage in either treatment arm.[63]

The Ludwig Breast Cancer Study Group randomized patients with Stage II disease (1 to 3 positive nodes only) to receive either cyclophosphamide, methotrexate and 5-FU, or the same drugs plus prednisone.[36] The four-year follow-up reports indicate no differences in DFS or OS between the two groups despite the statistically significant increased dosages of CMF given to the patients randomized to receive the continuous low-dose (7.5 mg/day) prednisone.

One may conclude from this series of randomized studies several points (Table 1):

1) Breast cancer response to cytotoxic therapy is heterogenous.
2) Chemotherapy results in increased DFS and OS for some subsets of patients with Stage II breast cancer.
3) Single agent chemotherapy compares favorably with placebo, and combination therapy compares favorably with single agent.
4) No clearly superior treatment regimen has emerged.
5) Long-term follow-up is necessary to assess a treatment program for breast cancer.

During the time many of the adjuvant trials were underway, prognostic factors other than node status and menopausal status were identified. Among the most important of these was the development of a sensitive and reproducible assay for estrogen receptors, and more recently, progesterone receptors in breast cancer tissue. The absence of estrogen receptors in breast cancer predicts earlier recurrence and shorter survival in locoregional breast cancer (Stage I, II)[4,33] but does not appear to predict the overall survival.[39]

Other factors such as thymidine-labelling index, DNA index, and S-phase determination by flow cytometry have been studied but are less widely applied.[40]

The introduction of tamoxifen into clinical practice for advanced metastatic disease, and the fact that it has few side effects, led to its adoption in combination with cytotoxic chemotherapy in locoregional breast cancer trials (Table 2). The NSABP B-09 trial began in 1977. L-PAM plus 5-FU (PF) was compared to these drugs plus tamoxifen 10 mg twice a day (PF + T).[19] Analysis at five years indicated a significant prolongation of DFS, but not OS, for the tamoxifen-treated group. Further analysis revealed that benefit was limited to women more than 50 years old with four or more positive nodes, and in this subgroup a survival advantage was noted. As expected, the advantages from tamoxifen correlate with hormone receptor levels. Somewhat surprising is the finding that women less than 49 years with negative hormone receptors ($<$ ∫mole/mg) were adversely affected by the addition of tamoxifen and had a statistically shorter survival, compared with the same group of patients treated with chemotherapy alone. Tamoxifen had no effect on women less than 49 years old whose tumor was positive for hormone receptors.

The Ludwig Cancer Group studied the addition of tamoxifen to CMF treatment and compared it to a group treated with tamoxifen and prednisone, and to a control group of premenopausal Stage II patients.[37] At four years, an improvement in DFS was seen in the CMF plus tamoxifen treatment group, but the beneficial effects of this combined therapy were restricted to estrogen receptor–negative patients. This study confirms that CMF has DFS advantages in disease-free survival over control in premenopausal women, but no additional benefit from tamoxifen was evident.

The Eastern Cooperative Oncology Group trial, beginning in 1978, demonstrated an improvement in DFS in postmenopausal women with negative hormone receptors treated with chemohormonal therapy compared to the control group. No advantages were seen for the combined therapy in premenopausal women, and the addition of prednisone increased toxicity.[57]

Although there seems a sound basis for combining endocrine and chemotherapy in the treatment of Stage II breast cancer, the results have been mixed, and therapeutic effects have been seen only in selected subsets of the treatment groups. Indiscriminate use of endocrine therapy is not justified on the basis that it is innocuous. Prednisone[57] and tamoxifen[22] have produced a toxic effect without therapeutic benefit in some groups of patients.

Although the results of early studies utilizing adjuvant hormonal therapy for Stage II breast cancer were disappointing, some recent studies have established a clear role for this form of treatment. The earliest studies were reported on oophorectomy or ovarian radiation in the treatment of premenopausal women. At the time these trials were conducted, hormone receptor assays were not available. Recent trials have used tamoxifen (Table

Table 2. Randomized Trials of Adjuvant Combined Therapy in Stage II Breast Cancer

Study	Reference	Patients	Treatment Arms	Follow-up Results
NSABPB-09	(22)	1891	2 yr PF vs 2 yr PF + T	5 yr improved DFS for ≥ 50 yr, ≥ 4 + nodes + hormone receptors[a,b]
Ludwig III	(36)	503	CMFP + T vs P + T vs control	4 yr improved DFS for CMFP + T vs P + T or control[c]
ECOG	(57)			
premenopausal		662	CMF vs CMFP vs CMFPT	4 yr no difference in DFS or OS[d]
postmenopausal		265	Control vs CMF + P vs CMFPT	4 yr improved DFS in ER negative patients in either arms vs control[e]

[a] DFS advantage seen in entire PF + T group but beneficial effects restricted to ≥ 50 years, ≥ 4 + nodes, positive receptors.
[b] > 49 years with negative hormone receptors treated with tamoxifen shorter DFS and OS than same group without tamoxifen.
[c] ER + patients no difference between CMFP + T vs P + T, in ER negative patients CMFP + T superior to P + T and control.
[d] Noted increased toxicity with addition of prednisone without therapeutic benefit.
[e] No improvement in DFS seen in ER positive patients on the CMFPT arm.

3), megestrol acetate, and aminoglutethimide, although other experimental antiestrogens are also undergoing clinical trials.[35]

The NSABP sponsored a randomized trial of 699 patients treated with either oophorectomy or no endocrine treatment following mastectomy for Stage II breast cancer.[45] No advantages in DFS or OS were seen in the oophorectomy group (Table 3). The Princess Margaret Hospital reported prolonged DFS and OS for premenopausal women over the age of 45 years treated with ovarian radiation and prednisone compared to either no treatment or ovarian radiation therapy alone.[39] Bryant et al. reported a DFS or OS advantage for women randomized to prophylactic oophorectomy following mastectomy for resectable breast cancer.[10] At the five-year analysis, these advantages were no longer significant.

Following the introduction of tamoxifen into clinical use for metastatic breast cancer, it has been used in a number of adjuvant trials. Riberio and Swindell reported on experience at Christie Hospital using adjuvant endocrine therapy for all operable breast cancers.[46,47] This study is flawed in a number of respects. However, when all patients are evaluated according to whether they were treated with tamoxifen or were controls, there was a significant DFS and OS advantage for the tamoxifen group compared to controls.[47]

The Toronto-Edmonton Breast Cancer Study Group reported a series of 366 postmenopausal women randomized to receive either tamoxifen or no further treatment.[44] The tamoxifen-treated group showed a significant improvement in DFS at a median follow-up of three years.

The Ludwig Breast Cancer Study Group entered postmenopausal Stage II patients into two studies. Women less than 65 were randomized after mastectomy to receive either CMF plus tamoxifen, prednisone plus tamoxifen, or no further therapy (the control group). Women aged 65 to 80 years were randomized to receive either prednisone plus tamoxifen or no therapy (control). Comparing the patients from both studies in the control versus the prednisone plus tamoxifen group, a significant increase in the three-year DFS but not OS was seen for the hormone-treated group,[36] but the beneficial effects were limited to those who were estrogen receptor–positive, and there was no decrease in the number of systemic metastases even in that group.

The Eastern Cooperative Oncology Group randomized elderly (over the age of 65) women to receive either tamoxifen or placebo.[14] At four year follow-up, there is a significant advantage in DFS for the tamoxifen group. Subgroups displaying significant benefit are those with four to ten positive nodes, those who were estrogen receptor–positive, and those with T_1 tumors.

The Danish Breast Cancer Cooperative Group treated patients with Stage II breast cancer with total mastectomy and axillary dissection, followed by radiotherapy to the chest wall and regional nodes. The patients were ran-

Table 3. Randomized Adjuvant Trials of Endocrine Therapy

Study	REF	No. Patients	Treatment	Results
NSABP	(45)	699	Oophorectomy vs control	No DFS or OS advantage[a]
Princess Margaret	(38)	705	Ovarian radiation (OR) vs OR + pred vs control	↑ DSF and OS in premenopausal > 45 yrs with OR + pred[b]
Blair Memorial	(10)	359	Oophorectomy vs control	10 yr DFS and OS > 50 yrs in oophorectomy group[c]
Christie Hospital	(47)	961	Premenopause: TAM vs OR Postmenopause: TAM vs control	No significant difference in DFS of OS[d]
Toronto-Edmonton	(44)	366	TAM vs control	Increased DFS at 3 yr in TAM group[e]
Ludwig	(36)	681	Pred + TAM vs control	Increased DFS, OS at 3 yr in TAM group[f]
ECOG	(14)	181	TAM vs placebo	Increased DFS at 4 yr in TAM group[g]
Danish	(41)	1650	TAM vs control	Increased DFS at 7 yrs in TAM group[h]
NATO	(5)	1285	TAM vs control	Increased DFS and OS at 6 years in TAM group[i]

[a]Control group: 161 patients on placebo, 207 on thiotepa
[b]No benefits to postmenopausal women or to premenopausal < 45 years
[c]No benefit in > 50 yr group. Differences not seen at 5 year analysis
[d]Receptor analysis was not done. Advantages seen only when all TAM treated patients compared to other treatments.
[e]Hormone receptor negative patients did not benefit from TAM.
[f]Hormonal treatment did not decrease incidence of systemic metastasis. No benefits seen for ER-negative patients.
[g]All patients > 65 yr. No advantage in OS. Subgroups benefiting: 4–10 + nodes, ER-positive, T₁ tumor
[h]No difference in OS. Subgroups benefiting: < 69 yrs, > 4 + nodes grade I-II histology, > 100 |mole/mg
[i]All subgroups benefited, including node-negative patients.

domized to receive tamoxifen or to the control group.[48] At 48-month follow-up, there was no significant difference between the two groups. Sub-
grouping on the basis of estrogen receptor content of the tumor showed that
the treated group enjoyed a significant improvement in DFS for those
patients whose tumor had greater than 100 ∫mole/mg estrogen receptor.
When two groups of patients were studied at seven years follow-up,[41] there
emerges a significant improvement in DFS for the tamoxifen group, but still
no difference in OS. The subgroups benefiting were those with high estrogen receptor values (> 100 ∫mole/mg), four or more positive nodes,
patients less than 69 years, and those with histologically low grade tumors.

The most important report on the use of adjuvant hormonal therapy has
been published for the Nolvadex Adjuvant Trial Organization (NATO) by
Baum et al.[5] Stage II premenopausal and Stage I pre- and postmenopausal
women were randomized to receive either tamoxifen or no treatment after
mastectomy. When analyzed at six years, there is a significant OS and DFS
advantage for the entire treatment group. The advantages were seen across all
the subgroups, and surprisingly, even in the hormone receptor–negative group.
There were no differences in relapse rates seen in the patients when grouped
according to estrogen receptor content.

Overall, the use of adjuvant hormonal therapy seems to have benefited
primarily those patients with an estrogen/progesterone receptor–positive tumor
(with the notable exception of the NATO trial). Several of the studies have not
had sufficient follow-up time to evaluate survival advantages. The patients who
primarily benefit from hormone therapy have high levels of hormone receptor.
The natural history of tumors rich in estrogen and progesterone receptors
favors longer survival, requiring prolonged follow-up to determine the beneficial effects.

From the various studies done in Stage II breast cancer, it is evident (see
Tables 1, 2, and 3) that results are heterogeneous and sometimes conflicting.
What does seem clear is that, for the vast majority of Stage II breast cancer
patients, adjuvant treatment is superior to no treatment. The selection of
appropriate therapy should be based on menopausal status and hormone receptor concentration. When available, patients should be entered into suitable
randomized clinical trials. Table 4 summarizes our treatment approach to
patients not enrolled in an experimental study.

Treatment of Node-Negative Breast Cancer

The presence of metastases in ipsilateral axillary lymph nodes remains the
best indicator of prognosis in women with locoregional breast cancer. Stage I
breast cancer is generally regarded as a relatively benign disease, despite the fact
that up to 30% of premenopausal patients will eventually develop a recurrence.
Estrogen receptor content has been used to select higher risk Stage I patients.[60]
Alternatively, the use of in vitro thymidine-labelling index as a measure of

**Table 4. Treatment Recommendations Based on Stage[a]
(after Primary Treatment)**

Stage I		Therapy
Premenopause	ER/PR negative	Consider adjuvant therapy[b]
	ER/PR positive	Probably not indicated
Postmenopause	ER/PR negative	Consider adjuvant therapy[b]
	ER/PR positive	Not indicated
Stage II		
Premenopause	ER/PR negative	Adjuvant combination chemotherapy
	ER/PR positive	Adjuvant combination chemotherapy[c]
Postmenopause	ER/PR negative	Adjuvant combination chemotherapy[d]
	ER/PR positive	Adjuvant tamoxifen[e]
Stage III, Localized IV		
All patients		Combined modality: Hormonal synchronization→chemotherapy and/or surgery and/or radiation therapy
Stage IV, and Recurrent Disease		
Premenopause	ER/PR negative	Combination chemotherapy
	ER/PR positive	Consider hormonal therapy[f]
Postmenopause	ER/PR negative	Combination chemotherapy
	ER/PR positive	Hormonal therapy

[a]Appropriate patients should be entered into clinical trials.
[b]Especially if other tumor characteristics are unfavorable.
[c]No indications for adding hormonal therapy to combination chemotherapy.
[d]NCI consensus statement less definite " . . . Considered but cannot be recommended as standard practice."[2]
[e]Duration at least 2 years.
[f]Depending upon presentation of disease, hormonal manipulation should be considered prior to combination chemotherapy.

tumor proliferative activity has been demonstrated to be a useful prognostic variable independent of nodal status and hormone receptor content.[40] Cell cycle distribution and DNA content of tumor cells have been shown to be important prognostic variables as well. Identification of higher risk Stage I (node-negative) patients would allow use of adjuvant therapy at a point where the tumor burden after surgery is low compared with Stage II patients. This group should benefit maximally from adjuvant therapy because of the low tumor burden.

Both the Milan[59] and the NSABP[17] reported a 25% ten-year relapse rate for Stage I patients. The Milan group observed a 37% relapse rate in a subgroup of Stage I patients with estrogen receptor–negative tumors at five years from mastectomy.[60] This group has conducted a randomized trial of node-negative and estrogen receptor–negative breast cancer patients to receive either cyclophosphamide, methotrexate, and 5-FU, or no further treatment. At three-year follow-up, the DFS rate was 50% in the control arm, but 94% in treated arm.[8] Advantages to treatment were seen in premenopausal and postmenopausal patients, and patients with tumors having a high thymidine-labelling index. Caffier has reported similar experience in patients treated with cyclophosphamide, methotrexate, and 5-FU at five years postmastectomy.[12] The DFS and OS are better in the treatment group but have not reached statistical significance. The Nissen-Meyer trial,[42] randomizing patients to receive either perioperative cyclophosphamide or no treatment, now at more than 20-year follow-up, continues to show a significant advantage for those patients treated with cyclophosphamide versus the control group. This advantage is equally apparent in the 600 node-negative patients. Senn et al.[52] have reported encouraging results with the adjuvant treatment of node-negative patients with melphalan, methotrexate, and 5-FU. At nine-year follow-up, the group reports an advantage in DFS out to five years, OS out to seven years, and both of these trends continue in the treatment group compared to controls. Node-positive patients treated on this protocol showed no advantages over the control group. The Arizona group treated 156 patients with Stage I breast cancer with doxorubicin and cyclophosphamide (3 cycles) in an uncontrolled study.[9] Only 1 of 58 patients with a T_1 primary and 15 of 98 patients with a T_2 primary have relapsed.

Although none of these studies provides definitive evidence of the value of adjuvant therapy in patients with Stage I breast cancer, all of the studies show a trend favoring treatment, and none of the studies report excessive toxicity. With analysis of thymidine-labelling index, DNA content, mitotic rates, tumor grade, hormone receptor analysis, and cell cycle distribution, patients at higher risk can be selected for treatment while those at low risk can avoid the toxicity (although minimal) of systemic chemotherapy. Long-term follow-up of these studies will be necessary to exclude development of late toxic effects such as leukemia.

ADVANCED LOCAL DISEASE (STAGE III, LOCALIZED STAGE IV)

Haagensen and Stout[28] identified the now familiar signs associated with locally advanced breast cancer. These signs include inflammatory carcinoma, internal mammary or supraclavicular node involvement, satellite skin nodules, skin ulceration, fixation of the tumor to the chest wall, and fixation of the axillary nodes. Although most breast cancer series report 10% or less of all breast cancer patients present with locally advanced breast cancer, these patients carry a poor prognosis because of the development of metastases, which leads to death in up to 80% of patients.[1] Within the group with locally advanced cancer is a subgroup comprising approximately 1% of the total of most series, which has been identified since 1924 as "inflammatory" carcinoma.

The presence of edema, wheals, and erythema involving more than one-third of the breast is diagnostic of inflammatory carcinoma.[27] Histologically, inflammatory carcinoma can be confirmed by the presence of dermal lymphatic tumor invasion in about 70% of patients.[13] Recognition of the poor response of locally advanced breast cancer to standard therapy lead Haagensen to develop criteria of inoperability for those patients.[28] Improvements in surgical technique, delivery and dosing of radiation, and postoperative radiation therapy failed to improve the outlook for this group of patients. Modest gains in response rate and local control have been made by treating patients with locally advanced breast cancer on aggressive protocols of induction chemotherapy followed by radiation therapy.[11,54]

Observations in the laboratory have been applied to the treatment of locally advanced breast cancer. Addition of estradiol to established cultures of the hormonally responsive human breast carcinoma cell line MCF-7 stimulates growth that is inhibited by the antiestrogen tamoxifen.[34] Further studies demonstrated that tamoxifen arrested cells in the G_1 phase of the cell cycle, and subsequent addition of estrogen induced a wave of DNA synthesis, and those stimulated cancer cells had an increased sensitivity to chemotherapeutic drugs.[61] Applying these laboratory observations, Lippman et al. reported a 65% response rate in both arms of a randomized study of advanced breast cancer patients treated with combination chemotherapy with or without hormonal synchronization.[53] Although the hormonal synchronization had no impact on the response rate in metastatic disease, the authors noted a response in 13 of 14 patients with inflammatory carcinoma. Since then, the study has been extended to patients with locally advanced breast cancer, and the results of the most recent update show a 93% response rate, with 53% of the patients without evidence of tumor. Seventy percent of those patients with a complete remission were found to be free of tumor pathologically after mastectomy or extensive biopsies. The treatment with hormonal synchronization and chemotherapy is continued until there is either a complete remission or no further improvement. At that point, the patient has extensive biopsies. If residual tumor is present, then a mastectomy is performed. If no evidence of residual cancer is found, the breast is treated with a standard course of radiotherapy. Following either mastectomy or radiation therapy, chemotherapy is continued with hormonal synchronization for a total of 12 months.

The simple combination of chemotherapy plus tamoxifen is not effective in achieving the high complete response rates seen with hormonal synchronization followed by chemotherapy.[23] The hormonal synchronization is achieved by treating the patient for one week with tamoxifen, and then priming the estrogen-starved cells with Premarin two days prior to chemotherapy (Table 5). The presumed mechanism is that the estrogen increases the fraction of the tumor cells that are undergoing cell division and renders them more susceptible to the chemotherapy.

It is interesting to note that the estrogen and progesterone receptor content of

Table 5.   Hormonal Synchronization and Combination Chemotherapy in Locally Advanced Breast Cancer*

Start				Restart
Cyclophosphamide (IV) Doxorubicin (IV)	Conjugated Estrogens (p.o.) (Premarin)	Methotrexate (IV) 5-FU (IV)	Tamoxifen (p.o.) (Nolvadex)	Cyclophosphamide Doxorubicin
Day 1	Days 5,6,7	Day 7	Days 8 through 14	Day 22

*This hormonal synchronization combination chemotherapy protocol (MICH 0786) is currently enrolling patients.   It cannot be recommended as "standard therapy."

the tumor seem to have no influence on the response rate in locally advanced breast cancer. The hormonal synchronization appears to work effectively even in hormone receptor–negative tumors by a yet unexplained mechanism.[53]

TREATMENT OF METASTATIC BREAST CANCER

Patients presenting with Stage IV carcinoma of the breast (except inflammatory carcinoma) and those who experience recurrence after treatment of early stage disease provide a therapeutic challenge to the medical oncologist. He or she must balance the natural history of the disease, the side effects of chemotherapeutic agents, use of hormonal manipulations, and the patient's quality and duration of life. Metastasis of cancer beyond the regional lymphatics continues to be fatal for nearly all patients.

It was observed at the beginning of the twentieth century that metastatic breast cancer could be put into temporary remission following oophorectomy. Since that time, a variety of additive and ablative hormonal therapies have been developed that are of use in selected women with metastatic breast cancer. The adjuvant hormonal studies notwithstanding, endocrine therapy has remained true to the original observation of only temporary responses in patients with advanced disease. Hormonally responsive tissues contain receptors for various steroid hormones, conferring specificity to that tissue. The hormone enters the cell, binding to the receptor, and subsequently influences gene expression as manifested by growth or differentiation. Prior to the development of a clinical assay for the determination of estrogen (and later progesterone) receptors, it was found that approximately one-third of patients treated with a hormonal maneuver (oophorectomy, adrenalectomy, etc.) would respond. With the widespread application of hormone receptor assays for both estrogen and progesterone, one may select patients more appropriately for consideration of hormonal manipulation. There is a direct correlation between the estrogen receptor content of the primary tumor and response to endocrine therapy.[21] This correlation is even better with the progesterone receptor. Selecting patients based on the presence of estrogen and progesterone receptors in the tumor improves the response rate from 30% in the unselected population to 60% (if a cutoff for "positive" is 10 ∫mole/mg).[30] It must also be remembered that the natural history of estrogen/progesterone receptor–positive tumors is favorable compared with estrogen/progesterone receptor–negative tumors.[21]

Surgical or ablative endocrine therapy has fallen into disuse since the development of effective substitutes for oophorectomy, adrenalectomy, and hypophysectomy. Ovarian function can be ablated by surgical removal, radiation, or chemotherapeutic regimens (including antiestrogens). Although the response rates to oophorectomy and tamoxifen are equivalent, the surgical procedure is seldom selected, except occasionally in premenopausal patients. Patients responding to oophorectomy, however, will often respond to tamoxifen.[51] Adrenalectomy has been in use in metastatic breast cancer since 1952 and response rates were similar to those seen in oophorectomy. The general indication for adrenalectomy was a previous response to oophorectomy and subsequent relapse.[51] Aminoglutethimide is a potent inhibitor of steroid synthesis and has replaced adrenalectomy in the treatment of metastatic breast cancer. Steroid replacement with hydrocortisone is necessary during aminoglutethimide treatment. A study of 147 women with metastatic breast cancer treated with aminoglutethimide and hydrocortisone revealed a 49% response rate and decreased plasma and urinary estrogen levels.[50] Aminoglutethimide has been demonstrated to be equally effective as surgical adrenalectomy in a randomized study, with a response rate in both arms of about 50%.[49]

Tamoxifen compares favorably with hypophysectomy,[31] which is seldom if ever used, and diethylstilbestrol (DES),[29] which is associated with thromboembolic and coronary artery disease.

Megestrol acetate (Megace), a potent progestational agent, has demonstrated effectiveness in palliative treatment of advanced breast cancer. This agent has minimal side effects. The response rate in unselected patients is about 30%.

Tamoxifen is generally the first choice for hormonal manipulation. It is well tolerated and free of major side effects. If a second hormonal manipulation is indicated, either megestrol acetate or aminoglutethimide with hydrocortisone replacement is chosen. There are no clear-cut differences in response rates to these agents (or with the surgical equivalents) and the choice is made on the basis of matching side effects to a particular patient.

Cytotoxic Chemotherapy of Advanced Breast Cancer

A complete discussion of the role of chemotherapy in treatment of advanced breast cancer is beyond the scope of this review and the reader should rely on standard texts for a detailed discussion.

Among the many agents that have demonstrated antitumor activity in breast cancer, doxorubicin has the highest rate of response, albeit with considerable toxicity. Other than doxorubicin, most drugs are not often used as single agents. Table 6 lists the active agents and approximate response rate. Response rates to commonly used combination therapies are superior to the individual agents, but the toxicity is increased (Table 7). It is controversial whether the simultaneous use of chemotherapy and hormonal therapy in metastatic breast cancer offers any advantages to the use of these agents sequentially.[32,58]

The approach to selecting appropriate therapy in women with advanced cancer of the breast should be based on menopausal status, sites of disease, symptoms, hormone receptor content, response to previous therapies, and associated medical conditions.

Symptomatic postmenopausal women with hormone receptor–rich tumors often respond to hormone manipulation. Tamoxifen is the drug chosen most often. If there is a response to the initial hormone treatment, a second or third

Table 6.   Drugs Active in the Treatment of Advanced Breast Cancer

Drug	Response Rate (%)
Cyclophosphamide	35
Melphalan	22
Chlorambucil	20
Thiotepa	30
5-FU	26
Methotrexate	34
Mitomycin-C	38
Doxorubicin	
No prior therapy	38–50
Prior therapy	27–38
Vincristine or vinblastine	20
Bisantrene or mitoxantrone (investigational)	22

manipulation is likely to be effective, while lack of response predicts that a subsequent response to hormonal therapy is unlikely (less than 10%). After exhaustion of the endocrine treatment options, cytotoxic chemotherapy is often considered. Chemotherapy is also appropriate for symptomatic patients with hormone receptor–negative tumors, and patients with hormone receptor–positive tumors with life-threatening disease. The site of metastatic disease was thought to be important (i.e., skin vs bone vs viscera); however, recent data suggest a much stronger correlation with hormone receptor content than with disease site.[55]

In postmenopausal women requiring cytotoxic therapy, a cyclophosphamide-containing program is usually chosen, reserving doxorubicin as the second or third line due to its serious side effects. With the pending FDA approval of mitoxantrone, the use of alternative anthracyclines may increase in

Table 7.   Combination Chemotherapy for Advanced Breast Cancer

Program	Response Rate (%)
CMF: cyclophosphamide, methotrexate, 5-FU	50–65
CMF + A: cyclophosphamide, methotrexate, 5-FU, doxorubicin	50–65
CMF + P: cyclophosphamide, methotrexate, 5-FU, prednisone	50–60
CMF + VP: cyclophosphamide, methotrexate, 5-FU, vincristine, prednisone	50–60
CAF: cyclophosphamide, doxorubicin, 5-FU	45–80
AC: doxorubicin, cyclophosphamide	50–80
VAC: vincristine, doxorubicin, cyclophosphamide	50
AM: doxorubicin, mitomycin-C	25–50

this group of women. Judicious use of radiotherapy and surgical resection are often indicated for isolated symptomatic metastases.

Premenopausal women with advanced disease have traditionally been treated with combination chemotherapy in favor of endocrine therapy, based on early studies comparing oophorectomy and chemotherapy in unselected patients. However, some encouraging results have emerged from studies on premenopausal women with estrogen–receptor positive tumors treated with either oophorectomy or tamoxifen.[3] These studies demonstrate that response rates to tamoxifen are equivalent to oophorectomy in premenopausal women.[24] There is appropriately little enthusiasm for concurrent combinations of hormonal and chemotherapy treatment in premenopausal women based on lack of convincing data in the adjuvant setting.[37] In those premenopausal women with hormone receptor–positive tumors, either tamoxifen or oophorectomy should be considered. As in the postmenopausal patient, a response to hormonal manipulation predicts response to a subsequent hormonal maneuver. In hormone receptor–negative patients and those who have no longer responded to hormonal therapy, combination chemotherapy is appropriate.

Table 6 presents a summary of our approach treatments based on stage, menopausal status, and hormone receptor status for breast cancer patients who are not enrolled in an experimental study. These recommendations are consistent with the consensus statement issued by the National Cancer Institute.[2] This table is merely a guide, however, and it is important to individualize treatment based on clinical judgment and desires of the patient. Consideration of experimental treatments should be given in all groups of patients and enrollment into clinical trials is encouraged.

REFERENCES

1. Adair T, et al.: Long-term follow-up of breast cancer patients. The 30 year report. Cancer 33:1145–1150, 1974.
2. Adjuvant Chemotherapy for Breast Cancer, National Institutes of Health Consensus Development Statement. Vol 5: No 12, 1985.
3. Ahmann DL, et al.: An evaluation of early or delayed adjuvant chemotherapy in premenopausal patients with advanced breast cancer undergoing oophorectomy. N Engl J Med 297:356–360, 1977.
4. Allegara, JC, Lippman ME, et al.: Association between steroid hormone receptor status and disease free interval in breast cancer. Cancer Treat Rep 63:1271–1277.
5. Baum M, et al.: Controlled trial of tamoxifen as single adjuvant agent in management of early breast cancer. Lancet 1:836–840, 1985.
6. Bonadonna G, et al.: Combination chemotherapy as an adjuvant treatment in operable breast cancer. N Engl J Med 294:405–410, 1976.
7. Bonadonna G, et al.: Ten-year experience with CMF based adjuvant chemotherapy in resectable breast cancer. Breast Cancer 5:95–115, 1985.
8. Bonadonna G, et al.: Current status of Milan adjuvant chemotherapy

trials for node-positive and node-negative breast cancer. NCI Monograph 1:45–49, 1986.

9. Brooks RJ, et al.: Adjuvant chemotherapy of axillary node-negative carcinoma of the breast using doxorubicin and cyclophosphamide. NCI Monograph 1:135–137, 1986.

10. Bryant AJ, Weir JA: Prophylactic oophorectomy in operable instances of carcinoma of the breast. Surg Gynecol Obstet 153:660–664, 1981.

11. Budzar AU, et al.: Management of inflammatory carcinoma of the breast with combined modality approach – An update. Cancer 47:2537–2542, 1981.

12. Caffier H. Adjuvant chemotherapy versus post-operative irradiation in node-negative breast cancer, in Jones SE, Salmon SE (eds): *Adjuvant Therapy of Cancer IV*. Orlando, Grune & Stratton, 1984, pp 417–424.

13. Camp E. Inflammatory carcinoma of the breast. Am J Surg 31:583–586, 1976.

14. Cummings FJ, et al.: Tamoxifen versus placebo: Double-blind adjuvant trial in elderly women with stage II breast cancer. NCI Monograph 1:119–123, 1986.

15. Fisher B, Slack NH, Bross DJ: Cancer of the breast, size of the neoplasm and prognosis. Cancer 24:1071–1080, 1969.

16. Fisher B, et al.: L-phenylalanine mustard (L-PAM) in the management of primary breast cancer. A report of early findings. N Engl J Med 292:117–122, 1975.

17. Fisher B, et al.: Ten year follow-up results of patients with carcinoma of the breast in a co-operative clinical trial evaluating surgical adjuvant chemotherapy. Surg Gynecol Obstet 140:528–534, 1975.

18. Fisher B, et al.: L-phenylalanine mustard (L-PAM) in the management of primary breast cancer. An update of earlier findings and a comparison with those utilizing L-PAM plus 5-fluorouracil (5-FU). Cancer 39:2883–2903, 1977.

19. Fisher B, et al.: The treatment of primary breast cancer with chemotherapy and tamoxifen: Correlation of quantitative estrogen levels with response to therapy. N Engl J Med 305:1–6, 1981.

20. Fisher B, et al.: Influence of the interval between primary tumor removal and chemotherapy on kinetics and growth of metastasis. Cancer Research 43:1488–1492, 1983.

21. Fisher B, et al.: Influence of tumor estrogen and progesterone receptor levels on the response to tamoxifen and chemotherapy in primary breast cancer. J Clin Oncol 1:227–239, 1983.

22. Fisher B, et al.: Adjuvant chemotherapy with and without tamoxifen in the treatment of primary breast cancer: 5-year results from the National Surgical Adjuvant Breast and Bowel Project Trial. J Clin Oncol 4:459–471, 1986.

23. Fouble B, et al.: Combined modality treatment of inflammatory breast cancer. Int J Radiat Oncol Bio Phys 12 (Supp 1):151, 1986.

24. Glick JH, et al.: Randomized clinical trial of tamoxifen plus sequential CMF vs tamoxifen alone in postmenopausal women with advanced breast cancer. Breast Cancer Res Treat 1:59–68, 1981.

25. Glucksberg H, et al.: Combination chemotherapy (CMFVP) versus L-phenylalanine mustard (L-PAM) for operable breast cancer with positive axillary nodes. Cancer 50:423–434, 1982.

26. Griswold DP: The potential for murine tumor models in surgical adjuvant chemotherapy. Cancer Chemother Rep 5:187–204, 1979.

27. Haagensen CD: *Diseases of the Breast*. Philadelphia, WB Saunders, 1971, pp 576–584.

28. Haagensen CD, Stout AP: Carcinoma of the breast II: Criteria of operability. Ann Surg 118:859–870, 1943.

29. Ingle JN, et al.: Randomized clinical trial of diethylstilbestrol versus tamoxifen in postmenopausal women with advanced cancer. N Engl J Med 304:16–21, 1981.

30. Kiang DT, et al.: Estrogen receptors and responses to chemotherapy and hormonal therapy in advanced breast cancer. N Engl J Med 299:1330–1334, 1978.

31. Kiang DT, et al.: Comparison of tamoxifen and hypophysectomy in breast cancer treatment. Cancer 45:1322–1325, 1980.

32. Kiang DT, et al.: A randomized trial of chemotherapy and hormonal therapy in advanced breast cancer. N Engl J Med 313:1242–1246, 1985.

33. Knight WA, et al.: Estrogen receptor as an independent prognostic factor for early recurrence in breast cancer. Cancer Res 37:4669–4671, 1977.

34. Lippman ME, et al.: The effects of estrogens and antiestrogens on the hormone responsive human breast cancer in long-term tissue culture. Cancer Res 36:4595–4601, 1976.

35. Lippman ME: Adjuvant systemic therapy of breast cancer, in *Important Advances in Oncology*, DeVita V, Hellman S, Rosenberg S (eds)., Philadelphia, J. B. Lippincott Company, 1985, pp 254–273.

36. Ludwig Breast Cancer Study Group: Randomized trial of chemo-endocrine therapy, endocrine therapy and mastectomy alone in postmenopausal patients with operable breast cancer and axillary node metastasis. Lancet 1:1256–1260, 1984.

37. Ludwig Breast Cancer Study Group: Adjuvant combination chemotherapy with or without prednisone in premenopausal breast cancer patients with metastasis in 1 to 3 axillary lymph nodes: A randomized trial. Cancer Res 45:4454–4459, 1985.

38. McGuire WL, et al.: Role of steroid hormone receptors as prognostic factors in primary breast cancer. NCI Monograph 1:19–23, 1986.

39. Meakin JW, et al.: Ovarian radiation and prednisone therapy following surgery and radiotherapy for carcinoma of the breast. Can Med J 120:1221–1229, 1979.

40. Meyer JS: Cell kinetics in selection and stratification of patients for adjuvant therapy of breast cancer. NCI Monograph 1:25–28, 1986.

41. Mouridsen HT: Adjuvant tamoxifen in postmenopausal high-risk breast cancer patients: Present status of Danish breast cancer cooperative trials. NCI Monograph 1:115–118, 1986.

42. Nissen-Meyer R, et al.: Treatment of node-negative breast cancer patients with short course of chemotherapy immediately after surgery. NCI Monograph 1:125–128, 1986.

43. Osborne CK, et al.: Adjuvant therapy of breast cancer: Southwest Oncology Group Studies 71-74. NCI Monograph 1:71-74, 1986.
44. Pritchard KI, et al.: A randomized trial of adjuvant tamoxifen in postmenopausal women with axillary node positive breast cancer, in Jones SE, Salmon SE (eds): *Adjuvant Therapy of Cancer IV*. Orlando, Grune & Stratton, 1984, pp 339-347.
45. Radvin RG, et al.: Results of a clinical trial concerning the worth of prophylactic oophorectomy for breast carcinoma. Surg Gynecol Obstet 131:1055-1064, 1970.
46. Ribeiro G, Palmer MK: Adjuvant tamoxifen for carcinoma of the breast: Report of clinical trial by Christie Hospital and Holt Radium Institute. Br Med J 286: 827-830, 1984.
47. Ribeiro G, Swindell R: The Christie Hospital tamoxifen (Nolvadex) adjuvant trial for operable breast carcinoma – 7-year results. Eur J Clin Oncol 21:897-900, 1985.
48. Rose C, et al.: Beneficial effect of adjuvant tamoxifen therapy in primary breast cancer patients with high oestrogen receptor values. Lancet 1:16-19, 1985.
49. Santen RJ, et al.: A randomized trial comparing surgical adrenalectomy with aminoglutethimide plus hydrocortisone in women with advanced breast cancer. N Engl J Med 305:545-551, 1981.
50. Santen RJ, et al.: Aminoglutethimide as treatment of postmenopausal women with advanced breast carcinoma. Ann Intern Med 96:94-101, 1982.
51. Schweitzer RJ: Oophorectomy/adrenalectomy. Cancer 46:1061-1065, 1980.
52. Senn HJ, et al.: Swiss adjuvant trial (OSAKO 06/741 with Chlorambucil) methotrexate, and 5-FU plus BCG in node-negative breast cancer patients: Nine year results. NCI Monograph 1:129-134, 1986.
53. Sorace RA, et al.: The management of non-metastatic locally advanced breast cancer using primary induction chemotherapy with hormonal synchronization followed by radiation therapy with or without debulking Surgery. World J Surg 9:775-785, 1985.
54. Sponzo RW, et al.: Management of non-resectable (stage III) carcinoma of the breast. J Rad Oncol Biol Phys 5:1475-1478, 1979.
55. Stoll BA: Clinical experience with tamoxifen in advanced breast cancer. Recent results. Cancer Res 71:207-211, 1980.
56. Tancini, G, et al.: Adjuvant CMF in breast cancer: Comparative 5-year results of 12 versus 6 cycles. J Clin Oncol 1:2-10, 1983.
57. Taylor SG, et al.: Combination chemotherapy compared to tamoxifen as initial therapy for stage IV breast cancer in elderly women. Ann Intern Med 104:455-461, 1986.
58. Taylor SG, et al.: Adjuvant CMFP versus CMFP plus tamoxifen versus observation alone in postmenopausal node positive breast cancer patients: Three year results of an Eastern Cooperative Oncology Group Study. J Clin Oncol 3:144-154, 1985.
59. Valagussa P, et al.: Patterns of relapse and survival following radical

mastectomy. Analysis of 716 consecutive cases. Cancer 41:1170–1178, 1978.

60. Valagussa P, et al.: Are estrogen receptors alone a reliable prognostic factor in node negative breast cancer, in Jones SE, Salmon SE (eds): *Adjuvant Therapy of Cancer IV*, Orlando, Grune & Statton, 1984, pp 407–416.

61. Weichselbaum RR, et al.: Proliferation kinetics of a human breast cancer line *in vitro* following treatment with 17 β-estradiol and 1-b-D-arabino-furanocytosine. Cancer Res 38:2339–2342, 1978.

62. Wittes, RE: Adjuvant chemotherapy—clinical trials and laboratory models. Cancer Treat Rep 70:87–103, 1986.

63. Wolmark N, Fisher B: Adjuvant therapy in primary breast cancer. Surg Clin North Am 65:161–179, 1985.

15. Breast Reconstruction

THOMAS R. STEVENSON

Following mastectomy, a woman often seeks information regarding breast reconstruction. When faced with such a patient, the reconstructive surgeon must consider the issues of patient selection, timing, and appropriate technique. Counseling consists of outlining the reconstructive alternatives and making recommendations. Final approval of the plan is made by the patient.

PATIENT SELECTION AND TIMING

Every woman who expresses an interest in breast reconstruction is a potential candidate. Certain medical criteria must be met before an operation is seriously considered.[6] The patient's age is noted, but advanced age does not preclude breast reconstruction. General physical health is evaluated. Evidence of cardiac, renal, or respiratory disease is sought and the underlying condition treated. Diabetes mellitus should be well controlled. Any infection (urinary tract, respiratory, or wound) should be cleared preoperatively.

The patient's psychological status plays an important role in any decision regarding reconstruction. Recovery is facilitated by a stable and supportive home environment. A severe or untreated thought disorder is a contraindication to reconstruction. Thorough preoperative teaching establishes patient rapport, builds confidence in the surgeon, and prepares the patient for the postoperative appearance of the breast. It must be understood that the goals of reconstruction are to improve clothing fit and restore a feeling of "wholeness" to the woman. However, every breast reconstruction is *just that*, a *reconstruction*. The patient must have realistic expectations. If she anticipates a normal breast on the operated side, she will be disappointed.

Breast reconstruction can be performed at the time of ablative surgery or as a delayed procedure. Immediate reconstruction will be discussed in a later section.[12] If reconstruction is to be delayed, a three-month wait following mastectomy is recommended. This allows the postoperative inflammation to subside. Patients receiving adjuvant chemotherapy are advised to await completion of the course before undergoing breast reconstruction.[4]

179

Occasionally, a patient with metastatic breast cancer will seek reconstruction.[4] Once such a patient has completed chemotherapy, radiation therapy, or both for the metastases, she is evaluated and the alternatives discussed. If the patient is comfortable and metabolically stable, reconstruction can be undertaken.

The patient who seeks reconstruction following breast or chest wall irradiation presents special problems. Irradiated skin may be woody, thin, or ulcerated. In such a case, it is usually necessary to select a reconstructive technique that provides transposition of uninvolved skin from a distant site to create or reinforce the reconstruction.

RECONSTRUCTIVE TECHNIQUES

Techniques Using Local Tissue

The primary requirement for breast reconstruction is the creation of a breast mound. Many patients who have undergone total or modified radical mastectomy have sufficient anterior chest wall skin and muscle to permit reconstruction using local tissues alone.

Reconstruction can be accomplished by placing a silicone gel implant in the subpectoral position (Figure 1).[2] Under general anesthesia, a portion of the mastectomy wound is opened and the pectoralis major muscle identified. A pocket is made beneath this muscle extending superiorly to the clavicle, inferiorly to the level of the inframammary fold (positioned symmetrically with the opposite breast), laterally to the anterior axillary line, and medially to the sternal border. An appropriate implant is inserted in this pocket and the wound is closed. The patient is usually able to leave the hospital on the first postoperative day.

Subcutaneous mastectomy may be performed to diminish the potential risk of cancer in a patient whose probability of developing the disease is high. The majority of the breast tissue can be removed with preservation of the nipple or areola. Reconstruction is usually accomplished by placement of a submuscular prosthesis, since adequate skin is almost always available (Figure 2).

Mastectomy requires removal of varying amounts of breast and anterior chest wall skin. If little redundancy remains in the skin or the patient is moderately obese, it may not be possible to insert an implant of adequate volume in a single operation. In consultation with the patient, the surgeon may elect to place the largest implant that can be accommodated in the subpectoral position. After waiting three to six months for the skin and muscle to stretch, a second operation is performed employing a larger implant.

Complications after breast reconstruction using prostheses can occur

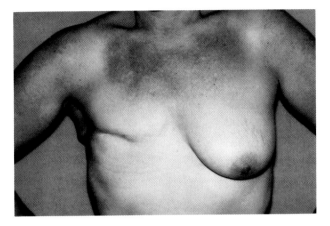

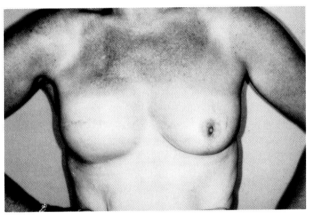

Figure 1. Breast reconstruction by submuscular prosthesis placement. *Above,* preoperative appearance following modified radical mastectomy; *below,* postoperative appearance after reconstruction using prosthesis placed
beneath pectoralis major muscle.

early or late in the patient's course. Early complications include hematoma
formation and postoperative infection. These are seen in less than 5% of
patients. Capsular contracture occurs in up to 26% of patients and results
from dense thickening of the scar surrounding the prosthesis.[7] Onset of the
contracture is usually within the first postoperative year. The patient notices
firmness and often a cephalad migration of the reconstructed breast. When
the symptoms are severe, treatment consists of open capsulotomy and
implant exchange. Recurrence of the contracture can be treated by repeat
capsulotomy. Rarely is it necessary to remove the prosthesis permanently
due to intractable capsular contracture.

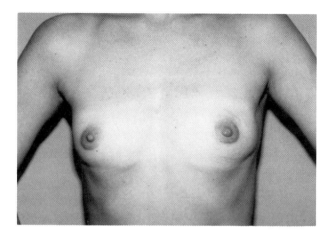

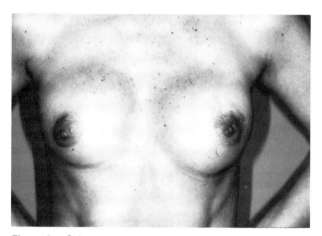

Figure 2. Subcutaneous mastectomy and immediate reconstruction. *Above,* preoperative appearance; *below,* patient seen six months postoperatively.

Tissue Expansion

Tissue expansion offers an alternative for reconstruction in the patient with a deficiency in chest wall skin and muscle (Figure 3). As exemplified by the abdomen in pregnancy, tissues have the capacity to stretch or expand under the influence of persistent pressure. The resultant increase in surface area is due to elasticity of the tissues, an apparent increase in the number of epidermal cells, and a thinning of the dermis.

The principle of tissue expansion finds application in the patient with a

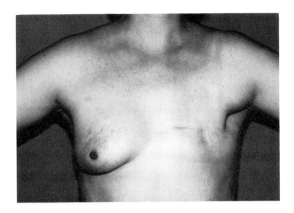

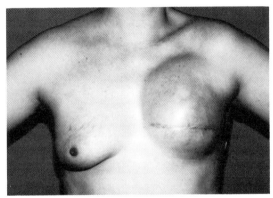

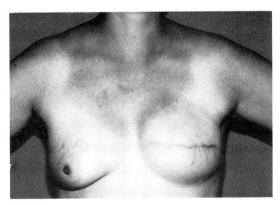

Figure 3. Breast reconstruction by tissue expansion. *Above,* preoperative appearance following modified radical mastectomy; *middle,* expander inserted and inflated to appropriate volume; *below,* permanent prosthesis placed.

deficiency of chest wall skin who desires breast reconstruction. A tissue expander can be placed either at the time of mastectomy or after the surgical wound has healed. Once expansion is complete, a permanent prosthesis is used to establish a breast mound.

The tissue expander itself consists of a collapsed silicone bag connected to a self-sealing reservoir. After placing the expander beneath the skin and muscle of the chest wall and waiting two to three weeks, the reservoir is entered percutaneously with a small-gauge needle and sterile saline is injected. Saline flows into the expander and increases its volume. The overlying tissues respond by expanding to accommodate the new volume. Injections are repeated on a weekly basis until sufficient additional skin is available to permit placement of an adequately sized permanent prosthesis.[11]

Latissimus Dorsi Musculocutaneous Flap

The problem of inadequate chest wall skin for breast reconstruction has also been addressed by transposition of tissue from a distant site to enclose a breast prosthesis. The latissimus dorsi musculocutaneous flap found early widespread usage in this manner.[1,10] This muscle takes origin from the spinous processes of the lower cervical and upper thoracic vertebrae, converging to insert on the posterior crest of the humerus. It is innervated by the lateral thoracic nerve and nourished by the thoracodorsal artery and vein. Skin overlying the latissimus dorsi receives its blood supply from the muscle and can be moved with it to augment the anterior chest skin.

The latissimus dorsi muscle, even when paralyzed, can be transposed successfully in most patients. Denervation of the muscle implies an injury to the thoracodorsal pedicle. A collateral artery and vein from the serratus anterior muscle also nourish the latissimus dorsi muscle, and the musculocutaneous flap usually can be based safely on these vessels.[3]

Breast reconstruction using the latissimus dorsi muscle begins with preoperative marking of the proposed new inframammary fold. A skin island is outlined over the latissimus dorsi of dimensions adequate to replace the breast skin removed at mastectomy. The musculocutaneous flap is elevated through the skin island incision, leaving only the thoracodorsal pedicle undivided. An incision is then made at the site of the new inframammary fold, ignoring the previous mastectomy incision. Skin flaps are elevated superiorly to the clavicle, medially to the sternum, and laterally to the anterior axillary line. Care is taken not to enter the back wound at this point. A dissection is carried high in the axilla and a tunnel made into the latissimus dorsi donor wound. The muscle and its skin island are brought through this tunnel into the anterior chest. A silicone breast prosthesis of adequate size is inserted deep to the flap, and the wound is closed over suction drains (Figure 4).

Complications of this procedure in the immediate postoperative period,

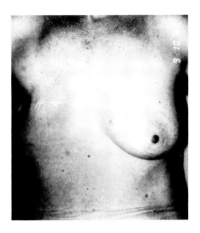

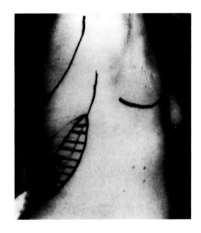

Figure 4. Latissimus dorsi musculocutaneous flap and implant for breast reconstruction. *Above,* appearance after modified radical mastectomy; *middle,* outline of skin island over latissimus dorsi muscle; *below,* postoperative appearance after breast reconstruction using latissimus dorsi musculocutaneous flap and prosthesis.

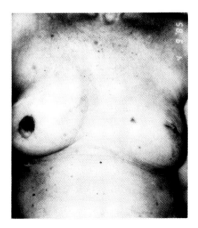

including hematoma and wound infection, are rarely seen. Transposition of the latissimus dorsi muscle causes a modest decrease in strength of the upper extremity with little functional impairment. Capsular contracture about the breast prosthesis does occur in up to 20% of patients, occasionally requiring revisional procedures.

Transverse Rectus Abdominis Musculocutaneous Flap

In an effort to avoid the complications of silicone prostheses used for breast reconstruction, other techniques have been devised using exclusively the patient's own tissues. Most popular among these techniques is the transverse rectus abdominis musculocutaneous (TRAM) flap.[8] Success of this flap is based on the observation that skin and subcutaneous tissue of the lower abdomen remain viable when left attached to one rectus abdominis muscle and its associated anterior rectus sheath. A musculocutaneous flap consisting of lower abdominal skin and one or both rectus abdominis muscles can be elevated and used for unilateral or bilateral breast reconstruction (Figure 5).

Specific features characterize the appropriate patient for breast reconstruction using the TRAM flap. The patient must not have had bilateral upper abdominal surgery with division of both superior epigastric arteries. Similarly, lower midline surgery precludes use of one half of the lower abdominal skin if the flap is based on a single rectus abdominis muscle. A very thin patient may not have enough lower abdominal skin and subcutaneous tissue to permit reconstruction. Smoking risks partial necrosis of the skin island. Recovery from this operation is more prolonged than that following prosthesis insertion and the patient must be able to curtail her activities for several weeks postoperatively.

The surgical procedure for unilateral breast reconstruction requires approximately five hours of operating time. A lower abdominal skin island is outlined preoperatively. Marks are placed on the chest at the site of the proposed inframammary fold. Transposition of the flap is facilitated by basing it on the muscle opposite the breast to be reconstructed. The abdominal skin incisions are made and the flap elevated on the appropriate rectus abdominis muscle. A chest wall incision is opened and undermining of the skin performed. The TRAM flap is passed subcutaneously into the chest wound and tailored to the shape of a breast. A portion of the flap is de-epithelialized and sutured superiorly to the pectoralis major muscle or clavicle, giving the reconstruction a more natural contour. The abdominal wall defect is repaired primarily or reinforced with plastic mesh. The skin incision is closed as in an abdominoplasty.

Postoperatively, the patient is maintained in a sitting position for several days. Infection and hematoma rarely complicate this procedure. There is some risk of partial flap necrosis, occurring in less than 5% of our patients.

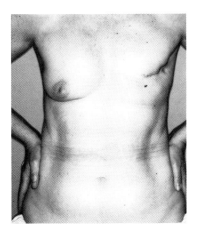

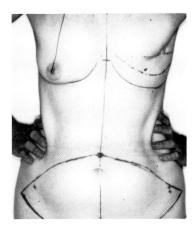

Figure 5. Transverse rectus abdominis muscu-locutaneous (TRAM) flap for breast reconstruction. *Above*, preoperative appearance after modified radical mastectomy; *middle*, skin island out-lined in lower abdomen; *below*, breast reconstructed using TRAM flap.

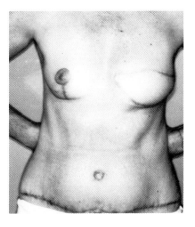

Heavy lifting is to be avoided for six weeks. Long-term structural stability of the abdominal wall closure has been questioned. It appears that fewer than 8% of patients will develop abdominal wall weakness requiring an additional operative procedure.

Immediate Reconstruction Following Mastectomy

It is possible to perform breast reconstruction at the time of total or modified radical mastectomy.[5] This avoids a second surgical procedure for reconstruction. A pocket can be developed beneath the pectoralis major muscle, serratus anterior muscle, and anterior rectus sheath.[9] An implant is placed in this closed space, preventing migration into a subcutaneous position. If the cavity is too restricted to accept an implant of adequate size, a tissue expander is inserted and later inflated to permit subsequent placement of a permanent prosthesis.

Immediate reconstruction has certain disadvantages. It does prolong the operative procedure. Many surgeons find it difficult to insert an implant of adequate size in the submuscular position and achieve satisfactory breast projection postoperatively. The patient does incur the risks of silicone implant placement, including infection and capsular contracture. Immediate reconstruction using the TRAM flap is not recommended since it is difficult to achieve a satisfactory position of the reconstructed breast postoperatively.

Nipple Reconstruction

When discussing reconstructive surgery, a patient may request information regarding reconstruction of the nipple. The reconstructed nipple, while insensate and nonfunctional, can provide an individual patient with a feeling of complete breast restoration.

Reconstruction of the nipple is delayed until the breast mound restoration is complete and postoperative swelling has diminished. A three-month interval between breast and nipple reconstruction is usually satisfactory. At the time of nipple reconstruction, small irregularities in breast contour can be corrected. For example, if a significant size discrepancy is apparent between the two breasts, an implant can be replaced with one of more appropriate size.

Nipple reconstruction requires restoration of the flat pigmented areola and the elevated papule. Selection of the proper nipple position is made on the basis of symmetry with the opposite nipple. When both nipples are absent, the surgeon must rely on standard measurements and his or her aesthetic judgment to determine the site for the new nipples. The procedure is most often performed under general anesthesia and in a single operative procedure (Figure 6). Skin from the upper medial thigh is harvested as a full thickness graft and used to recreate the areola. This skin tends to be darkly

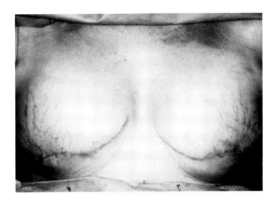

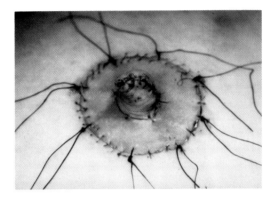

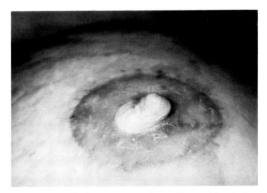

Figure 6. Nipple reconstruction. *Above*, site of nipple reconstruction has been selected; *middle*, areola graft in place and local skin being fashioned to simulate papule; *below*, appearance of reconstructed nipple three weeks postoperatively.

pigmented and retains its color well. The papule can be reconstructed by using a portion of the opposite papule. Alternatively, local skin at the site of the new nipple can be elevated at a deep dermal layer, trimmed appropriately, and used to simulate the elevated papule. This local skin remains light in color, although the shape is usually satisfactory.

SELECTING THE APPROPRIATE TECHNIQUE

After considering the options and weighing the risks, the patient must ultimately select the reconstructive technique to be employed. If she desires the procedure requiring the minimum hospital stay and shortest recovery period, she usually selects reconstruction by placement of a submuscular prosthesis. However, should she be concerned about the possibility of capsular contracture around an implant, the TRAM flap reconstruction is often chosen. In general, the patient will ask the plastic surgeon for a recommendation regarding reconstruction. Such a recommendation is made on an individual basis, taking all available information into account.

FOLLOW-UP AND RESULTS

Postoperatively, patients are seen on a weekly basis until the wound has healed. The reconstructed breast assumes a stable appearance within three months, although subtle changes occur for up to eighteen months postoperatively. Each patient is seen on a yearly basis to evaluate the reconstruction and examine the opposite breast.

Should a suspicious lesion be detected on the reconstructed side, it is treated as a potential recurrence and early biopsy is performed. In the event of local recurrence, treatment by irradiation or chemotherapy may be accomplished without removal of the prosthesis if the tumor is physically separated from the immediate site of reconstruction.

The satisfied patient is one who feels relieved from the necessity of wearing an external prosthesis, fits her clothing comfortably, and is free of discomfort in the operated breast. After reconstruction, the majority of patients share a sense of "completeness" in body image.

SUMMARY

After mastectomy for cancer of the breast, virtually every patient considers reconstruction. The majority of these are operative candidates who could benefit from evaluation and breast restoration. It is incumbent on the plastic surgeon to provide support for the patient as well as information regarding the reconstructive options and potential postoperative results. Once given this information, the patient can make an intelligent decision regarding her subsequent course.

REFERENCES

1. Bostwick J, Vasconez LO, Jurkiewicz MJ: Breast reconstruction after a radical mastectomy. Plast Reconstr Surg 61:682, 1978.
2. Bostwick J: *Aesthetic and Reconstructive Breast Surgery*. St. Louis, C. V. Mosby, 1983, pp 287–378.
3. Fisher J, Bostwick J, Powell RW: Latissimus dorsi blood supply after thoracodorsal vessel division—The serratus collateral. Plast Reconstr Surg 72:502, 1983.
4. Gargan TJ, Come SE, Satwicz PR: Breast cancer chemotherapy—Perioperative considerations in breast reconstruction. Plast Reconstr Surg 75:430, 1985.
5. Georgiade GS, Riefkohl R, Cox E, et al.: Long-term clinical outcome of immediate reconstruction after mastectomy. Plast Reconstr Surg 76:415, 1985.
6. Gilliland MD, Larson DL, Copeland EM: Appropriate timing for breast reconstruction. Plast Reconstr Surg 72:335, 1983.
7. Gruber RP, Kahn RA, Lash H, et al.: Breast reconstruction following mastectomy: A comparison of submuscular and subcutaneous techniques. Plast Reconstr Surg 67:312, 1981.
8. Hartrampf CR, Scheflan M, Black PW: Breast reconstruction with a transverse island flap. Plast Reconstr Surg 69:216, 1982.
9. Jarrett JR, Cutler RG, Teal DF: Aesthetic refinements in prophylactic subcutaneous mastectomy with submuscular reconstruction. Plast Reconstr Surg 69:624, 1982.
10. Maxwell GP: Latissimus dorsi breast reconstruction. Clin Plast Surg 8:373, 1981.
11. Radovan C: Breast reconstruction after mastectomy using the temporary expander. Plast Reconstr Surg 69:159, 1982.
12. Wellisch DK, Schain WS, Noone RB, et al.: Psychosocial correlates of immediate versus delayed reconstruction of the breast. Plast Reconstr Surg 76:713, 1985.

16. Management Dilemmas: The Contralateral Breast and the Role of Prophylactic Mastectomy

MARY K. EAST

The frequency of bilateral breast cancer and its clinical significance is of importance in the logical treatment of breast cancer and the nature of follow-up of the patient after treatment. This chapter will review the current literature regarding the incidence of bilaterality, both by clinical occurrence and by histologic study of random biopsies or autopsy specimens, the usefulness of contralateral breast biopsy at the time of treatment of a breast cancer, as well as a schedule for the follow-up of the contralateral breast.

The factors that influence a decision regarding prophylactic mastectomy will be discussed, including family history and the presence of abnormal histology on breast biopsy, including in situ carcinoma and epithelial proliferative changes of hyperplasia or atypical hyperplasia.

The types of prophylactic mastectomy will be discussed in terms of success in removing breast tissue and what is known about its effectiveness in decreasing the risk of breast cancer.

INCIDENCE OF BILATERAL BREAST CANCER

Women with cancer in one breast are at an increased risk for developing cancer in the opposite breast, generally given to be three to five times the rate of women in the general population developing their first breast cancer. In the literature, the overall frequency of the development of contralateral breast cancer varies between 1% to 14%[19] or from 3 to 10 cases per 1000 woman-years of follow-up,[5,35] a risk four to seven times the rate of women in the general population developing their first primary.[35] The figure 7% is a commonly accepted average estimate of frequency of bilateral breast cancer.

Robbins and Berg performed a prospective twenty-year study of 1458 patients and detected 94 cases of contralateral breast cancer for a frequency rate of 6.5% and an incidence of 7 cases per year per 1000 patients at risk.[35] Fisher reported on 1578 women enrolled in Protocol 04 of the National Surgical Adjuvant Breast Project (NSABP) and followed for ten years.[10] Sixty-six instances of metachronous breast cancers were encountered for an incidence of 3.7% invasive and 0.5% noninvasive cancer. Except for a peak of 1.75% in the second postoperative year, the annual incidence based on patients at risk was constant and slightly less than 1%. Leis followed 787 patients with potentially curable breast cancer for ten years or more without routine mammograms or contralateral biopsies with the development of 70 cancers (8.0%).[19]

ANALYSIS OF STUDY DIFFERENCES

The incidence of bilateral breast cancer depends on the length of follow-up and whether the cancer was detected clinically, by mammography, or by histologic studies of random biopsy, prophylactic mastectomy, or autopsy specimens. The age of the patients at the time of diagnosis of the first cancer and the duration of observation will influence the frequency, as it would be expected that a series including a larger number of young women with favorable breast cancers followed for several decades would have a higher incidence of bilateral breast cancer than a series of middle-aged and elderly women. The method of following the second breast will influence the incidence figures: Contralateral breasts followed only by physical exam will have fewer and more delayed cancers diagnosed than those followed closely by mammography, and especially those followed by contralateral breast biopsy or prophylactic mastectomy. The inclusion of carcinoma in situ, which may not become invasive during the lifetime of the patient, also leads to higher incidence figures.

One of the difficulties in assessing the incidence of bilateral breast cancer is the certainty with which a cancer arising in the contralateral breast can be determined to be a new primary cancer and not a metastasis from the first primary. Certain histologic criteria can be applied:[13] A carcinoma in the contralateral breast can be considered an independent primary if it is of distinctly different histologic type from the carcinoma of the other side; if the second lesion is distinctly of a higher degree of differentiation; if contiguous in situ carcinoma is seen with the second lesion; and if there is no clinical evidence of local or regional spread or of distant metastasis. Despite these guidelines, it may be difficult to determine whether a lesion is an independent primary or a metastasis, and this may influence the rate of bilaterality in some studies.

Synchronous vs. Metachronous

The number of synchronous bilateral breast cancers, that is, those found at the same time as the index cancer, varies with the aggressiveness of examination: Higher frequency rates are obtained with contralateral breast biopsy, particularly if in situ cancers are included. As the availability and quality of mammography has improved, there has been a trend toward an increase in the number of cancers found simultaneously in both breasts. The reported frequency of synchronous disease has varied between 0.2% and 2.0%, with an average of 0.5%.[19] As mammography has become available to guide biopsies of the contralateral breast, rates of synchronous cancer are found in the range of 2.4%[5] to 3.6%.[19] Higher rates of synchronous cancers are found by investigators who do biopsy of the contralateral breast at the time of treatment of the initial breast cancer. These biopsies are either directed at physical or mammographic abnormalities or are random biopsies of the upper outer quadrant.

Contralateral Breast Biopsy

Urban,[41] who has been a major proponent of contralateral biopsies, performed 954 biopsies in 1204 patients over a ten-year period. The amount of breast parenchyma removed was estimated to be 20% to 25% of the breast. His study detected a 12.5% incidence of simultaneous carcinoma in the contralateral breast when the original lesion was a noninfiltrating carcinoma. Of these cancers, 47% were invasive and 53% were noninvasive. Others have reanalyzed this data in terms of patients who actually had potentially curable breast cancer and found the rate of bilaterality to be 9%, of which half are invasive.[13]

Not all studies, however, have shown contralateral biopsies to be useful. Fenig[8] found cancer in 23 mirror image biopsies of the contralateral breast in 314 patients with breast cancer, for an incidence of 7%. All of these patients were subsequently shown to have benign axillary lymph nodes at the time of operation. King, et al.[17] studied 109 patients with contralateral biopsy of the upper outer quadrant and mirror image quadrant who had no clinical or mammographic evidence of suspicious lesions. Malignant disease was found in only five biopsies, of which only one was invasive cancer. They concluded that the yield was too low to recommend this approach as a routine procedure.

Some investigators are now advising a more selective policy of biopsy of the contralateral breast. Pressman[29] originally reported on random contralateral biopsies in 83 patients with ten positive for noninfiltrating in situ carcinoma (none with invasive carcinoma) for an incidence of 12%. He subsequently modified his selection criteria to eliminate all patients older than 65 years of age, all those with Stage III or Stage IV disease, and those with Stage II disease with axillary node enlargement. He reported on a series of 258 eligible patients out of a total of 610 patients.[30] Forty-three contralateral breast cancers were detected for an incidence of 16.7%. In 11 of these 43 patients, the biopsy was directed by clinical or mammographic suspicion of malignancy; all of these were infiltrating carcinomas. In 32 patients with cancer found by a contralateral biopsy obtained in a truly random fashion, four infiltrating cancers and 28 in situ cancers were detected. It should be noted that infiltrating cancer subsequently developed in five patients in whom the biopsy performed at the time of treatment was negative. Their total incidence of bilateral breast cancer was 19.7%.

The incidence of bilateral breast cancer is even higher if the material studied is the entire breast, either from a prophylactic mastectomy or from material obtained at autopsy. In a study of 84 consecutive autopsies of women with a clinical diagnosis of invasive breast cancer,[23] 33% were judged to have primary invasive lesions in the contralateral breast, 35% had in situ lesions, and 16% had metastases. Only about one-third of the invasive breast cancers had been suspected clinically. Sixty-one percent of the lesions were found to be multifocal and 65% multicentric (defined as separate foci in more than one quadrant). On review of the available histologic slides of the initial primary, 20% of lesions were found to be multicentric; 96% of these were associated with a contralateral primary cancer.

Advantages and Disadvantages of Contralateral Breast Biopsies

The obvious discrepancy between the figures of bilateral preclinical invasive or in situ carcinoma obtained by these more complete studies and the estimated 6% to 7% lifetime risk of developing a second primary may indicate that progression of premalignant changes to invasive cancer is an unpredictable event.[1,35] It is apparent that many in situ cancers never become invasive cancers of clinical significance.[10]

The decision regarding advisability of a contralateral breast biopsy at the time of treatment of the initial cancer depends on the benefits obtained versus the cost. The advantage of a random contralateral breast biopsy would be whatever increase in survival is obtained if a contralateral breast cancer could be found and treated at an earlier stage than if it was found by physical exam or mammography. This increase in survival is probably small, depending on the stage of the initial primary. The disadvantages of a contralateral breast biopsy are the large number of negative biopsies and the fact that the biopsy makes future physical examinations and mammography more difficult. Primary cancers that have lobular in situ changes is the circumstance most likely to produce a positive contralateral biopsy (20% to 33%).[41] Lesser reported that women who had lobular carcinoma in situ associated with infiltrating ductal carcinoma had a threefold increase in the likelihood of contralateral cancer being found on contralateral biopsy, most of which was lobular carcinoma in situ.[21]

Based upon the data presented in the above reports, as well as our own experience, we do not routinely perform a biopsy of the contralateral breast if there are no clinically evident abnormalities on physical examination or mammogram. In contrast, if the lesion appears to be lobular carcinoma in situ, biopsy of the upper outer quadrant, even in the absence of a clinically apparent lesion, usually is done.

Technique

If a contralateral breast biopsy is to be done, it is recommended that the biopsy be performed in the upper outer quadrant, as that is the most frequent site of cancer regardless of the site in the initial breast. In situ disease occurs most frequently in the subareolar area, and the biopsy should include some of this area. Fracchia[13] recommends the biopsy be performed through a circumareolar incision placed in the upper outer quadrant. Two triangular-shaped wedges of breast tissue are removed in a diamond-shaped manner. One apex of the excised wedge of tissue extends toward the axillary tail and the other points toward the subareolar area.

FACTORS INFLUENCING THE DEVELOPMENT OF CONTRALATERAL BREAST CANCER

Not all studies agree on the significance of risk factors in the development of contralateral breast cancer. Factors that have been found to increase the risk of bilateral breast cancer are premenopausal status; a family history of breast cancer, although some studies do not support this hypothesis; and characteristics of the first cancer, such as size, degree of anaplasia, location and clinical stage, multicentricity, and histologic type.

Lobular carcinoma, and particularly lobular carcinoma in situ (LCIS), is known to have a particularly high incidence of bilaterality, with an incidence of simultaneous breast cancer of 23%[24] to 33%[41] on contralateral breast biopsy. A statistically significant association has been seen with a tubular histologic type.[10]

Age as a Factor

Some studies have shown a definite correlation between age at first primary and risk of developing a second breast cancer. Robbins and Berg[35] reported that women in their series who developed clinically apparent cancer before the age of 50 years had almost twice the risk of a second tumor per year of exposure as women entering their series after the age of 60 years.

Chaudary[5] showed that the risk of developing a second cancer in women younger than 40 years was three times that observed in women who developed their first breast cancer after the age of 40. Adami[1] found a marked age-dependent trend in risk, with a pronounced decline at about the age of 50. He calculated cumulative risk figures for the development of a contralateral cancer of 13.3% for women younger than 50 years and 3.5% for women older than 50 years at time of first diagnosis.

Family History

There has also been a correlation proposed between development of second primaries and family history. A study by Anderson[4] of 699 sisters of patients with breast cancer indicated that patients with a family history of breast cancer developed both the first and second primaries at a younger age. Women with a family history of breast cancer whose first primary developed while premenopausal had a probability of developing a second by their twentieth postoperative year of 35% to 38%. With postmenopausal diagnosis, the probabilities ranged from 11% with a second-degree relative to 26% for women with mothers having breast cancer. Fisher, in his study of bilateral breast cancer, however, noted only a slight correlation with family history (in the range of 1.5% to 2.1%).[1]

Multicentricity

The concept of multicentricity is similar to that of bilateral breast cancer, as it implies that conditions influencing the development of malignancy are present throughout both breasts. Multicentricity is usually defined as foci of in situ or invasive carcinoma found in the same breast but in different quadrants than that involved by the clinically dominant invasive carcinoma, although some studies have used a separation by a certain distance, usually at least 5 cm, and other studies require only the presence of normal ducts separating tumor sites. This lack of uniformity in definition, variation in specimen preparation technique, and methods of study have produced a range of multicentric breast cancer from 12% to 75%.

The problem of the multicentricity of breast cancer gained practical importance when limited extent of excision was proposed. Rosen[32] determined the incidence of multifocal cancer remaining in 203 breasts removed by mastectomy after simulated quadrantectomy for invasive breast cancer; two or three sections for microscopic study were obtained from each of the remaining quadrants. Noninvasive cancer was found in 12% of breasts and invasive cancer in 20% of breasts, with higher rates of invasive cancer found with larger primaries (greater than 2 cm). Patients with primary carcinomas in the subareolar part of the breast had a higher incidence of additional carcinoma (eight of ten patients).

Fisher[11] found multicentric foci of invasive and in situ carcinomas in two and three quadrants in 11.6% and 5.8% of cases (although a limited number of tissue blocks were examined from each specimen); he noted a significant correlation of multicentricity with large tumor size, invasion of the nipple, and lobular infiltrating carcinoma. Fisher[11] points out that despite the frequent finding of multicentricity on histologic studies, the occurrence of two clinical cancers in the same breast is very rare, estimated to be 0.1%.

In an interesting study, Egan[7] correlated poor survival from apparently limited breast cancer to the frequency of multicentricity. He reported on a study of 118 breasts removed for unilateral breast cancer. Eight percent were Stage 0, 52% were Stage I, and 40% were Stage II. The breasts were frozen and sliced in serial sections, and detailed radiographs of each section were used to select areas for microscopic examination. This detailed examination took five years and required a separate histopathology laboratory and a full-time pathologist and two technologists. Distinct multiple sites of carcinoma were found in 60% of breasts. Most of the cancer was invasive; intraductal cancer was found in only four breasts and lobular carcinoma in situ in three breasts. All patients were followed for at least ten years. Those patients with a breast with a single site of a single histologic type had the lowest mortality with a 78% ten-year survival rate. Those with breasts with single site of multiple histologic types had a 50% ten-year survival, and those with multiple sites of multiple types had a 47% ten-year survival.

Holland and associates[15] studied breasts in terms of those qualifying for published randomized studies of breast-conserving surgery and radiation therapy, excluding known multifocal tumors on clinical or mammographic exam as well as those labeled diffuse invasive cancers, which were mainly lobular invasive carcinomas consisting of numerous tumor foci distributed fairly evenly in a large area. They found that if tumors less than 4 cm in size were removed with a 2-cm margin, 14% of the breasts would have residual invasive cancer and 28% noninvasive cancer. Tumors removed with a 4-cm margin (roughly equal to a quadrantectomy) would have an incidence of 5% invasive and 5% noninvasive cancer in the remaining breast.

It is of interest to see what the recurrence rate is of breast cancer treated by local excision either with or without postoperative radiation. The five-year results of the NSABP B-06 trial[9] showed a recurrence rate of 28% in cancers treated by segmental mastectomy alone compared with 8% in those treated with postoperative radiation. Thus, radiation apparently eradicated the residual tumor foci or delayed their growth in 20% of these patients. Recurrences were almost all within the same region of breast as the primary excision; survival appeared unrelated to local recurrence. It is still uncertain whether radiation therapy is an effective treatment for noninvasive cancer; the additional recurrences seen in the next five to ten years of follow-up may be attributable to delayed growth but not eradication of intraductal cancer.

The relation of multicentricity to the development of contralateral breast cancer was analyzed by Lesser, et al.[21] Their study found that women with bilateral cancer were more likely than those with unilateral cancer to have multicentric lesions. Approximately one-third of women with multicentric lesions in the mastectomy specimen of the initial cancer developed contralateral carcinoma. Tulusan[40] reported that 45% of patients with multicentric ductal cancer in the ipsilateral breast had the occurrence of contralateral breast cancer, of which one-third was invasive. Only 15% of patients without multicentricity had bilateral disease.

INFLUENCE OF THE CONTRALATERAL BREAST CANCER ON SURVIVAL

There are conflicting reports regarding the prognostic significance of the occurrence of contralateral breast cancer. Some investigators have found a contralateral breast cancer to have an adverse influence; others report the prognosis to be unaffected or even improved.

Robbins and Berg[35] analyzed survival among matched patients in whom second breast cancers did or did not develop. They concluded that the development of a second breast cancer almost halved the survival in a group of patients relative to their matched controls who had only a single breast cancer, although their study was done before mammography was available to monitor the second breast. A recent study from Memorial Sloan-Kettering Cancer Center reported the five-year and ten-year relapse-free survival rate of patients with bilateral invasive disease presenting metachronously to be less than those with unilateral disease (60% and 51% for unilateral disease compared to 54% and 38% for bilateral disease).[13]

Senofsky[39] reported that second breast cancers detected in the period 1977 through 1984 showed a considerable improvement in stage compared with those in years 1969 through 1975. The recent group showed 33% Stage 0, 22% Stage I, 30% Stage II, 4% Stage III, and 4% Stage IV. There was also earlier detection of the second breast cancer: 1.5 years in the more recent group and 4.75 years in the earlier group. This finding of earlier cancers in the contralateral breast contrasts to the findings of NSABP Protocol 04.[10] Despite close follow-up, second cancers measured only one centimeter less than the first, averaging 2.4 cm; no significant difference in pathologic nodal status was noted between the first and second cancers or that of patients with unilateral disease. No difference in survival rate, however, was seen between those who developed a second cancer and those with unilateral disease. A study of patients with bilateral breast cancer at the M.D. Anderson Hospital revealed no significant difference in the disease-free, 20-year survival rate between patients with unilateral tumors and those with bilateral simultaneous or consecutive tumors.[37]

Other studies report improved survival. A study from the University of Iowa of 104 bilateral invasive breast cancers compared survival in those with synchronous lesions (26 patients) and those with metachronous lesions (78 patients).[2] The five-year and ten-year survival in those with synchronous lesions was 39% and 20% compared to 92% and 74% in those with metachronous lesions.

RECOMMENDATIONS FOR FOLLOW-UP

It is clear from the above data that there is a significant risk of breast cancer occurring in the contralateral breast. The risk is further increased by several factors, primarily premenopausal status and a strong family history. It is also important to consider the stage of the breast cancer and expected survival, since the value of a prophylactic mastectomy is less if the patient dies from the initial cancer before the cancer in the contralateral breast becomes clinically significant. Another factor to be considered is the probability of detecting the second cancer and treating it at a time at which cure can be attained; this may be influenced by the patient's facility with self-examination technique and whether her breasts are clinically and mammographically easy to study. In any individual patient, it may be difficult to assess each of these factors. In general, prophylactic mastectomy of the contralateral breast should be reserved for premenopausal women with Stage I breast cancer with a strong family history of breast cancer, particularly if she is unreliable in her follow-up or in the technique of breast self-examination, and if anxiety about cancer is significant.

We believe that the majority of women can be observed with cautious and careful follow-up, including efforts to ascertain that adequate breast self-examination is performed each month, with biannual examination by a physician, at least initially, and annual mammography. The woman's abilities at self-examination, her reliability in complying with recommendations, and her emotional response influence the adequacy of a policy of careful follow-up.

CONSIDERATIONS FOR PROPHYLACTIC MASTECTOMY IN WOMEN WITHOUT INVASIVE CARCINOMA

The question of prophylactic mastectomy is also commonly raised with women who do not have known invasive breast cancer but who do have other risk factors. The physician needs to be informed about the importance of various risk factors to estimate for the patient her risk of developing cancer. The determination of risk is often an educated guess rather than established scientific fact. The etiology of breast cancer is complex, representing a poorly understood interplay of reproductive, hormonal, genetic, and environmental factors.

Risk Factors for Development of Breast Cancer

Risk factors for the development of breast cancer have been analyzed by the American Cancer Society in a large-scale prospective study begun in 1959.[38] Their analysis of risk factors in 578,000 women found that most are relatively modest and that these risk factors could account for only approximately a quarter of the breast cancers. A family history of breast cancer and a history of previous breast biopsy were found to be the most important risk factors (relative risk in the 2 to 3 range). Less important risk factors were: no live birth by age 30, menopause after age 50, and menarche before age 12, with a relative risk of 1 to 2 compared with women with no risk factors. It is important to note that known risk factors could account for only 21% of breast cancer risk among women aged 30 to 54 and 29% among women aged 55 to 84. The conclusion of this study was that three-fourths of all breast cancer cannot be attributed to known specific causes.

Correlation of Risk with Family History

A review of the increase in risk of development of breast cancer in a woman with a history of breast cancer in close relatives is given in Chapter 6, Epidemiology of Breast Cancer. The highest risk appears to be present in those women with both mother and sister with breast cancer,[36] especially if the relative had bilateral breast cancer,[4] and especially if the disease had occurred premenopausally.[3,25]

Correlation of Risk with "Fibrocystic Disease"

The relationship between fibrocystic changes and cancer has been a matter of controversy. Fibrocystic changes include adenosis, fibrosis, cystic lobular ducts, and intraductal epithelial proliferation. Only the latter has been shown to be a significant risk factor for subsequent development of carcinoma. Several older prospective studies reached the conclusion that the incidence of breast cancer in patients who had such a diagnosis was between 2.5 and 5 times the expected incidence. However, subdividing the histology of the fibrocystic pattern according to the degree and character of epithelial proliferation has brought progress in the prognostic evaluation. A significant increase in the risk for malignancy is found to be present only in cases of abnormal and atypical epithelial proliferation. Only certain of the proliferative alterations predispose to development of cancer: significant increase in the incidence rate was found in ductal hyperplasia (1.8) and atypical epithelial hyperplasia (4.2). These account for approximately 26% and 4%

of the biopsy specimens of fibrocystic disease.[6] Combining age and a family history of breast cancer with the histologic characteristics of the biopsy specimen yields even more meaningful information. Women over 55 who have proliferative lesions have a risk of 2.2 times the general population. Women at highest risk are those with atypical lesions and a positive family history; their risk is 11 times that of women with no proliferative lesions and no familial incidence.[6] The absolute risk for cancer in women with atypical hyperplasia and a family history of breast cancer (mother, sister, or daughter) is 20% during 15 years of follow-up compared with 8% for women with proliferative disease lacking atypia.[6]

Page and co-workers[27] recently published a long-term follow-up study on a consecutive series of women with atypical hyperplastic lesions. Of a total of 10,542 biopsy specimens in their study, 377 atypical lesions were identified (3.6%). Of these, two-thirds were atypical ductal hyperplasia (ADH) and one-third were atypical lobular hyperplasia (ALH). Eighteen of the 150 women with atypical ductal hyperplasia developed breast cancer during the follow-up period, which averaged 17.5 years. Ten of the cancers were on the same side as the ADH; eight were on the contralateral side. The interval until development of invasive carcinoma averaged 8.2 years. Sixteen of the 126 women with ALH developed invasive breast cancer at an average of 12 years after the original diagnosis. Eight of the cancers were of invasive ductal type; two were invasive lobular; one was atypical medullary; one was mixed; and three were predominantly in situ cancers. Ten of the cancers were ipsilateral to the biopsy; three were contralateral, and two were bilateral. This study tabulated risk for ADH and ALH with and without family history. The risk of invasive cancer with ALH or ADH is approximately four times that of the general population; the addition of positive family history doubles the level of risk over that of ALH or ADH alone.

Carcinoma in Situ

The level of risk with atypical hyperplastic lesions is approximately one-half that found in LCIS or DCIS, as reported in a previous series by the same co-workers.[26] On review of biopsy specimens initially thought to be benign, a total of 28 cases of DCIS were found that were treated with biopsy only. Seven of these women subsequently developed invasive breast cancer within three to ten years after biopsy. All seven invasive cancers developed in the same breast and six in the same quadrant. In contrast, 18 of these women remained free of neoplasm over a mean follow-up interval of 16 years, thereby reflecting the lack of predictability of this finding.

In a similar study published by Rosen,[34] 10,000 consecutive breast biopsies were reviewed with the finding of 99 patients with LCIS and 30 with DCIS, treated only with biopsy. Of the 15 patients with DCIS available for follow-up, 10 developed recurrent carcinoma in the same breast as the initial lesion, with a mean follow-up interval of 9.7 years; there were no contralateral carcinomas in this series or in the study of Page.

Lobular Carcinoma in Situ

LCIS is regarded more as a marker for the risk of development of invasive cancer rather than as a precursor lesion per se. Approximately 30% of women with LCIS on biopsy will develop invasive cancer, which may take 20 to 25 years to develop. Consideration of the treatment choices for LCIS must also take into consideration the incidence of multicentricity and invasive cancer associated with this lesion. One analysis[33] of mastectomy specimens of breasts removed for LCIS revealed infiltrating cancer in 2 of 59 breasts (4%), a rate consistent with other studies of LCIS. Residual LCIS was found in 30 patients, 24 of whom had the lesion in quadrants other than the biopsy site, showing the multicentric nature of the lesion. The treatment options for LCIS are three: close observation after biopsy, watching for the development of abnormalities in either breast; total mastectomy on the basis of the 4% incidence of invasive cancer found in mastectomy specimens with LCIS; and bilateral mastectomies on the basis of the risk present in both breasts. Consideration of risk factors, extent of LCIS, age, and the late occurrence of carcinoma influence the decision. Our choice has been that of careful observation, with frequent physical examinations by the patient and physician, and annual mammography in an attempt to detect the development of invasive cancer at an early stage and thereby spare mastectomy in the majority of women who would not develop invasive cancer.

Intraductal Carcinoma

In contrast to LCIS, DCIS is more widely regarded as a precursor lesion because of the high risk for the development of invasive cancer of ductal type in the ipsilateral breast in a shorter time than that of LCIS. Decisions regarding the treatment of DCIS are based on this premise, as well as the incidence of multicentricity and residual invasive cancer found in breasts removed for DCIS. Rosen found residual DCIS in 30 of 50 breasts removed for DCIS on biopsy.[33] In 20 of these, the residual DCIS was limited to the biopsy site and in 10 extended to other quadrants. Residual infiltrating carcinoma was found in 6% of breasts removed because of DCIS on biopsy. Lagios[18] also studied breasts removed for DCIS. He studied 53 breasts extensively with combined mammographic and serial subgross histologic examination, and found multicentricity in 14% of patients with tumors 2.5 cm or less, as compared to 46% in patients presenting with tumors greater than 2.6 cm. He reported occult invasive cancer in 21%, almost all occurring in larger lesions; there was no instance of occult invasion in lesions less than 2.5 cm.

The treatment options for DCIS include wide local excision with and without irradiation, and mastectomy with or without axillary node dissection. The choice among these alternatives ideally should be based on the natural history of DCIS, but most of the data on DCIS is derived from retrospective pathologic analyses and not prospective studies. There have been few prospective studies published of DCIS treated with lumpectomy alone or with irradiation.

Between 1955 and 1979, 34 patients at the M.D. Anderson Hospital with intraductal carcinoma were treated with local excision and radiation therapy. With a follow-up time of 3 to 17 years, there has been only one recurrence, which was in the axilla only.[22] Recht reported on 40 women with intraductal carcinoma treated with excisional biopsy and irradiation with a median follow-up of 44 months.[31] Four patients had a recurrence for a recurrence rate of 10%. In two cases, the recurrence consisted of only intraductal carcinoma; in the other two, both intraductal and invasive cancer were found. Two of the recurrences were in the site of the primary or area of boost and two were considered as occurring at the edge of the boost. Three of the recurrences occurred in four patients who presented with a nipple discharge and a central primary.

Recently, Fisher has published the results of treatment of 78 cases of DCIS identified after pathologic review of 2072 specimens obtained from the NSABP Protocol 06.[12] This compared total mastectomy to lumpectomy with and without irradiation, with all patients subjected to axillary lymph node dissection. Recurrence occurred in 5 of 22 women (23%) with DCIS treated with lumpectomy alone and 2 of 29 (7%) treated with lumpectomy and irradiation. All exhibited recurrence in the immediate vicinity of the initial cancer. This study concluded that local treatment of DCIS be further studied, and a randomized clinical trial of patients with DCIS has been started by the NSABP.

The necessity for axillary lymph node dissection in patients treated for DCIS is controversial. The rate of lymph node involvement is 1% to 2%;[34] the detection of these patients would allow their treatment by adjuvant chemotherapy. Proponents for axillary dissection also state that dissection of level I of the axillary contents ensures complete removal of the axillary extension of the breast, if a mastectomy is done. Others point up that the number of women actually benefiting from axillary dissection is small. It has been our practice to perform axillary dissection with DCIS. We are currently analyzing the incidence of axillary nodal metastases with DCIS and may move toward a policy of not performing axillary dissections in patients treated with lumpectomy.

ADVICE REGARDING PROPHYLACTIC MASTECTOMY

The question of prophylactic mastectomy is most pertinent for women with combinations of family history of breast cancer and biopsy-proved changes of epithelial hyperplasia, atypical hyperplasia, or LCIS. For any individual woman, the decision is strongly influenced by her desire for breast conservation as opposed to her anxiety about the development of cancer. Other considerations are the ease of physical examination of the breast, which is decreased secondary to scarring in women with multiple biopsies or women with very lumpy breasts. Those women with dense breasts on mammography are also at a disadvantage. There are no clear-cut recommendations, except for the extremes. Women with a sister or mother with bilateral, premenopausal cancer who have had a breast mass biopsy that showed the development of hyperplastic epithelium would be advised to consider bilateral prophylactic mastectomies. Conversely, prophylactic mastectomies in the woman without family history and without worrisome pathological changes on biopsy, who may desire mastectomies to avoid the risk of cancer or development of future breast masses should be discouraged. For the many women in between these two extremes, an intelligent estimate of risk for her particular combination of risk factors combined with her emotional response will be the factors involved in the decision; in most situations, the risk is bilateral and bilateral mastectomies will be required.

In those women who choose prophylactic mastectomies, the next decision is between the types of mastectomies. The most conservative choice is total mastectomy, which removes all breast tissue, and which can then be followed by reconstructive techniques as described in Chapter 15. Another choice is subcutaneous mastectomy, which has been proposed as a means of substantially reducing the risk of breast cancer with the potential of retaining fairly normal appearance of the breast. The majority of experience has been obtained in the past 15 years. The technique, which has been described in Chapter 15, involves the removal of most of the breast parenchyma, usually by an inframammary approach, with the preservation of the nipple and areola. The controversial nature of subcutaneous mastectomy arises in the amount and significance of breast parenchyma left under the nipple-areola complex, which is necessary to prevent sloughing, and at the far ends of the dissection, particularly the infraclavicular area and the tail of Spence toward the axilla, which may be difficult to reach from an inframammary incision. Goldman and Goldwyn demonstrated in cadavers and in living women that 10% to 15% of breast tissue remains with the completion of a meticulous subcutaneous mastectomy.[14]

The rate of complications and patient satisfaction also weigh in the decision regarding the usefulness of subcutaneous mastectomy. One of the chief problems has been a high incidence of capsule formation around the prosthesis, which has been considerably lessened by the placement of the prosthesis submuscularly rather than subcutaneously. Woods and Verheyden of the Mayo Clinic reported a capsule formation rate of less than 5% when the prosthesis was placed submuscularly.[43] Other considerations are the occasional unsatisfactory aesthetic result found with breasts which have moderate to severe ptosis. A concomitant mastopexy may be needed to achieve a successful result.

The success of subcutaneous mastectomy in preventing the occurrence of breast cancer is difficult to analyze because of the relatively small series reported and the short follow-up available. Another difficulty in analyzing the data is the difference in the extent of the mastectomy and the meticulousness of breast tissue removal, depending on the surgeon. Perhaps the most important factor in analyzing the results, however, is outlined by Humphrey[16] in his discussion of Pennisi's report from the Subcutaneous Mastectomy Data Evaluation Center.[28] Pennisi reported on the results of 1244 patients with an average follow-up of seven years. Six patients had developed cancer (an incidence of 0.5%), although in two patients the cancer arose in the axillary nodes within one year of the procedure and probably represented unrecognized invasive cancer removed by the subcutaneous mastectomy. Humphrey, in his invited comments on these results, points out that this low rate of cancer can be judged only in terms of the indications that prompted the procedure and the fact that most of these women were in the age range of 30 to 50 years and were unlikely to develop cancer during the time period of observation anyway, and that much longer follow-up will be needed to prove the effectiveness of the procedure.

Perhaps the largest series in one institution is that of the Mayo Clinic. Although they have not fully reported their conclusions, they have seen the development of invasive cancer in 2 patients among the first 600 patients who have been followed for three or more years. They note that another ten years may be necessary to accumulate sufficient data to prove the success of the procedure.[42]

Until more complete follow-up data is available, it remains our choice to advise women contemplating prophylactic mastectomies to undergo total mastectomies as the best available assurance against the development of breast cancer.

SUMMARY

Breast cancer is a concern for all women, for 1 of every 11 women in the United States will develop the disease and approximately one-third to one-half of these women will die within ten years of discovery. Better diagnostic procedures and enhanced patient awareness may lead to an earlier diagnosis and, it is hoped, improved survival; however, prevention of the cancer would be desirable, but at this time it can only be achieved through total removal of the breasts. Unfortunately, over three-fourths of the breast cancers occur in women for whom no risk factor is identified. This chapter has reviewed the published literature on the three major risk factors that can be identified: history of cancer in the opposite breast, family history of breast cancer, and biopsy-proved changes of the breast extending along a spectrum toward invasive carcinoma. Reports in the literature of the risk of cancer may be very different, even with the same risk factor, highlighting the difficulty in studying large groups as well as the difficulty in defining the significance of in situ cancer, and even the difficulty in deciding what is atypical hyperplasia, in situ cancer, and invasive cancer. Even more difficult has been deciding how these risk factors combine in any individual to make an intelligent estimate of her risk.

Coloring all of these estimates of risk is the individual woman's unique perception of the importance of her breasts as opposed to her anxiety about the development of breast masses and cancer. For the clinician caring for this patient, these factors must be respected and allowed to influence the decision. Firm guidelines in this area are not possible; the most that can be done is to present the patient with the best estimate of her risk and help her to make the decision within her personal framework.

REFERENCES

1. Adami HO, Bergstrom R, Hansen J: Age at first primary as a determinant of the incidence of bilateral breast cancer. Cancer 55:643–647, 1985.
2. Al-Jurf AS, Jochimsen PR, Urdaneta LF, et al.: Factors influencing survival in bilateral breast cancer. J Surg Oncol 16:343–348, 1981.
3. Anderson DE: Genetic study of breast cancer: Identification of a high risk group. Cancer 34:1090–1097, 1974.
4. Anderson DE, Badzioch MD: Risk of familial breast cancer. Cancer 56:383–387, 1985.
5. Chaudary MA, Millis RR, Hoskins EO, et al.: Bilateral primary breast cancer: A prospective study of disease incidence. Br J Surg 71:711–714, 1984.
6. Dupont WD, Page DL: Risk factors for breast cancer in women with proliferative breast disease. N Engl J Med 312:146–151, 1985.
7. Egan RL: Multicentric breast carcinomas: Clinical-radiographic pathologic whole organ studies and 10-year survival. Cancer 49:1123–1130, 1982.
8. Fenig J: The potential for carcinoma existing synchronously on a microscopic level within the second breast. Surg Gynecol Obstet 141:394–396, 1975.
9. Fisher B, Bauer M, Margolese R, et al.: Five-year results of a randomized clinical trial comparing total mastectomy and segmental mastectomy with or without radiation in the treatment of breast cancer. N Engl J Med 312:665–673, 1985.
10. Fisher ER, Fisher B, Sass R, et al.: Pathologic findings from the National Surgical Adjuvant Breast Project (Protocol No. 4) XI. Bilateral breast cancer. Cancer 54:3002–3011, 1984.

11. Fisher ER, Gregorio RM, Fisher B: The pathology of invasive breast cancer: A syllabus derived from the findings of the National Surgical Adjuvant Breast Project (Protocol No. 4). Cancer 36:1–85, 1975.
12. Fisher ER, Sass R, Fisher B, et al.: Pathologic findings from the National Surgical Adjuvant Breast Project (Protocol No. 6) I. Intraductal carcinoma. Cancer 547:197–208, 1986.
13. Fracchia AA, Robinson D, Legaspi A, et al.: Survival in bilateral breast cancer. Cancer 55:1414–1421, 1985.
14. Goldman LD, Goldwyn RM: Some anatomical considerations of subcutaneous mastectomy. Plast Reconstr Surg 51:501–505, 1973.
15. Holland R, Veling SH, Mravunac M, et al.: Histologic multifocality of Tis, T1-2 breast carcinomas. Cancer 56:979–990, 1985.
16. Humphrey LJ: Invited comment. Subcutaneous mastectomy: An interim report on 1244 patients. Ann Plast Surg 12:245–347, 1984.
17. King RE, Terz JJ, Lawrence W: Experience with opposite breast biopsy in patients with operable breast cancer. Cancer 37:43–45, 1976.
18. Lagios MD, Westdahl PR, Margolin FR, et al.: Duct carcinoma in situ: Relationship of extent of noninvasive disease to the frequency of occult invasion, multicentricity, lymph node metastases, and short-term failures. Cancer 50:1309–1314, 1982.
19. Leis HP: Managing the remaining breast. Cancer 46:1026–1030, 1980.
20. Leis HP, Cammarato A, LaRaja R, et al.: Bilateral breast cancer. Breast 7:13–17, 1981.
21. Lesser ML, Rosen PR, Kinne DW: Multicentricity and bilaterality in invasive breast carcinoma. Surgery 91:234–240, 1982.
22. Montague ED: Conservation surgery and radiation therapy in the treatment of operable breast cancer. Cancer 53:700–704, 1984.
23. Nielsen M, Christensen L, Andersen J: Contralateral cancerous breast lesions in women with clinical invasive breast carcinoma. Cancer 57:897–903, 1986.
24. Newman W: In situ lobular carcinoma of the breast: Report of 26 women with 32 cancers. Ann Surg 157:591–599, 1963.
25. Ottman R, King M, Pike MC, et al.: Practical guide for estimating risk for familial breast cancer. Lancet 2:556–558, 1983.
26. Page DL, Dupont WD, Rogers LW, et al.: Intraductal carcinoma of the breast: Follow-up after biopsy only. Cancer 49:751–758, 1982.
27. Page DL, Dupont DW, Rogers LW, et al.: Atypical hyperplastic lesions of the female breast: A long-term follow-up study. Cancer 55:2698–2708, 1985.
28. Pennisi VR, Capozzi A: Subcutaneous mastectomy: An interim report on 1244 patients. Ann Plast Surg 12:340–345, 1984.
29. Pressman PI: Bilateral breast cancer: The contralateral biopsy. Breast 5:29–33, 1980.
30. Pressman PI: Selective biopsy of the opposite breast. Cancer 57:577–580, 1986.
31. Recht A, Danoff BS, Solin LJ, et al.: Intraductal carcinoma of the breast: Results of treatment with excisional biopsy and irradiation. J Clin Oncol 3:1330–1343, 1985.

32. Rosen PR, Fracchia AA, Urban JA, et al.: "Residual" mammary carcinoma following simulated partial mastectomy. Cancer 35:739-747, 1975.
33. Rosen PR, Senie R, Schottenfeld D, et al.: Noninvasive breast carcinoma: Frequency of unsuspected invasion and implications for treatment. Ann Surg 189:377-382, 1979.
34. Rosen PR, Braun DW, Kinne DE: The clinical significance of preinvasive breast carcinoma. Cancer 46:919-925, 1980.
35. Robbins GF, Berg JW: Bilateral primary breast cancers: A prospective clinicopathologic study. Cancer 17:1501-1527, 1964.
36. Sattin RW, Rubin GL, Webster LA, et al.: Family history and the risk of breast cancer. JAMA 2353:1908-1913, 1985.
37. Schell SR, Montague ED, Spanos WJ, et al.: Bilateral breast cancer in patients with initial stage I and II disease. Cancer 50:1191-1194, 1982.
38. Seidman H, Stellman SD, Mushinski MH: A different perspective on breast cancer risk factors: Some implications of the nonattributable risk. CA 32:301-314, 1982.
39. Senofsky GM, Wanebo HJ, Wilhelm MC, et al.: Has monitoring of the contralateral breast improved the prognosis in patients treated for primary breast cancer? Cancer 57:597-602, 1986.
40. Tulusan AH, Ronay G, Egger H, et al.: A contribution to the natural history of breast cancer. V. Bilateral primary breast cancer: Incidence, risks and diagnosis of simultaneous primary cancer in the opposite breast. Arch Gynecol 237:85-91, 1985.
41. Urban JA, Papachristou D, Taylor J: Bilateral breast cancer: Biopsy of the opposite breast. Cancer 49:1968-1973, 1977.
42. Woods JE, Arnold PG, Fisher J, et al.: Subcutaneous mastectomy in the treatment of breast disease. Am J Surg 146:683-684, 1983.
43. Woods JE, Verheyden CN: Pitfalls and problems with subcutaneous mastectomy. Mayo Clin Proc 55:687-693, 1980.

17. Dilemmas in Breast Cancer: Occult Carcinoma and Paget's Disease of the Breast

MICHAEL K. MCLEOD

There are several unusual dilemmas in the management of breast cancer that any clinician or health care professional involved in the care of patients with breast carcinoma is apt to encounter. Many of these "special" situations are addressed elsewhere in this book. In this chapter the problematic issue of occult breast carcinoma will be discussed. In considering the predicament of occult breast carcinoma, five clinical situations will be similarly reviewed and discussed: management of breast carcinoma presenting as axillary nodal metastases in the absence of a clinically evident primary; carcinoma in the patient who presents with an incidental, serous nipple discharge in the absence of a palpable breast mass; carcinoma occurring in a benign fibroadenoma; hemorrhage into the breast resulting from trauma obscuring underlying carcinoma; and finally, Paget's disease of the breast.

The fundamental goal in each of these discussions is to make general recommendations based on a review of the literature that may be helpful and relevant to any clinician who is interested in the care of patients with diseases of the breast.

OCCULT CARCINOMA

Adenocarcinoma of the Breast Presenting as Axillary Adenopathy

The underlying cause of axillary adenopathy is nonspecific or inflammatory in roughly 70% of cases, based on data from a series by Pierce et al.[50] The most common malignancy found in axillary nodes submitted for pathologic evaluation was lymphoma in 13.9%. The next most common malignancy diagnosed was Broders' grade 4 adenocarcinoma in 6.9%. Three out of five such metastatic adenocarcinomas were demonstrated to be from the ipsilateral breast. In the remaining two lesions the source was unknown, but presumed to be from the breast. Melanoma was diagnosed in 1.4% of these axillary nodes, as was squamous cell carcinoma of the lung (also 1.4% of the cases).

In addition to melanoma and squamous cell carcinoma of the lung, other primary sites of origin to be considered when axillary nodal metastases are shown to contain metastatic adenocarcinoma are thyroid, renal cell, stomach, pancreas, colon, and ovary. Axillary nodal metastases have also been found to arise from primary liver cancer.[9,15]

Although adenocarcinoma of the breast is clearly the most common primary source for adenocarcinoma metastatic to an axillary node, these other sources must be looked for and ruled out. Past medical history and a careful review of systems are critical in this regard, in that a disappearing primary malignant melanoma,[8] as well as a squamous cell lesion arising from the head and neck area may be easily missed if pertinent, previous signs and symptoms are not elicited. Furthermore, it has been recommended that the measurement of estrogen receptor protein in the axillary node or mass in question may also be helpful in making a diagnosis.[23] This remains true despite the fact that estrogen receptor protein has been measured in several ovarian cancers, endometrial tumors, renal carcinomas, and to a smaller extent, in some adenocarcinomas of the colon. It should also be noted that there are benign lesions in axillary nodal tissue that may simulate metastatic breast carcinoma. These include heterotopic glands, endometriosis, and nevus cell aggregates.[57]

Halsted was the first to describe axillary nodal metastases preceding clinically apparent breast cancer in three patients.[25] Following Halsted's report in 1907, there have been over 200 cases reported of breast carcinoma presenting initially as a mass in the axilla.* The overall incidence of breast adenocarcinoma presenting as axillary nodal metastases in the absence of a palpable breast tumor is reported to be 0.3% to 0.9%, or less than 1%.[12,16,24,37,57,67] The rarity of this clinical situation is summarized in Table 1.

Table 1. Incidence of Axillary Nodal Metastases Heralding a Clinically Occult Adenocarcinoma of the Breast

Author	Year	Incidence	Percentage
Davidoff[12]	1954	6/800	0.75%
Owen[45]	1954	25/5451	0.46
Fitts[16]	1963	11/1300	0.85
Vilcoq[67]	1982	11/1250	0.80
Haagensen[24]	1986	28/8000	0.35
Total		81/16801	0.48%

*2,5,8–10,12,14–16,21,23–25,29,30,34,37,41,45,49,51–53,57,63,67–70

Workup for Extramammary Source of Axillary Adenopathy

The question of how extensive a workup should be and what studies it should include in order to satisfactorily rule out an extramammary source for axillary nodal metastases is pertinent and perhaps controversial. Feuerman et al.[15] addressed this question in a reported series of 21 patients who presented with carcinoma in axillary lymph nodes as the first manifestation of their cancer. Ten of these patients ultimately underwent mastectomy, and seven of these ten, or one-third of the entire group, had pathologic documentation of a primary breast carcinoma. These investigators concluded from their experience that once an extramammary carcinoma reached the axillary lymph nodes, it was very late in its clinical course. Usually by the time axillary nodal metastasis was evident, there were unequivocal signs and symptoms pointing to the extramammary primary. They recommended that a workup should consist of a careful history and physical examination, sigmoidoscopy, chest X-ray, gastrointestinal series, and intravenous pyelogram. If this workup failed to identify a primary focus, then the ipsilateral breast should be presumed to be the source until proven otherwise.

On the other hand, Osteen et al.[44] reported that in their series of 67 cases of systemic metastases with unknown primaries, radiographic contrast studies were useful only when they were indicated by appropriate signs or symptoms (for example, a positive stool guaiac). Liver scans were not helpful when serum liver function studies were normal. However, bone scans were useful for identifying unrecognized systemic metastases. These investigators concluded that a "limited" workup produced almost identical results to one that was more elaborate, comprehensive, and costly.

The Role of Mammography

Most of the reported series on patients with axillary metastases were published before the 1980s, and for the most part have extended over a period from 1907 to 1986. During this time, computerized axial tomography (CT) and mammography have been introduced and refined. In particular, the technique of mammography has improved considerably over the last decade and has played an increasingly major role in the evaluation of patients with suspected breast lesions. Therefore, after a careful history and physical examination, bilateral mammography should be the first screening test performed.

The above facts notwithstanding, the utility of mammography in the management of patients who present with sentinel axillary nodal metastases has been quite variable. Ashikari et al.[2] reported that 22/25 (88%) of their patients with breast cancer presenting with axillary adenopathy had negative mammograms. Feigenberg et al.[14] reported that 6/7 (86%) of their patients had negative mammograms. Patel et al.[49] reported that 47% of the mammograms obtained in their series were positive and that 75% of these had histologically documented breast carcinoma. However, they also reported that 44% of their patients with negative mammograms were subsequently shown by histologic evaluation to have breast carcinoma as the source of the axillary nodal metastases. Table 2 summarizes the findings of several series on mammographic findings in this group of patients.

It is difficult to know what percentage of patients presenting with axillary nodal metastases will have their breast carcinoma identified on currently available bilateral mammography. In view of the minuscule morbidity and the relative inexpensiveness, however, it seems reasonable to consider this the first study to obtain. Further routine workup should include chest X-ray, bone scan, and standard biochemical and hematologic blood profiles, including liver function studies, after careful head and neck, thyroid, pelvic, and rectal examinations. If the patient's history, review of systems, and remaining physical examination are negative and the above studies are all within normal limits, then available wisdom would suggest that additional studies are not likely to be worthwhile. For example, routine total body CT scans in these patients cannot be justified in light of available information.

Fitts et al. have recommended that when the histologic picture of the axillary nodal metastasis is consistent with a breast primary, then a limited workup is appropriate.[16] It has been shown that the pattern observed in the axillary node need not bear any resemblance to the primary carcinoma in the breast, so this recommendation may not be helpful,[53] especially since the majority of adenocarcinomas seen in axillary nodal metastases are Broders' class 3 and 4 (moderately to poorly differentiated).[45,50,70]

Sentinel presentations. Among the approximately 250 reported cases of breast adenocarcinoma presenting initially with sentinel axillary nodal metastases, only one was reported to occur in a man.[45] The mean ages ranged from 47 to 56 years and were largely similar to the ages of patients with frank breast carcinoma with axillary nodal metastases. These patients presented with axillary masses that had been present for weeks to several months before their evaluation. Breslow[5] reported on six patients who simi-

Table 2. Summary of Findings on Mammography Among Patients with Axillary Nodal Metastases Heralding a Clinically Occult Adenocarcinoma of the Breast

Author	Year	Number of Positive or Suspicious Mammograms	Percentage
Vilcoq[67]	1982	0/11	0%
Patel[49]	1981	8/17	47
Ashikari[2]	1976	3/25	12
Feigenberg[14]	1976	1/7	14
Westbrook[69]	1971	10/17	59
Gershon-Cohen[21]	1955	5/5*	100%

*These were regular X-rays of the breast in contrast to the technique of modern mammography

larly presented with "occult" carcinoma of a second breast primary two to nine years following radical mastectomy for the management of a previous contralateral breast carcinoma. All were treated with a second radical mastectomy. Four out of six had histologic documentation of a second breast primary and 4/6 (66%) were alive for six or more years following their second mastectomy. The incidence of bilateral breast carcinoma is 5.8% to 6.5%.[24,56] Therefore, the possibility of a second breast primary presenting in such an unusual fashion should be kept in mind. This is in contradistinction to the occurrence of so-called crossover axillary nodal metastases (metastases to the contralateral axilla) which can occur, especially when the breast primary is extensive. The incidence of crossover metastases is reported to be approximately 4%.[13,24] In spite of the above, I am not aware of any case of primary breast carcinoma (no previous breast cancer) presenting initially with axillary nodal metastases only to the contralateral axilla.

The majority of patients presenting with sentinel axillary nodal metastases from occult breast carcinoma have been treated with mastectomy. Many have been managed with a combination of mastectomy and radiation therapy. Table 3 summarizes the larger series in which mastectomy was a major component of therapy. As can be seen from the data cited in Table 3, the five-year survival rate in this group, when treatment included mastectomy, ranged from 28% to 79%.

Pathologic assessment of all mastectomy specimens has failed to confirm adenocarcinoma of the breast in between 25% to 30% of the cases (Table 4). The reasons most often cited for this are as follows. First, a small cancer may be overlooked on routine sectioning. Second, the breast primary may regress completely leaving no detectable evidence. Third, the breast primary may be "occult" but located in the contralateral breast. Fourth, the breast primary may arise from either heterotopic glandular tissue (glands within the axillary node) or breast tissue that is in the axillary fat and therefore

Table 3.   Result and Survival Data for Treatment Which Included or Consisted Primarily of Mastectomy Among Patients with Axillary Nodal Metastases Heralding a Clinically Occult Adenocarcinoma of the Breast

Author	Year	No. Patients	No. With Mastectomy	5 Year Survival
Haagensen[24]	1986	28	13*	62%
Patel[49]	1981	29	29	28
Ashikari[2]	1976	42	34	79
Westbrook[69]	1971	18	12†	61
Feuerman[15]	1962	21	10	36
Owen[45]	1954	25	18‡	50

*Excludes patients treated with mastectomy plus postoperative radiation therapy (4 patients).
† All received radiation therapy in combination with mastectomy.
‡All except one patient were treated with postoperative radiation therapy
All others represent series in which mastectomy was the only form of therapy.

mistaken for nodal metastasis, when in fact it represents the primary breast cancer. Fifth, the patient may not have adenocarcinoma of the breast. It is important to note, however, that in no report to date has a patient presenting with sentinel axillary nodal metastases who was treated with mastectomy and was not found to have a breast cancer in the mastectomy specimen ever been subsequently shown to have an extramammary source for their axillary nodal adenocarcinoma. Indeed, failure to identify adenocarcinoma of the breast in the ipsilateral breast following mastectomy does not rule out breast cancer.[15] In support of this is the observation that patients who have been treated and followed for breast carcinoma metastatic to axillary nodes, and in whom there has been no pathologic confirmation of a breast primary in their mastectomy specimen, appear to have a five-year survival rate that approximates that of women with overt breast carcinoma and axillary nodal metastases.

"Occult" cancer. The largest reported series in the literature on the use of radiation therapy in the treatment of patients with axillary nodal metastases due to probable subclinical "occult" breast cancer is that reported by Vilcoq et al.[67] In this series, 11 patients were treated with 5000-6000 rads over a five- to six-week period to the ipsilateral breast, and axillary and supraclavicular lymph nodes. Ten of 11 patients (91%), 4/5 (80%), and 3/4 (75%) were alive and disease-free 5, 10, and 15 years following treatment. Three patients (27%) had local recurrence at 6, 11, and 14 years following treatment. The latter two patients were salvaged with mastectomies. The former patient was reirradiated but subsequently died of widespread distant metastases. The only complications were moderate fibrosis in two patients with some limitation of movement of the upper arm. One of these patients also developed moderate edema of the upper extremity on the irradiated side. An overall survival in this series of 82% (9/11), combined with a local recurrence rate of 27%, suggests that radiation therapy without mastectomy or axillary node dissection may be a reasonable alternative for the management of these patients.

Table 4. **Percentages of Histologically Proven Adenocarcinoma from Mastectomy Specimens Among Patients with Axillary Nodal Metastases Heralding a Clinically Occult Adenocarcinoma of the Breast**

Author	Year	No. Mastectomy	No. Histologically Confirmed Carcinoma
Patel[49]	1981	29	16 (55%)
Rosen[57]	1980	8	8 (100%)
Westbrook [69]	1971	12	6 (50%)
Fitts[16]	1963	7	5 (71%)
Feuerman[15]	1962	10	7 (70%)
Gershon-Cohen[21]	1955	5	5 (100%)
Owen[45]	1954	25	25 (100%)
Kaplan[30]	1954	4	3 (75%)

The expected five-year survival rate for women with adenocarcinoma of the breast and positive axillary nodes is approximately 30% to 45%.[15,16,24,26,68] This has been reported to be as low as 20% to 30%,[30] and as high as 60%.[12] Nevertheless, comparative survival data in patients with "occult" breast carcinoma and axillary nodal metastases ranges from 50% to 80% (see Table 3). There are two studies on this group of patients that report less favorable survival data. Feuerman et al. and Patel et al. report five-year survival rates of 36% and 28% respectively.[15,49] Considering all of the available data, it is probably reasonable to conclude that patients who present with only sentinel axillary nodal metastases from primary breast adenocarcinoma have a more favorable prognosis than do patients with overt breast carcinoma and positive axillary nodes.

Possible explanations. The fact that all demonstrable cancers in one small series of eight cases of occult breast cancer with axillary nodal metastases were histologically noninvasive carcinomas may provide some insight into why the above may indeed be true.[57] The incidence of axillary nodal metastasis in patients with preinvasive breast cancer (intraductal or lobular in situ) is reported to be 1%.[58] It is therefore possible that patients with occult breast cancer have a higher proportion of cancers that are noninvasive or preinvasive when compared to patients with overt breast carcinoma and axillary nodal metastases. If this is true, then the expectation would be that these patients would have a more favorable outcome or prognosis. The observation that invasion through the basement membrane can occur before it is detectable by light microscopy has been already demonstrated by electron microscopy.[46] This is therefore consistent with the implication that patients with clinically occult carcinoma of the breast may present with axillary nodal metastases but, more often than not, have early preinvasive or noninvasive lesions and, consequently, a more favorable prognosis.

An algorithm for the management and treatment of patients who present with sentinel axillary nodal metastases from an unrecognized adenocarcinoma of the breast is summarized in Figure 1. A preliminary workup should consist of a careful history and physical examination combined with a chest X-ray, bilateral mammography, biochemical and hematologic blood profiles, including liver function studies (LFTs), a bone scan, and measurements of estrogen and progesterone receptor levels from the axillary node biopsy specimen. If this preliminary evaluation uncovers any pertinent positive findings, then optional studies should be performed as appropriate to the findings observed. Optional studies to be considered are chest, abdominal, and pelvic CT scans, gastrointestinal contrast studies and endoscopy, and thyroid scanning or needle biopsy. If an extramammary source for the axillary nodal metastases is not identified or suspected following such an approach, then the patient should be managed for what is most likely a carcinoma of the

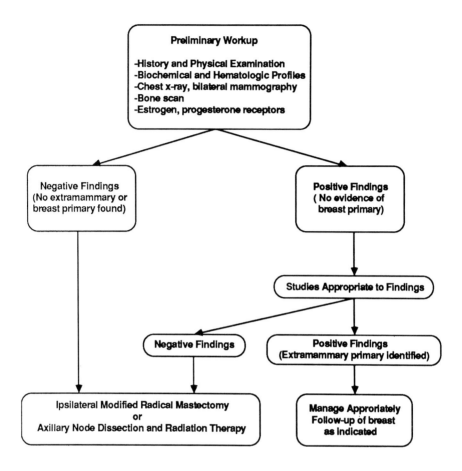

Figure 1. Algorithm for the management and treatment of patients with sentinel axillary nodal metastases from an unrecognized adenocarcinoma of the breast.

ipsilateral breast. Treatment should consist of either a modified radical mastectomy or an axillary node dissection followed by radiation therapy to the ipsilateral breast.

Whether radiation therapy should be directed to the axilla and the supraclavicular nodal area in lieu of, or in addition to, axillary nodal dissection and radiation therapy to the ipsilateral breast has not been established.

Carcinoma of the Breast Presenting as a Nipple Discharge in the Absence of a Palpable Mass and with a Benign- or Normal-Appearing Mammogram

There is nothing unusual about a bloody nipple discharge associated with an underlying palpable breast mass. Excisional biopsy of the palpable mass will allow the distinction to be made between a benign intraductal papilloma and an adenocarcinoma of the breast. A nonbloody, serous nipple discharge, however, with no palpable breast mass and a benign- or normal-appearing mammogram represents a diagnostic dilemma and sets the stage for another relatively obscure presentation of carcinoma of the breast.

Recently I was asked to see an active 50-year-old woman referred to the University of Michigan Breast Care Center for the evaluation of an intermittent, serous left nipple discharge with no palpable mass or other discernible breast abnormality. The patient's past medical history was negative for breast disease. She had no symptoms prior to the onset of an occasional, nonbloody nipple discharge noted several months prior to her seeking medical advice. The patient's family physician obtained a smear of the nipple discharge and sent it for cytologic evaluation, which revealed carcinoma. Her family history and remaining history and physical examination were noncontributory to the case. Accompanying bilateral mammograms revealed two areas of benign-appearing calcifications in the left breast, one in the subareolar region and the other in the upper outer quadrant. On my examination I could not appreciate any breast masses, skin changes, or adenopathy; however, the responsible duct was easily identified with gentle massage and found to be in the 3 o'clock position (upper outer quadrant of the areolar complex). I arranged for a ductogram by one of our mammographers. This study revealed a small intraductal lesion that was not coincident with, but was in close proximity to, the subareolarly located area of calcification. Subsequent wide local excisional biopsy of this lesion along with the subareolar calcification revealed, on permanent section, multiple foci of intraductal adenocarcinoma with several different histologic patterns, including comedo, medullary, and papillary. The patient elected to have an axillary node dissection with breast irradiation instead of a modified radical mastectomy and is currently undergoing radiation therapy.

In the original descriptions of nipple discharge, these were usually all associated with a palpable mass and, therefore, were not associated with any delays or dilemmas in diagnosis.[27] Subsequently, it became apparent that a very small percentage of carcinomas of the breast could present with only a nipple discharge and no palpable mass.[33] A method for cannulization of the mammary duct demonstrated to be responsible for the nipple discharge was first described by Hicken.[28] Problems with the toxicity of the then available contrast media prevented the widespread use of this technique until 1969.[20] Threatt and Appelman from The University of Michigan introduced their technique of performing a ductogram and illustrated its ability to identify an intraductal lesion.[66]

In many respects, access to state-of-the-art mammography performed by a specialty group of physicians here at the University of Michigan Medical Center made the management of the case previously presented appear rather routine in retrospect. But the situation becomes more difficult when no lesion can be identified. Haagensen describes his experience with two such patients in whom the diagnosis was missed or delayed.[24] In such an instance, careful reexamination in a month's time to identify the responsible duct is considered reasonable. Of course, the problem is compounded when the surgeon does not use ductograms because of his or her concerns regarding the potential risk of inflammation and infection, and the consideration that by injecting contrast under pressure there is an additional theoretical risk of disseminating cancer cells into the bloodstream and lymphatics. For these reasons, and the belief that ductograms are inexact, Haagensen employs a method of "meticulous surgical exploration of the subareolar areas guided by a pressure point that produced the discharge in patients who [have] only a nipple discharge," in the management of such patients.[24]

Finally, the point to be emphasized here is that while the diagnosis in a woman presenting with a spontaneous nipple discharge not associated with a discernible breast lesion is statistically more than likely to be that of a benign intraductal papilloma, this assumption cannot be relied upon. A determined effort should be made to identify the culpable duct by gently, in a circumferential manner, massaging the subareolar region to appreciate a trigger point that will elicit the discharge. This will allow the performance of a surgical exploration and excision of the involved ducts and lobules for biopsy. An alternative approach would be to obtain a ductogram to look for an intraductal papilloma or papillary carcinoma. If a lesion is found, the study will facilitate localization and excisional biopsy. If no lesion is identified by ductogram, and no trigger point or responsible duct can be identified, then in the absence of any findings on mammography, one is forced to follow the patient and reexamine her in one month's time. In this setting, the nipple discharge should also be sent for cytologic evaluation.[9]

Unsuspected Carcinoma in a Clinically Benign Appearing Adenofibroma

Adenofibromas represent one of the two major classes of fibroepithelial tumors of the breast. Cystosarcoma phyllodes is the second. Adenofibroma is the third most common neoplasm of the breast, following the so-called fibrocystic breast disease and carcinoma.[24] The incidence of adenofibroma in an autopsy series of 225 patients was 9%.[19] This included lesions that were only evident microscopically. Adenofibromas are most prevalent in women in their twenties; however, the mean age for occurrence is reported to range from 34 to 45 years. The natural history of adenofibroma is usually that of a painless, incidentally discovered, slow-growing mass in the breast of a premenopausal woman. The finding of a coexistent carcinoma in an adenofibroma is exceedingly unusual. Only when a carcinoma is found solely within the adenofibroma, and not in the adjacent surrounding tissue, can this diagnosis be confirmed. The common type of neoplasia observed to arise in these lesions is lobular carcinoma in situ (LCIS).[7,18,22,39] The largest series on this topic has been reported by Fondo et al.[18] In their report of 14 cases of breast carcinoma found in clinically innocuous adenofibromas, 6 were found to contain LCIS only within the excised adenofibroma. The remaining patients had LCIS also in the surrounding breast tissue or associated with intraductal and terminal duct carcinomas in both the adenofibroma and the remaining breast. Three of their patients were treated with local excision and the remaining 11 were treated with mastectomy, 3 of whom were treated with radical mastectomy. Only one of the patients treated with radical mastectomy had both infiltrating and intraductal carcinomas in both the excised adenofibroma and the remaining breast. The remaining patients, with one exception, were treated with a modified radical mastectomy for either LCIS in the adenofibroma alone, in the adenofibroma and surrounding breast, or LCIS associated with an intraductal and/or infiltrating duct carcinoma in the adenofibroma and remaining breast. The one exception was treated with a simple mastectomy. Among these 11 patients, LCIS was found in adjacent breast tissue in 73%. Four patients were evaluated and treated for bilateral disease and all 4 contained either LCIS (2) or ductal carcinoma (2). In their entire group of patients, the incidence of bilateral carcinomas was 4/14 (29%).

There are no data that I am aware of to argue against treating a patient with an infiltrating carcinoma in an excised adenofibroma, especially when also present in adjacent breast tissue, with some form of total mastectomy. Admittedly, if a single focus of cancer is found entirely within the excised adenofibroma, and nowhere in adjoining breast tissue, then alternatively irradiating the breast is theoretically reasonable. However, the management of noninvasive carcinoma within an adenofibroma is less well established and remains controversial. There is some evidence that the likelihood of noninvasive carcinoma to progress to invasive carcinoma is sufficient (for intraductal lesions) to argue for managing these situations with mastectomy.[4]

The management of LCIS remains quite controversial. This is no less true for LCIS within an adenofibroma. There are many experienced and astute clinicians who believe that LCIS is a benign lesion. Haagensen, for example, considers these lesions benign "lobular neoplasia," and therefore, presumably he and those who adhere to this point of view would be comfortable to closely follow a patient with such a lesion. There is some evidence, however, that there is a 10% to 15% risk that invasive carcinoma will develop in such a breast.[39] In view of the fact that a total mastectomy is probably curative for this lesion, an alternative approach is to manage these patients with a simple or total mastectomy. Because the risk of subsequent contralateral invasive carcinoma is real and in view of the high incidence of bilaterality in the series reviewed here, serious consideration should be given to also obtaining a contralateral upper outer quadrant or mirror image biopsy during the management of patients with such lesions.

Breast Carcinoma Obscured by Hemorrhage Associated with Trauma

The typical scenario in this circumstance is to be asked to evaluate a slightly obese woman with large and pendulous breasts who describes being struck in her breast with a ball or by a child during play and now is complaining of a discolored area on her breast with an underlying mass. On examination she is found to have an area of ecchymosis with a mass beneath or immediately adjacent to the area of ecchymosis.

The point to be made here is that with a good history and a reliable patient it is reasonable initially to observe such a patient if there are no other findings on history and physical examination to raise your index of suspicion. If the mass is still present on repeat examination a month later, however, then an excisional biopsy with removal of the mass should be performed. In the vast majority of cases this will confirm fat necrosis as suspected.[11] Nevertheless, as recommended by Haagensen, biopsy is necessary to rule out bleeding from an underlying carcinoma that has bled from being traumatized. It is roughly similar to the clinical situation encountered when one is following a patient on chronic anticoagulation with warfarin, for example, who develops gastrointestinal bleeding. The burden of proof falls on the physician to rule out an underlying malignancy.

PAGET'S DISEASE OF THE BREAST

In 1856, Velpeau described a lesion of the breast that would only later become associated with carcinoma of the breast. This association was first made by Sir James Paget.[47] In his classic article published in 1874, Paget described a series of women, ranging in age from 40 to 60 years or more, who initially developed an eruption on the nipple and areola. This process gave the appearance of eczema or psoriasis of the nipple and areola and was always associated with a copious clear, yellowish, and viscid exudate. Tingling, itching, and burning were common. In each case, breast carcinoma followed within two years and often within one year of the patient's presentation.

Paget's disease of the breast constitutes approximately 1% to 3% of all breast carcinomas.[1,17,24] In reported series, the patients' ages range from 28 to over 80 years with an average age of 54 to 60 years.[24,35,48] The disease occurs primarily in women but has been reported in men.[36,62]

Histopathology and Histogenesis of Paget's Disease

The characteristic pathologic finding is the presence of large cells with abundant pale cytoplasm and prominent, irregular, hyperchromatic nuclei in the epidermis of the nipple. These cells are called Paget cells and occur either individually or in poorly defined groups and often cluster in the suprabasilar portion of the epidermis of the nipple.[24,35] Ultrastructurally, mature Paget cells show hemidesmosomal attachments with the basal lamina of the epidermis, variable desmosomal attachments between themselves and keratinocytes, and the formation of an abnormal microvillous surface over portions of its surface.[36,62]

Although Paget cells can on occasion contain melanin in their cytoplasm and can resemble junctional melanomas,[24] the work of Sagebiel[60] supports the epithelial origin of these cells, and the possibility of Paget cells originating from an "altered melanocyte" has been discarded. Paget cells have been shown to express carcinoembryonic antigen (CEA) and apocrine epithelial antigen (AEA).[31,42] These antigens were also found in the cells of ductal carcinomas of the breast associated with Paget's disease as well as with extramammary Paget's disease. Paget cells have also been shown to express specific cytokeratin antigens by utilizing two monoclonal cytokeratin antibodies that typically react to simple glandular epithelium and not to surrounding epidermal cells.[32] Furthermore, the milk protein casein has been detected in well-differentiated carcinomas of the breast, in neoplastic cells from the ducts of a breast with Paget's disease of the nipple, and finally, in the typical intraepidermal Paget cell.[6] Therefore, despite the work of Sumitomo,[65] in which the specific expression of CEA by Paget cells is questioned, the above body of data strongly supports the fact that Paget cells are neoplastic cells of glandular origin, i.e., adenocarcinoma cells probably of ductal origin.

Paget cells infiltrating the epidermis of the nipple and the epithelial surfaces of nipple and mammary ducts are known to be associated with underlying intraductal or invasive adenocarcinoma of the breast. This clinical observation has given rise to two prevailing theories regarding the origin of the Paget cell. The epidermotropic theory suggests that Paget cells are neoplastic cells that arise from an intraductal carcinoma and, because of their peculiar proclivity, migrate through ducts to invade ductal epithelium and the nipple epidermis. In similar fashion, they invade the epithelium of lactiferous ("milk") ducts. This epidermotropic theory dictates, therefore, that in all cases of Paget's disease of the breast there is an underlying ductal carcinoma. However, Ashikari et al.[1] have described the absence of any identifiable ductal carcinoma in 2.8% (6/214) of their cases of histologically proved Paget's disease of the breast. This represented 6.25% of their cases of Paget's disease in which there was no palpable tumor. This phenomenon has also been described by others.[24]

The second theory regarding the histogenesis of Paget's disease of the breast suggests that Paget cells are neoplastic cells which arise de novo in the nipple epidermis independent of any underlying breast carcinoma. This spontaneous in situ neoplastic transformation is supported by others who have documented both mammary and extramammary Paget's disease without dermal invasion or associated underlying carcinoma.[35,59,60] These two theories on the histogenesis of Paget's disease, the migratory "epidermotropic" versus the in situ spontaneous appearance, are thought to be both valid and not necessarily mutually exclusive by Azzopardi.[3]

There is compelling reason for discussing the origin of the Paget cell and Paget's disease at such great length, simply because rational recommendations for therapy are quite dependent upon which of these views one emphasizes or adopts. The epidermotropic theory implies that in every case of Paget's disease of the breast there is an underlying breast carcinoma, which in many instances may be occult, and therefore dictates the use of standard therapy for carcinoma of the breast. On the other hand, the theory of de novo intraepidermal origin does not in itself imply an underlying breast cancer, and therefore favors the consideration of using alternative forms of therapy. Alternative therapy, for example, might include simple local excision with careful follow-up. This point will be elaborated on further when recommendations for therapy are discussed.

Signs and Symptoms of Paget's Disease

The early symptoms and signs of Paget's disease include pain, itching, or burning in the nipple. Subsequently, redness, roughening, and thickening of the nipple skin implies further progression of the infiltrative process. Finally, erosion and spread of involvement onto the areola and skin of the breast are seen and suggest a longstanding process. It should be kept in mind that breast carcinoma in the absence of Paget's disease can infiltrate and involve the areola without involving the nipple. Involvement of the areola without involvement of the nipple is not Paget's disease. It should also be kept in mind that bilateral nipple lesions cannot be assumed to be benign, since bilateral Paget's disease has been described.[64] Therefore, any patient who presents with pain, itching, burning, bleeding, redness, thickening, or an eczematoid or psoriasiform lesion of the nipple should be managed with a biopsy within weeks of presentation. If the patient presents with an erosive or ulcerating lesion of the nipple, then a biopsy should be performed immediately. Furthermore, a pathologic report of dermatitis or inflammation mandates a repeat biopsy.[38] Maier et al.[38] described a patient who was treated for 48 months with a topical salve. Treatment was based on a pathologic report of dermatitis following biopsy. The patient subsequently died of metastatic disease 16 months after a repeat biopsy confirmed Paget's disease. Biopsy of the nipple lesion should entail a wedge or ellipse of tissue from, and perpendicular through, the nipple. This can be performed with local anesthesia.

Theoretically, Paget's disease should be a lesion that lends itself to a very early presentation. In fact, its benign appearance and innocuous presentation has resulted in considerable delay by both patient and physician in seeking and rendering appropriate care. Haagensen has recently reported a median delay of 21 months for patients with Paget's disease before the diagnosis has been made. This finding is supported by the literature, in that patients with Paget's disease have had their symptoms on an average of 10 to 21 months prior to diagnosis.[38,43,49,54]

Patients with Paget's disease of the breast fall into three clinical categories: those with with nipple symptoms or signs only; those with nipple symptoms or findings and an underlying breast mass, which is most commonly located immediately beneath the nipple; or those with a breast mass only. This third group of patients has a routine clinical presentation with a palpable breast mass, no discernible nipple symptoms or signs, but on subsequent examination of the tissue are shown to have Paget's disease. The relative distributions of patients among these categories are summarized in Table 5. Ashikari et al.,[1] in their series of 214 patients with Paget's disease, did not separate out which patients among those with breast masses had a breast mass without nipple symptoms or signs. Paone et al.,[48] in their series of 50 patients, did not separate out which patients among those with nipple changes had an underlying breast mass. Nevertheless, approximately 40% to 45% of patients with Paget's disease present with only nipple symptoms or signs, approximately 30% to 50% present with both nipple changes and an underlying breast mass, and from 10% to 20% present with a palpable breast mass only.[1,24,48]

Impact of a Breast Mass on Survival

Data illustrating the relationship of prognosis in patients with Paget's disease of the breast and their clinical presentation is summarized in Table 6. This data dramatically illustrates the prognostic significance of the presence of an underlying breast mass in a patient with Paget's disease. The incidence of axillary nodal involvement is 0% to 20% and the mean five-year survival rate is 90% when no breast mass is present at the time of diagnosis. On the other hand, the incidence of axillary nodal involvement is 50% to 77% and the mean five-year survival rate is 33% when a breast mass is present at the time of diagnosis. Another index of the prognostic significance related to the presence of an underlying breast mass is the relative incidence of invasive carcinoma observed in each clinical circumstance.

Table 5.   Paget's Disease of the Breast: Clinical Presentations

Author	Year	No. Pts.	Nipple Only	Nipple & Breast Mass	Breast Mass Only
Maier[38]	1969	137	56 (42%)	67 (49%)	14 (10%)
Ashikari[1]	1970	214	96 (40%)	*	*
Paone[48]	1981	50	*	*	5 (10%)
Haagensen[24]	1986	182	83 (46%)	54 (30%)	45 (24%)
Total		583	235 (40%)	121 (38%)†	64 (20%)†

*Categories combined in these reports.
†Subtotals. Percentages based on combining data only from series with complete data recorded.

Table 6.   Paget's Disease of the Breast: Relationship of Clinical Presentation

Author (Total No. Pts.)	No Breast Mass Present			Breast Mass Present		
	No. Pts.	(%) + Axilla	5 Yr Sur	No. Pts.	(%) + Axilla	5 Yr Sur
Maier[38] (88)	40	20%	70%	48	*	38%
Ridenhour[54] (20)	8	0	100	12	67	25
Rissanen[55] (26)	13	0	83	13	77	0
Ashikari[1] (209)	96	14	92	113	65	45
Nance[43] (53)	21	0	94	32	50	41
Paone[48] (50)	19	0	100	31	65	45
Haagensen[24] (182)	36	8	81*	56	63	54

*10-year survival data
†Data not provided

Nance et al.[43] reported a 10% incidence of invasive carcinoma in patients with no underlying breast mass. On the other hand, there was a 94% incidence of invasive carcinoma in patients with an underlying breast mass. Moreover, Ashikari et al.[1] reported incidences of 34% and 91% for invasive carcinoma in the absence and presence, respectively, of an underlying breast mass.

Clearly there is a profound negative effect on survival by the presence of a breast mass in patients with Paget's disease.[17,40,61] Available data suggest that the delay in diagnosis is not, per se, the major factor in determining prognosis or survival. In fact, it is the presence or absence of axillary nodal involvement that appears to be the major determinant.[38] Nonetheless, as best as can be determined, it is widely accepted that early diagnosis does correlate with "early" disease and obviates axillary nodal involvement and systemic dissemination. Therefore, the importance of aggressively pursuing the diagnosis and having a high index of suspicion when evaluating a patient with persistent nipple symptoms cannot be overemphasized.

Treatment of Paget's Disease

The standard treatment of patients with Paget's disease of the breast has been mastectomy; it must still be considered to be the form of therapy against which all others must be compared, primarily because of the lack of data on other modes of therapy. Several authors have employed radiation therapy following either biopsy only, local excision, or mastectomy.[40,55] The numbers of patients and relatively small doses of radiation employed make it difficult to draw meaningful conclusions regarding the use of radiation therapy in the management of Paget's disease.

Lagios et al.[35] have described their experience with six patients without clinical or mammographic evidence of a breast mass. These authors advocate the in situ theory of the histogenesis of Paget's disease. In their series, four patients had disease confined to the nipple only, and two had underlying carcinoma of ductal origin. Five patients were treated conservatively. Four underwent total excision of the affected nipple-areolar complex, and three of these also underwent mammographically directed biopsy or blind four-quadrant breast biopsies. The sixth patient was treated with a modified radical mastectomy. Other than that the disease involved the lactiferous duct to a depth of 15 mm, no reason is offered for the decision to perform a mastectomy in this patient. Nevertheless, of the five patients treated conservatively, all were without evidence of disease with an average follow-up of 50 months. This experience suggests that mastectomy may not be necessary in all cases of Paget's disease.

An algorithm recommended for use in the management of patients with nipple symptoms suggestive of Paget's disease of the breast is presented in Figure 2.

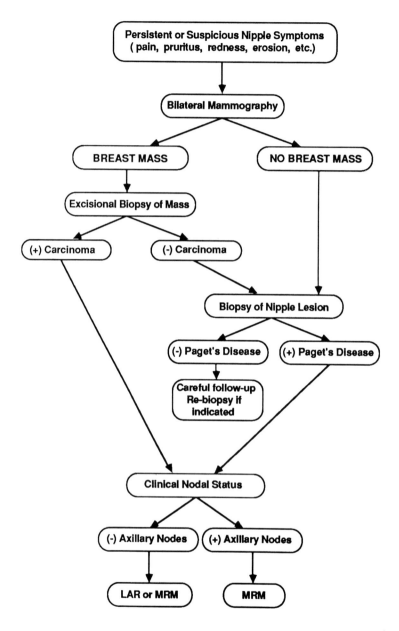

Figure 2. Algorithm for the management and treatment of patients with nipple symptoms suggestive of Paget's disease of the breast.

REFERENCES

1. Ashikari R, Park K, Huvos AG, Urban JA: Paget's disease of the breast. Cancer 26:680–685, 1970.
2. Ashikari R, Rosen PP, Urban JA, et al.: Breast cancer presenting as an axillary mass. Ann Surg 183:415–417, 1976.
3. Azzopardi JG: *Problems in Breast Pathology*. Saunders, London, 1979, pp 258–260.
4. Betsill WL, Rosen PP, Lieberman PH, et al.: Intraductal carcinoma: Long-term follow-up after "treatment" by biopsy alone. JAMA 239:1863–1867, 1978.
5. Breslow A: Occult carcinoma of second breast following mastectomy. JAMA 226:1000–1, 1973.
6. Bussolati G, Pich A, Alfani V: Immunofluorescence detection of casein in human mammary dysplastic and neoplastic tissues. Virchows-Arch Pathol Anat 365:15–21, 1975.
7. Buzanowski-Konakry K, Harrison EG, Jr, Payne WS: Lobular carcinoma arising in fibroadenoma of the breast. Cancer 35:450–456, 1975.
8. Cameron HC: Some clinical facts regarding mammary cancer. Br Med J 1:577–582, 1909.
9. Cogswell HD: Hidden carcinoma of the breast. Arch Surg 58:780–89, 1949.
10. Copeland EM, McBride CM: Axillary metastasis from unknown primary sites. Ann Surg 178:25–7, 1973.
11. D'Orsi CJ, Feldhaus L, Sonnenfeld M: Unusual lesions of the breast. Radiol Clin North Am 21:67–80, 1983.
12. Davidoff RB: Occult carcinoma of the breast. Geriatrics 9:128–129, 1954.
13. Devitt JE, Michalchuk AW: Significance of contralateral metastasis in carcinoma of breast. Can J Surg 12:178–180, 1969.
14. Feigenberg Z, Zer M, Dintsman M: Axillary metastases from an unknown primary source. Isr J Med Sci 12:1153–58, 1976.
15. Feuerman MD, Attie JN, Rosenberg B: Carcinoma in axillary lymph nodes as an indicator of breast cancer. Surg Gynecol Obstet 114:5–8, 1962.
16. Fitts WT, Steiner GC, Enterline HT: Prognosis of occult carcinoma of the breast. Am J Surg 106:460–3, 1963.
17. Freund H, Moydovnik M, Laufer N: Paget's disease of the breast. J Surg Oncol 9:93, 1977.
18. Fondo EY, Rosen PP, Fracchia AA, et al.: The problem of carcinoma developing in a fibroadenoma. Cancer 43:563–567, 1979.
19. Frantz VK, Pickren JW, Melcher GW, et al.: Incidence of chronic cystic disease in so-called 'normal breast'. Cancer 4:762, 1951.
20. Funderburk WW, Syphax B: Evaluation of nipple discharge in benign and malignant diseases. Cancer 24:1290, 1969.
21. Gershon-Cohen J, Ingleby H, Hermel MB: Occult carcinoma of the breast: Value of roentgenography. Arch Surg 70:385–89, 1955.
22. Goldman RL, Friedman NB: Carcinoma of the breast arising in fibro-

adenomas, with emphasis on lobular carcinoma – A clinico-pathologic study. Cancer 23:544–550, 1969.

23. Grundfest S, Steiger E, Sebek B: Metastatic axillary adenopathy. Arch Surg 113:1108–1109, 1978.

24. Haagensen CD: *Diseases of the Breast.* 3rd Ed. Philadelphia, WB Saunders, 1986.

25. Halsted WS: Results of radical operation for cure of carcinoma of the breast. Ann Surg 46:1, 1907.

26. Harrington SW: Surgical treatment of carcinoma of the breast. J Mich Med Soc 47:41, 1948.

27. Hart D: Intracystic papillomatous tumors of the breast, benign and malignant. Arch Surg 14:793, 1927.

28. Hicken NF: Intracystic papilloma of the breast. Surgery 7:724, 1940.

29. Jackson AS: Carcinoma of the breast in the absence of clinical breast findings. Ann Surg 127:177–179, 1948.

30. Kaplan IW, Reinstine H: Occult carcinoma of the breast. Am Surg 20:575–82, 1954.

31. Kariniemi AL, Forsman L, Wahlstrom T, et al.: Expression of differentiation antigens in mammary and extramammary Paget's disease. Br J Dermatol 110:203–10, 1984.

32. Kariniemi AL, Ramaekers F, Lehto VP, et al.: Target cells express cytokeratins typical of glandular epithelia. Br J Dermatol 112:179–83, 1985.

33. Kilgore AR, Fleming R, Ramos MM: The incidence of cancer with nipple discharge and the risk of cancer in the presence of papillary disease of the breast. Surg Gynecol Obstet 96:649, 1953.

34. Klopp CT: Metastatic cancer of axillary lymph nodes without a demonstrable primary lesion. Ann Surg 131:437–39, 1950.

35. Lagios MD, Westkahl PR, Rose MR, et al.: Paget's disease of the nipple. Alternative management in cases without or with minimal extent of underlying breast carcinoma. Cancer 54:545–551, 1984.

36. Lancer HA, Moschella SL: Paget's disease of the male breast. J Am Acad Dermatol 7:393–6, 1982.

37. Larsen RR, Sawyer KC, Sawyer RB, et al.: Occult carcinoma of the breast. Am J Surg 107:553–5, 1964.

38. Maier WP, Rosemond GP, Harasym EL, et al.: Paget's disease of the female breast. Surg Gynec Obstet 128:1253-1263, 1969.

39. McDivitt RW, Stewart FW, Farrow JH: Breast carcinoma arising in solitary fibroadenoma. Surg Gynecol Obstet 125:572–576, 1969.

40. McGregor JK, McGregor DD: Paget's disease of the breast. Surgery 45:562–568, 1959.

41. McNair TJ, Dudley HA: Axillary lymph-nodes in patients without breast carcinoma. Lancet 1:713–4, 1960.

42. Nadji M, Morales AR, Girtanner RE, et al.: Paget's disease of the skin: A unifying concept of histogenesis. Cancer 50:2203–2206, 1982.

43. Nance FC, DeLoach DH, Welsh RA, et al.: Paget's disease of the breast. Ann Surg 171:864–874, 1970.

44. Osteen RT, Kopf G, Wilson RE: In pursuit of the unknown primary. Am J Surg 135:494–498, 1978.
45. Owen HW, Dockerty MB, Gray HK: Occult carcinoma of the breast. Surg Gynecol Obstet 98:302–8, 1954.
46. Ozzello L, Sampitak P: The epithelial-stromal junction of intraductal carcinoma of the breast. Cancer 26:1186–1198, 1970.
47. Paget J: On disease of the mammary areola preceding cancer of the mammary gland. Classic articles in colonic and rectal surgery. Dis Colon Rectum 23:280–1, 1980.
48. Paone JF, Baker RR: Pathogenesis and treatment of Paget's disease of the breast. Cancer 48:825–829, 1981.
49. Patel J, Nemoto T, Rosner D, et al.: Axillary lymph node metastasis from an occult breast cancer. Cancer 47:2923–2927, 1981.
50. Pierce EH, Gray HK, Dockerty MB: Surgical significance of isolated axillary adenopathy. Ann Surg 145:104–7, 1957.
51. Polson C: Case of unrecognized carcinoma of breast. J Pathol Bacteriol 30:572, 1927.
52. Primrose A: Secondary manifestations of malignant disease. Ann Surg 76:312, 1922.
53. Rabinovitch J, Rabinovitch P, Pines B: Silent carcinomas of the breast. Am J Surg 85:179–83, 1953.
54. Ridenhour CE, Perez-Mesa C, Hori JM: Paget's disease of the nipple. Cancer Bull 21:15–16, 1969.
55. Rissanen PM, Holsti P: Paget's disease of the breast. Oncology 23:209–216, 1969.
56. Robbins GF, Berg JW: Bilateral primary breast cancers. Cancer 17:1501–1527, 1964.
57. Rosen PP: Axillary lymph node metastases in patients with occult non-invasive breast carcinoma. Cancer 46:1298–1306, 1980.
58. Rosen PP, Braun D, Kinne DW: The clinical significance of preinvasive breast carcinoma. Cancer 46:919–925, 1980.
59. Sagami S: Electron microscopic studies in Paget's disease. Med J Osaka Univ 14:173–187, 1963.
60. Sagebiel R: Ultrastructural observations on epidermal cells in Paget's disease of the breast. Am J Pathol 57:49–64, 1969.
61. Salvadori B, Farigelli G, Roberto ST: Analysis of 100 cases of Paget's disease of the breast. Tumori 62:529–536, 1976.
62. Satiani B, Powell RW, Mathews WH: Paget disease of the male breast. Arch Surg 112:587–592, 1977.
63. Shore BR: Obscure case of breast carcinoma. Am J Cancer 15:221, 1931.
64. Sinha MR, Prassad SB: Bilateral Paget's disease of the nipple. J Indian Med Assoc 80:2, 1983.
65. Sumitomo S, Tatemoto Y, Fukui S, et al.: False positive reaction for carcinoembryonic antigen in Paget cells. Virchows-Arch Cell Pathol 49:395–9, 1985.
66. Threatt B, Appelman HF: Mammary duct injection. Radiology 108:71, 1973.

67. Vilcoq JR, Calle R, Ferme F, et al.: Conservative treatment of axillary adenopathy due to probable subclinical breast cancer. Arch Surg 117:1136–38, 1982.
68. Weinberger HA, Stetten D: Extensive secondary axillary lymph node carcinoma without clinical evidence of primary breast lesion. Surgery 29:217–222, 1951.
69. Westbrook KC, Gallager HS: Breast carcinoma presenting as an axillary mass. Am J Surg 122:607–611, 1971.
70. Ximenes J, Brown HW: Occult carcinoma of the breast. Two case reports and review of the literature. Int Surg 47:159–165, 1967.

18. Breast Cancer Management in Pregnancy and Young Women

KAREN S. GUICE
KEITH T. OLDHAM

Fortunately, breast cancer in young women is rare. Fewer than 2% of all breast cancers occur in women under 30 years of age. Because breast cancer is a common malady, however, the overall magnitude of this problem merits specific discussion. Several important aspects of diagnosis, management, and prognosis are different for young women when compared with older women. These differences will be emphasized in this discussion. Special considerations such as pregnancy, familial disease, and childhood breast cancer will also be reviewed.

EPIDEMIOLOGY

Breast cancer is the most common malignancy in women in the United States. It is estimated that 123,000 new cases of breast cancer occurred in 1986 in this country;[13,44] of these, between 2000 and 2500 cases occurred in women 30 years of age or less. This represents only 1% to 2% of all breast cancers.[20,30,37,42,43]

Additionally, until recently, breast cancer has been the single largest cause of death among women who die of malignant disease.[16,44] Approximately 40,000 deaths from breast cancer occur annually in the United States.[44] The American Cancer Society's statistics for U.S. women in 1983 indicate that breast cancer was the cause of 19% of all cancer-related deaths in the 15 to 34 year old age group and 29% of the cancer-related deaths in the 35 to 54 year group.[44]

Breast cancer in childhood is even less common. In 1972 Nichini reviewed the medical literature and estimated that approximately 50 cases of breast cancer had been reported during the previous half-century in children and adolescents.[28]

In women younger than the age of 35, the overwhelming majority of breast lesions are benign.[31] The differentiation of benign lesions is beyond the scope of this discussion; however, in the adolescent female, the infrequent occurrence of breast carcinoma has led to an appropriate reluctance to embark on a diagnostic course that includes surgical biopsy. Skiles and Seltzer reviewed 635 breast biopsies in women less than 20 years of age: Only two (0.3%) were positive for primary breast carcinoma.[45] Beyond 20 years of age, breast cancer occurs with sufficient frequency to mandate a pathologic evaluation of any persistent or suspicious discrete breast nodule.

RISK FACTORS

The probability of an American woman developing breast cancer in her lifetime is estimated to approximate 1 in 11. Epidemiologic studies have related a number of factors, such as family history and reproductive status, to the risk of development of breast cancer. In general, these risk factors do not appear to be different in young women, although several observations relative to ovarian function and pregnancy are age-related.

The family history, in particular, is a critical and generally accepted predictor of breast cancer, which becomes an important consideration in the management of young women. Haagensen reports that a positive family history is strongly correlated with the occurrence of both early and bilateral breast cancer.[16] Anderson and Badzioch found a threefold increase in risk when one first-degree relative has had unilateral premenopausal breast cancer. This risk increases ninefold when the relative has had bilateral cancer. When two first-degree relatives have had unilateral premenopausal breast cancer, the risk increases 15 times. If bilateral, this risk soars 50-fold and has given rise to the concept that for certain high-risk patients prophylactic simple mastectomy is a reasonable alternative.[1]

The pathogenesis of familial breast cancer remains unclear. Several investigators have measured plasma levels of steroidal hormones in kinships in attempts to identify patients at increased risk. No significant relationship of plasma estrogen or progesterone levels to risk has emerged in these young women with a positive family history.[4,14] There is currently no serum screening test that is a helpful predictor of risk.

Ovarian function and pregnancy appear to be related to the risk of developing breast cancer. Pregnancy prior to 18 years of age is associated with a diminished risk of subsequent breast cancer.[5,16] Women who have their first pregnancy after 35 years of age have a slightly higher risk of subsequently developing breast cancer.[5] It has been theorized that women who are older at the time of the initial prelactation breast proliferation are more likely to have abnormal or environmentally damaged breast epithelium, which could become the source of dysplasia or carcinoma. This is an attractive but unproven hypothesis. Postmenopausal and celibate women also appear to be at slightly higher statistical risk for the development of breast cancer. Early lactation appears to be associated with a slightly diminished risk. The reasons for these epidemiological observations are not known.[16]

Oral contraceptives are not generally thought to be a risk factor in the development of breast cancer, in spite of close and continuing scrutiny.[33,39,40,46] A recent study by Pike, however, reported an increased risk when oral contraceptives were initiated before the first full-term pregnancy.[35] The risk in this report increased with the duration of oral contraceptive use, such that six years of use more than doubled the likelihood of developing breast cancer. Drife has observed that unopposed estrogen, either exogenously administered or endogenously produced, stimulates breast epithelial proliferation similar to uterine endometrial proliferation, where the risk of malignancy is widely recognized.[11] The relationship of this observation to the pathogenesis of breast cancer is speculative.

CHILDHOOD BREAST CANCER

Prepubertal breast cancer is rare to the extent that it may be considered a medical curiosity. McDivitt and Stewart reported seven patients in 1966, which remains the largest single experience.[26] The total number of such cases in the medical literature is estimated between 20 and 50 by Oberman[31] and by McDivitt and Stewart.[26]

Childhood breast cancer usually presents clinically as a unilateral subareolar nodule. It is usually nontender and not rapidly enlarging. This is clearly difficult to differentiate from the normal pattern of pubertal breast development. It is common to see a normal girl nine or ten years of age with a nodule beneath one nipple. This is often slightly tender and it may be several months before the contralateral breast begins to develop. Biopsy or excision of the breast at this stage of development may lead to serious breast deformity or no breast development at all. This is a procedure only to be undertaken with great care after careful consideration.

In general, we recommend that a nodule be followed clinically for several months prior to any intervention. Usually symmetric bilateral breast development occurs and nothing further is required. If the lesion becomes clinically suspicious, or there is overwhelming concern on the part of the family, the biopsy can be done. It is worthwhile to attempt fine needle aspiration with cytologic evaluation prior to excisional biopsy. If the nodule is cystic and disappears following aspiration, and the cytologic diagnosis is benign, the possibility of carcinoma is virtually eliminated. The fine needle aspiration with cytologic examination will eliminate the need for biopsy should malignant cells be identified. In that case, definitive treatment would be planned. If a biopsy becomes necessary, it is best done through a limited circumareolar incision with removal of minimal tissue for diagnosis. This must be done carefully to minimize the potential cosmetic deformity.

In addition to its rarity, most prepubertal breast cancer has a relatively indolent natural history.[16,31] This, too, should slow the hand of the surgeon. Most cases of childhood breast cancer have a characteristic secretory growth pattern, which is readily identifiable and is typically associated with slow growth and infrequent metastases.[31,32] Delay in diagnosis has been frequent in the childhood reports, but it does not necessarily lead to a poor result. In the McDivitt and Stewart experience, the time interval from discovery of a breast nodule to biopsy was as much as five years.[26] Only one of these seven children had a local recurrence; the other six remained free of disease up to 15 years postoperatively. Haagensen has reported a case involving a girl who had excision of a breast cancer at the age of 16 after the nodule had been documented for the preceding 11 years.[16] Although the lesion proved to be an infiltrating ductal carcinoma histologically, local excision alone proved adequate and she remained free of disease for 25 years and through two pregnancies.

Although this indolent clinical course is the rule, not all breast cancer in children behaves in this fashion.[8,31,36] Both regional and disseminated metastatic disease are reported as well as the occurrence of aggressive inflammatory carcinoma.[7,28] Oberman and Stephens concluded that the clinical course of children with breast cancer is related more to the histologic type of cancer rather than the age of the patient.[32] Carcinomas with a secretory pattern have a more benign clinical course, whereas tumors of either epithelial or mesenchymal origin without the secretory growth pattern behave more aggressively.

Mammography in children is not helpful. The density of normal developing breast tissue makes interpretation unreliable, and because the effects of irradiation are cumulative, efforts should be made to minimize the exposure in children and young women. We have abandoned its use in children and adolescents.

Treatment of children with breast cancer has generally consisted of total excision; procedures from simple excisional biopsy to radical mastectomy have been described.[7,8,19,26,28,36] No experience is large enough to allow definitive conclusions. Our approach is to select treatment based upon microscopic findings and extent of nodal disease. Therefore, biopsy of a persistent and suspicious lesion, if positive, is followed by excision of the primary tumor and axillary node dissection. The role of adjuvant chemotherapy and irradiation in children with breast cancer is not defined.

DIAGNOSIS

Early diagnosis of cancer remains the primary objective of any physician who cares for women with breast disease. This is, of course, because prognosis is dependent upon the stage of disease at the time treatment is begun. Early detection of breast cancer permits treatment before spread of disease to local or regional sites. Self-examination is without question the most common and useful method of detecting breast tumors.[7,25] In one study by Lesnick, 84% of breast tumors were detected by the patient, while only 14% were discovered by a physician on routine examination.[24] Efforts at public education have clearly been helpful in this regard. Given the simplicity and importance of self-examination in both old and young women, we emphasize its use in every adult woman.

Screening mammography has proved to be a rapid, relatively inexpensive tool for the detection of some occult breast cancers. In general, mammographic screening is advised for women beyond 40 years of age. Below this age threshold, the yield is low. Diagnostic accuracy becomes limited because of breast density, and the cumulative risks of multiple diagnostic irradiations mount. For these reasons, screening mammography in young women is generally reserved for those at high risk, for preoperative exam of the contralateral breast in a woman with known breast cancer, and for limited examination in certain clinical settings.

Microscopic examination of a biopsy specimen is the "gold standard" for establishing the diagnosis of breast cancer. Fine needle aspiration and cytological examination can, however, be very reliable in experienced hands and, if positive, may obviate the need for surgical biopsy.[3] If aspiration cytologic examination is negative, and the lesion is suspicious or the patient is at high risk, excisional biopsy is mandatory. We routinely perform excisional biopsy using local anesthesia in patients who are 15 years of age or older. In the unusual biopsy in a child below 15 years of age, or when special circumstances would make local anesthesia difficult, general anesthesia is used. Most biopsies in our hospital are performed on an outpatient basis even if general anesthesia is required. If carcinoma is suspected, and if at least one gram of neoplasm is available, a portion of the tissue specimen is frozen for subsequent estrogen and progesterone receptor assay.

In Egan's 1975 report, the overall incidence of malignancy among surgical breast biopsies was 6% in women less than 39 years of age. This increased to 26% in women between 39 and 62 years of age, and was 62% among women older than 62 years.[12] Preoperative planning has become very important, because wide local excision at the time of biopsy may be sufficient therapy for the selected patients who can be managed with "lumpectomy" and irradiation.

TREATMENT

The treatment of breast cancer is primarily dependent upon histological and clinical staging rather than the age of the patient. Clinical staging is determined independently of age. We currently use the Columbia Clinical Classification. Histological staging is discussed in detail below.

In the last decade, a number of treatment alternatives to the Halsted radical mastectomy have emerged. Most of the emphasis has been directed at minimizing surgical morbidity by preserving or reconstructing the breast. Procedures such as lumpectomy, tylectomy, segmental breast resection, and partial or simple mastectomy are all performed, and the results compare favorably with historical alternatives. It is important to emphasize that, for breast salvage procedures to be practical, a primary tumor must be small to permit wide local excision without creating a significant cosmetic defect. Similarly, multifocal disease precludes breast preservation. When combined with appropriate adjuvant chemotherapy and irradiation, preservation of the breast can be achieved with survival equal to that of more extensive classical surgical procedures.

The axillary lymph node dissection is a critical surgical component of all breast-saving procedures, not primarily as a curative extirpative procedure, but as a means of obtaining accurate nodal staging information for subsequent decisions regarding adjuvant chemotherapy. Therapy for women with breast cancer is now highly individualized, taking into account patient preferences, social situation, risk factors, and hormone receptor status in addition to the clinical stage of the disease and microscopic pattern.

Evolution of the collaborative breast care center concept has aided considerably in these efforts. In many ways, adult breast cancer groups, comprising specialists from surgery, diagnostic radiology, radiation oncology, pathology, and medical oncology, resemble the groups that have been in place for some time in the pediatric oncology community. Specific details of the diagnostic and management aspects of breast cancer are presented elsewhere in this text.

PROGNOSIS

Although a number of authors have reported a poorer survival for young women who develop breast cancer, it is not clear that age is the critical variable.[34,42] Conflicting reports in the literature make it difficult to evaluate the relationship of age and prognosis with certainty.

Schwartz and Zeok reported a ten-year follow-up of 111 women 30 years of age or younger from the Philadelphia County Medical Society Breast Cancer Registry who had histologically proved carcinoma of the breast.[42] Sixty-six (59.5%) were clinically classified as Stage A, twenty-one (18.9%) as Stage B, ten (9.2%) as Stage C, and seven (6.3%) as Stage D. Seven patients (6.3%) could not be classified retrospectively. Of the patients with clinical Stage A disease, 40.9% had negative lymph nodes, while 39.4% had at least one node positive for metastatic carcinoma. Of the patients with Stage B carcinoma, 9.5% had negative lymph nodes, and 85% had at least one positive node. Overall ten-year survivals for patients with Stage A, B, C, and D were 40.9%, 28.6%, 20%, and 0% respectively. When the histologic picture of the lymph nodes is taken into consideration, 66.7% of the Stage A women with negative axillary nodes were alive at ten years. This is very similar to the results reported for older women. These authors concluded that the survival rate in young women with breast cancer is equivalent to that of older women when the cancer is early (clinical Stage A), with uninvolved regional lymph nodes. Once the regional lymph nodes became involved, the prognosis for these young women was worse than for older patients. Regardless of clinical stage, the ten-year survival rate if lymph nodes are positive is poor, comprising only 16% of subjects in this series of young women. If metastatic disease is extensive (four or more positive axillary nodes), both young and older groups of women do equally badly.

In a similar ten-year study of young women from Sweden, 91 cases of breast cancer were reviewed.[50] The authors found no difference between the survival rate of young women and older women regardless of axillary lymph node status. Norris and Taylor reported 135 women less than 30 years of age at the time of diagnosis from the Armed Forces Institute of Pathology.[29] When only infiltrating ductal carcinoma was considered, the actuarial five-year survival rate in these young women was 56% and 37% at ten years. Patients without axillary metastases had survival rates of 81% at five years and 74% at ten years. They concluded that young patients had a poor prognosis for the following reasons: 1) about 10% of the series consisted of pregnant or lactating women, and this may be associated with a higher probability of axillary nodal disease; 2) the overall incidence of axillary nodal disease was higher in young women (57%) compared with a control group of older women (49%); 3) contralateral carcinoma developed in 17% of the patients; 4) for reasons that were unclear, women without advanced disease (only one or two lymph nodes positive), did more poorly than expected. On the positive side, women under 30 were found to have a relatively high proportion of low grade, infrequently metastasizing tumors. Medullary, intraductal, juvenile, papillary, and well-differentiated tumors represented 24% of the total series, and these women did as well as older women with similar neoplasms.

Noyes and colleagues reviewed the cases of 125 young women treated at the M.D. Anderson Hospital between 1945 and 1977.[30] They found that overall disease-free survival in these young women was poorer than that of older women with similar cancers. Young women with negative lymph nodes, and those with lesions less than 5 cm in diameter, had significantly diminished survival when compared with older women with comparable lesions.

In summary, an estimation of prognosis for a given patient is inexact. Clinical stage and, to a lesser extent, pathological type, are much more important than a patient's age. Several more recent measures of biologic activity, such as nuclear DNA content, thymidine labelling index, and S-phase fraction, promise to be good indicators of growth rate, and therefore of prognosis; however, these methods are not available clinically at this time. Currently, extent of axillary nodal metastases is the single most important determinant of outcome, and should be paramount when planning therapy and counseling young patients.

BREAST CANCER IN PREGNANCY

Breast cancer during pregnancy or lactation is not common but is invariably a cause of great concern. The fetus, as well as the mother, needs consideration, and therefore, decisions regarding diagnosis, treatment, and adjuvant therapy become more difficult. Delay of maternal treatment or termination of pregnancy become significant and emotional issues that must be resolved. We will briefly summarize some of our approaches to these issues.

Incidence of Breast Cancer in Pregnancy

Between 1% and 4% of all breast cancers are discovered in women who are pregnant or lactating.[2,38,48,49] The average age among these patients is 34 years.[49] Stated differently, approximately 1 of every 5000 pregnant women will develop breast cancer during gestation or lactation.[48] Pregnant and lactating women may be more susceptible to breast cancer for reasons related to the dramatic breast epithelial proliferation prior to beginning lactation, because of persistent estrogen and progesterone stimulation, and because the immunologic status of the mother is apparently altered.[11,22,23,49] Each of these factors has been suggested by way of explaining the oncogenesis of breast cancer, but none has convincing scientific support.

Breast duct epithelial proliferation begins shortly after conception and persists for the first half of pregnancy. It involves the stimulation of intraductal epithelial cells to form additional lobular ducts and expanded lobules. Following delivery, lactation is initiated and controlled hormonally by the pituitary. When lactation is terminated, atrophy of lobular mammary epithelium occurs. Whether these normal physiologic changes predispose a woman to the development of breast cancer is not known.[2,10,22,23,38,48] Rapidly proliferating epithelium may be at increased risk for carcinogen-induced or environmental injury, but evidence for this in breast cancer is circumstantial.

Diagnosis of Breast Cancer in Pregnancy

Delay in diagnosis and treatment of breast cancer is common in pregnant patients.[10] It was recently reported that physicians are slower to respond to a breast mass in pregnant patients; an average delay of more than two months between discovery of a nodule and initiation of treatment occurred when there was a coexistent pregnancy.[2] It is important, therefore, for physicians providing obstetrical care to remain aware and responsive to a breast mass in this setting. The assumption cannot be made that all masses are benign or related to impending lactation.

Diagnostic alternatives for breast masses arising during pregnancy may include mammography. Although we do not use screening mammography in pregnant women because of the low yield in this age group, selected women may benefit from mammographic evaluation when a breast mass appears. Proper shielding and modern film screen techniques with minimal radiation scatter make mammography relatively safe during pregnancy.[37] Mammograms are somewhat less helpful in this setting for specific masses because the increased breast tissue density that is normal with pregnancy makes interpretation difficult.[49] We occasionally use mammography during pregnancy and believe that it can be done safely.

Most often, our approach to a suspicious breast mass in a pregnant woman is to proceed as rapidly as possible with surgical excision and microscopic evaluation. This is best done under local anesthesia to minimize the risk to the fetus. Fine needle aspiration with cytologic examination can be done prior to biopsy and, if positive, will allow definitive surgical excision without preliminary diagnostic biopsy. General anesthesia is not necessarily contraindicated, but does have specific risks to the fetus. Byrd and colleagues reported only one fetal death in 134 breast biopsies performed in pregnant women using general anesthesia.[6]

Treatment of Breast Cancer in Pregnancy

Haagensen and Stout once wrote that the pregnant woman with breast cancer was incurable and therefore not a surgical candidate.[17] Although Haagensen later reversed this opinion, it remains true today that the treatment of pregnant women with breast cancer is altered in ways that may not be desirable.[15]

Clinical staging of the pregnant patient is the same as the staging of the nonpregnant patient. Risk to the fetus from standard imaging studies for evaluation of metastatic disease, however, is considerable. Fetal development is characterized by three phases: fertilization to implantation (days 0 to 10); organogenesis (days 11 to 56); and growth (more than 57 days).[18] The highest risk of radiation-induced fetal injury occurs during organogenesis,[49] often before a woman is aware of her pregnancy. If at all possible, irradiation during this period should be avoided or minimized. Radiation-induced fetal injury is manifested by a variety of congenital anomalies, particularly those involving the central nervous system. Because the central nervous system continues to develop well into the postnatal period, it remains at some risk for injury throughout gestation. This was clearly and tragically illustrated among the Japanese infants who were exposed in utero to large doses of radiation at the time of the 1945 Hiroshima bombing.[21,49] Subsequently, it has become clear that there is a relationship between in utero radiation exposure and the development of childhood leukemia.[49] Additionally, chromosomal abnormalities, such as trisomy 21, have been linked to fetal irradiation. There are very little data regarding the human threshold levels for radiation-induced fetal injury.

With these potential problems in mind, the physician caring for a pregnant woman with breast cancer still must properly stage the extent of disease prior to treatment. We currently recommend that a pregnant patient with breast cancer at least consider the option of terminating the pregnancy, particularly if she is in the first trimester. If a pregnancy is to be continued, it is highly desirable, and usually possible, to perform the imaging evaluation, computerized tomography, liver-spleen scan, and bone scan, at a time other than the first two months when the risk to the fetus is greatest. For women later in pregnancy, diagnostic radiation is less of a risk and is used judiciously where therapeutic decisions for the mother's treatment must be made.

Surgical therapy for pregnant women should be prompt and simple. For the majority of women with surgically resectable breast tumors, we recommend mastectomy. A decision to terminate the pregnancy is not mandatory. With careful general anesthesia, the risk to the mother and the fetus is slight.[49] Some breast cancers in pregnant women appear to respond favorably to elimination of the fetus and placenta. If the diagnosis of breast cancer is made close to the projected delivery date, a decision to allow a normal conclusion of the pregnancy is reasonable. Some authors have advocated cesarean section with mastectomy at the time of delivery to eliminate a second anesthesia.[49] If necessary, serial amniocentesis with lecithin/sphingomyelin ratios will allow reliable estimations of fetal lung maturity, minimizing the risk to the fetus and allowing optimal timing of the procedure.

In women with locally advanced breast cancer early in pregnancy, we recommend termination of the pregnancy. Late in pregnancy, the delivery should be performed as soon as possible. Therapy for the postpartum patient should be no different than under other circumstances. Pregnant patients with axillary nodes positive for metastatic disease require chemotherapy. The risk of chemotherapy to the fetus is clear and significant.[41,47] Therefore, we recommend termination of the pregnancy either by therapeutic abortion or, when feasible, delivery of the child prior to chemotherapy. In the event that these options are not available, chemotherapy can still be used, although it carries substantial risk. Animal studies have demonstrated a spectrum of congenital malformations associated with chemotherapeutic agents given during gestation.[49] At least two clinical reports of pregnant patients receiving chemotherapy substantiate these concerns in humans.[27]

The decision regarding termination of pregnancy is generally based upon many factors. The biologic behavior of the breast cancer is not necessarily affected whether the pregnancy is terminated or allowed to continue. The need for irradiation or adjuvant chemotherapy, however, places the fetus at significant risk for injury or developmental anomaly. In these situations, termination of the pregnancy becomes desirable.

Alternative surgical treatments offered to nonpregnant patients, such as quadrantectomy or lumpectomy followed by local irradiation, exceed safe irradiation limits for the fetus. Therefore, these are not reasonable choices in the pregnant patient who elects to continue her pregnancy. Only if the fetus is to be aborted should this treatment option be considered.

Prognosis in Breast Cancer in Pregnancy

Several authors have reported poorer survival rates in women with gestational breast cancer when compared with nonpregnant women. Overall five-year survival rates vary between 19% and 48%.[2,6,49] Upon careful examination, however, it appears that survival correlates most strongly with the clinical and pathological staging of the disease; particularly important is the axillary lymph node status. The presence of axillary metastases is a highly unfavorable finding in both pregnant and nonpregnant women. Pregnant women do have more advanced disease when initially diagnosed. Among women with gestational breast cancer and negative lymph nodes, the five-year survival is between 65% and 85%, which compares favorably with women with nongestational breast cancer.[2,6,38]

SUMMARY

Breast cancer in the young or pregnant patient is an uncommon occurrence with several areas of specific diagnostic and therapeutic concern. Prompt evaluation, accurate clinical and histological staging, and cooperative multimodal therapy yield good results in both pregnant and young women. Individualized treatment plans will allow most of these women to achieve the same success we see in older women with breast cancer.

REFERENCES

1. Anderson DE, Badzioch MD: Survival in familial breast cancer patients. Cancer 58:360, 1986.

2. Applewhite RR, Smith LR, DiVincenti F: Carcinoma of the breast associated with pregnancy and lactation. Am Surg 39:101, 1973.
3. Barrows GH, Anderson TJ, Lamb JL, et al.: Fine-needle aspiration of breast cancer. Relationship of clinical factors to cytology results in 689 primary malignancies. Cancer 58:1493, 1986.
4. Boffard K, Clark GMG, Irvine JBD, et al.: Serum prolactin, androgens, oestradiol and progesterone in adolescent girls with or without a family history of breast cancer. Eur J Cancer Clin Oncol 17:1071, 1981.
5. Brinton LA, Hoover R, Fraumeni JF Jr: Reproductive factors in the etiology of breast cancer. Br J Cancer 47:757, 1983.
6. Byrd BF, Bayer DS, Robertson JDC, et al.: Treatment of breast tumors associated with pregnancy and lactation. Ann Surg 155:940, 1962.
7. Byrne MP, Fahey MM, Gooselaw JG: Breast cancer with axillary metastasis in an eight and one-half-year-old girl. Cancer 31:726, 1973.
8. Close MB, Maximov NG: Carcinoma of breast in young girls. Arch Surg 91:386, 1965.
9. Diekamp U, Bitran J, Ferguson DJ: Breast cancer in young women. J Reprod Med 17:255, 1976.
10. Donegan WL: Mammary carcinoma and pregnancy. Maj Prob Clin Surg 5:448, 1979.
11. Drife JO: Breast cancer, pregnancy, and the pill. Br Med J 283:778, 1981.
12. Egan RL: Breast biopsy priority: Cancer versus benign preoperative masses. Cancer 35:612, 1975.
13. Feldman AR, Kessler L, Myers MH, et al.: The prevalence of cancer. Estimates based on the Connecticut Tumor Registry. N Engl J Med 315:1394, 1986.
14. Fishman J, Fukushima D, O'Connor J, et al.: Plasma hormone profiles of young women at risk for familial breast cancer. Cancer Res 38:4006, 1978.
15. Haagensen CD: The treatment and results in cancer of the breast at the Presbyterian Hospital, New York. Am J Roentgenol 62:328, 1949.
16. Haagensen CD: Diseases of the Breast. Philadelphia, WB Saunders Co., 1986.
17. Haagensen CD, Stout AP: Carcinoma of the breast: Criteria of operability. Ann Surg 118:859, 1032, 1943.
18. Hall EJ: Radiobiology for the Radiologist. Philadelphia, Harper and Row, 1978, pp 397–410.
19. Hartman AW, Magbish P: Carcinoma of breast in children. Case Report: Six-year-old boy with adenocarcinoma. Ann Surg 141:792, 1955.
20. Host H, Lund E: Age as a prognostic factor in breast cancer. Cancer 57:2217, 1986.
21. Jablon S, Kato H: Childhood cancer in relation to prenatal exposure to atomic-bomb radiation. Lancet 2:1000, 1970.
22. Janerich DT: Pregnancy, breast cancer risk, and maternal-fetal genetics (letter). Lancet 1:327, 1979.

23. Janerich DT: The influence of pregnancy on breast cancer risk: Is it endocrinological or immunological? Med Hypotheses 6:1149, 1980.
24. Lesnick GJ: Detection of breast cancer in young women. JAMA 237:867, 1977.
25. Ligon RE, Stevenson DR, Diner W, et al.: Breast masses in young women. Am J Surg 140:779, 1980.
26. McDivitt RW, Stewart FW: Breast carcinoma in children. JAMA 195:144, 1966.
27. Murray CL, Reichert JA, Anderson J, et al.: Multimodal cancer therapy for breast cancer in the first trimester of pregnancy. JAMA 252:2607, 1984.
28. Nichini FM, Goldman L, Lapayowker MS, et al.: Inflammatory carcinoma of the breast in a 12-year-old girl. Arch Surg 105:505, 1972.
29. Norris HJ, Taylor HB: Carcinoma of the breast in women less than thirty years old. Cancer 26:953, 1970.
30. Noyes RD, Spanos WJ, Montague ED: Breast cancer in women aged 30 and under. Cancer 49:1302, 1982.
31. Oberman HA: Breast lesions in the adolescent female, in Sommers SC, Rosen PP (eds), *Pathology Annual 1979*. New York, Appleton-Century-Crofts, 1979, pp 175–201.
32. Oberman HA, Stephens PJ: Carcinoma of the breast in childhood. Cancer 30:470, 1972.
33. Oral contraceptive use and the risk of breast cancer in young women. MMWR 33:354, 1984.
34. Patterson WB: The prognosis of young women with breast cancer. Int J Radiat Oncol Biol Phys 4:699, 1978.
35. Pike MC, Henderson BE, Casagrande JT, et al.: Oral contraceptive use and early abortion as risk factors for breast cancer in young women. Br J Cancer 43:72, 1981.
36. Ramirez G, Ansfield FJ: Carcinoma of the breast in children. Arch Surg 96:222, 1968.
37. Rickert RR, Rajan S: Localized breast infarcts associated with pregnancy. Arch Pathol 97:159, 1974.
38. Rosemond GP: Carcinoma of the breast during pregnancy. Clin Obstet Gynecol 6:994, 1963.
39. Rosner D, Lane WW, Brett RP: Influence of oral contraceptives on the prognosis of breast cancer in young women. Cancer 55:1556, 1985.
40. Sattin RW, Rubin GL, Wingo PA, et al.: Oral-contraceptive use and the risk of breast cancer. N Engl J Med 315:405, 1986.
41. Schapira DV, Chudley AE: Successful pregnancy following continuous treatment with combination chemotherapy before conception and throughout pregnancy. Cancer 54:800, 1984.
42. Schwartz GF, Zeok JV: Carcinoma of the breast in young women. Am J Surg 131:570, 1976.
43. Seltzer MH, Skiles MS: Diseases of the breast in young women. Surg Gynecol Obstet 150:360, 1980.
44. Silverberg E, Lubera J: Cancer statistics, 1986. CA 36:9, 1986.

45. Skiles MS, Seltzer MH: Adolescent breast disease. J Med Soc NJ 77:891, 1980.
46. Stadel BV, Rubin GL, Webster LA, et al.: Oral contraceptives and breast cancer in young women. Lancet 2:970, 1985.
47. Sweet DL, Kinzie J: Consequences of radiotherapy and antineoplastic therapy for the fetus. J Reprod Med 17:241, 1976.
48. Torres JE, Nickal A: Carcinoma of the breast in pregnancy. Clin Obstet Gynecol 18:219, 1975.
49. Wallack MK, Wolf JA, Bedwinek J, et al.: Gestational carcinoma of female breast. Curr Prob Cancer 7:1, 1983.
50. Wallgren A, Silfversward C, Hultborn, A: Carcinoma of the breast in women under 30 years of age. A clinical and histopathological study of all cases reported as carcinoma to the Swedish Cancer Registry, 1958-1968. Cancer 40:916, 1977.

19. New Horizons in the Treatment of Breast Cancer

JOHN E. NIEDERHUBER
STEPHEN V. DESIDERIO

A number of features characteristic of breast cancer suggest directions for future investigations. Included among these are its responsiveness to therapy, its striking endocrine dependence, and its obvious heterogeneity. As the most common cause of cancer death in women, breast cancer disturbingly lacks a disease-free survival plateau.[27] This means that the risk for developing metastatic disease, although decreasing with time, continues well beyond 15 years. This aspect of the disease may be in part responsible for the difficulty of defining optimal therapy for any subset of breast cancer patients. Nevertheless, a number of advances have been made during the past ten years. Most notable for their impact on mortality are the successful treatment of micrometastases following control of the primary tumor [10,11,26,28,29,63,82] and the decreasing mortality in women over 50 years of age undergoing routine yearly screening mammography.[75]

This review addresses four general questions: 1) What new techniques can be developed to better identify patients at increased risk for recurrence? 2) What advances can be made toward defining optimal adjuvant therapy? 3) What is the future role of endocrine therapy in the adjuvant and advanced disease settings? 4) What new developments in molecular genetics hold promise for improving the diagnosis and treatment of breast cancer?

DETERMINING RISK

Recurrent breast cancer is known as a responsive tumor, with 60% to 70% of patients showing significant benefit from chemotherapy and hormonal therapy.[36] In addition, numerous studies throughout the world have consistently demonstrated that multiple-drug chemotherapy used in an adjuvant setting can result in a 25% reduction in mortality during the period of follow-up.[10,11,26,28,29,63,82] These improvements in overall survival using adjuvant chemotherapy have been most dramatic in premenopausal women. As a result, it is of paramount importance to determine 1) which women with Stage I disease will benefit from potentially toxic therapy, 2) which women with a poor prognosis (Stage II disease) deserve even more aggressive treatment, and 3) which women should receive therapy that includes endocrine manipulation.

At present, the natural history of breast cancer for a given patient is determined by neoplastic involvement of the axillary lymph nodes, the size of the primary tumor, the presence of steroid-hormone receptors, the patient's age or menopausal status, and the microscopic pattern of the tumor. In the adjuvant setting, the principal way of selecting patients at risk for relapse, and therefore to receive chemotherapy, has been according to the pathologic assessment of axillary node metastases. Clearly, this is an imperfect approach, and as many as a third of women without evidence of nodal disease go on to develop recurrence and eventually die of breast cancer.

Several areas of investigation hold promise for identifying better prognostic risk factors. These include the development of more sensitive assays for steroid hormone receptors, for cellular DNA content, and for tumor-specific antigens.

Predictive Value of Steroid Hormone Receptors

During the past 15 years, it has clearly been shown that the measurement of estrogen receptor content in a breast carcinoma can identify patients who are most likely to respond to endocrine therapy.[17,19,60] The extensive documentation of steroid hormone receptor levels has also suggested that the presence or absence of receptors may provide important prognostic information.[2,13,45,56] As a result, future investigations will need to address two important questions regarding the role of steroid hormone receptors in determining prognosis: 1) Does the level of estrogen receptor and progesterone receptor in the primary tumor correlate with survival? 2) Would patients whose primary tumor is positive for estrogen receptor and progesterone receptor benefit from adjuvant endocrine therapy? Stated another way, does the determination of estrogen and progesterone receptor levels have a place in the management of patients with primary breast cancer similar to its well-documented role in the treatment of metastatic disease?

The first observation regarding the use of estrogen receptors as a prognostic factor was published in 1977. In a recent review of this topic, McGuire discussed two studies of Stage I breast cancer with significant numbers of patients: a report from the Milan Cancer Institute and his own study from the San Antonio Receptor Data Base.[59] The Milan study, which was based on 464 patients with negative axillary lymph nodes, demonstrated that estrogen receptor–negative patients had a significantly ($p < .001$)

shorter relapse-free survival. The study of 1,647 patients in the San Antonio data base led to the conclusion that two factors significantly influenced disease-free survival of Stage I patients: estrogen receptor status and tumor volume. These observations differed from a similar analysis of factors predicting disease-free survival and overall survival for Stage II breast cancer. The analysis of Stage II patients indicates that the number of axillary nodes involved, the size of the tumor, and the level of progesterone receptor are most critical for predicting disease-free survival.[25]

As a predictor of the outcome of adjuvant treatment in Stage II patients, progesterone receptor levels appear to have greater significance than estrogen receptor levels.[13] Two studies support this conclusion. First, the National Surgical Adjuvant Breast Project (NSABP) trial B-09 showed that in premenopausal women with Stage II disease a difference in disease-free survival and overall survival existed between patients treated with chemotherapy and those treated with chemotherapy plus tamoxifen. This difference in survival was observed only in patients with either estrogen receptor–negative/progesterone receptor–negative or estrogen receptor–positive/progesterone receptor–negative assays. A somewhat surprising observation was the apparent adverse effect of tamoxifen treatment in patients who were progesterone receptor–negative.[25]

In the postmenopausal group, the addition of tamoxifen to chemotherapy was of significant benefit when the tumor was estrogen receptor–positive, progesterone receptor–positive. If, however, the tumor lacked progesterone receptors, then no benefit was found.[25,64] Two other trials have also shown that the presence of progesterone receptors is of predictive value in assessing the usefulness of tamoxifen as an adjuvant treatment in Stage II breast cancer patients.[13,16,59,64]

While considerable evidence supports the usefulness of steroid-binding assays for determining steroid hormone receptor levels, there are some patients with significant levels of estrogen receptor and progesterone receptor in their tumors that do not respond to endocrine therapy. Because the binding assays are performed on homogenates of tissue, they cannot discriminate between receptor derived from normal or nonmalignant breast cells and that actually derived from invasive cancer. In addition, because stromal cells are generally receptor-negative, a tumor with a heavy stromal content may yield a spuriously low receptor value. Even when all of the steroid hormone receptor of the sample is derived from cancer cells, a low or moderate determination could be the result of a small proportion of the cells containing a high concentration of receptor or a high proportion of the cells containing a low concentration of receptor.

Thus, there are a number of advantages of using receptor-specific monoclonal antibodies and immunocytochemical methods to determine both the content and distribution of the steroid receptors.[18,32,38,42,50,66,68] Recent reports indicate a strong correlation between the distribution of stained cells and their overall staining intensity, on the one hand, and the quantitative estrogen receptor steroid binding assay value, on the other.[18] Monoclonal antibodies to estrogen receptors have the advantage of direct antigenic recognition of the receptor molecules. They recognize the receptor protein independent of the presence or absence of estradiol in the receptor binding site. Recently techniques have been developed which bind the monoclonal antiestrogen receptor antibodies to beads, which are then used in an enzyme immunoassay to measure the amount of receptor protein.[42,50]

These new studies appear to indicate that the prognostic value of the immunocytochemical monoclonal antibody assay and the proportion of immunocytochemical-positive tumor cells are each independent of lymph node status.[18] Direct evaluation of this assay indicates that consideration of the lymph node status along with the estrogen receptor immunocytochemistry of the tumor stratifies the patient population into distinct risk groups.

Predictive Value of Cell Kinetics

A number of studies have suggested that the doubling time of breast cancer cells is a strong prognostic indicator.[31,35,58,61,77,84] The proliferative characteristics of these cells have generally been quantitated by the in vitro thymidine labeling index (TLI).[61,77,84] For the determination of TLI, fresh tissue slices are incubated with tritiated thymidine in the presence of floxuridine and hyperbaric oxygen. The tissue slice is then fixed, processed, and thin sections are autoradiographed. The TLI is determined by counting the percentage of nuclei labeled.[62] Normal breast epithelium and benign proliferative epithelium were shown to have a median TLI of 0.2% to 0.65%.[3] Invasive breast cancer was found to have a median TLI of 5.2%. The TLI appeared to decrease with patient age and to be lower in tumors lacking significant levels of estrogen receptor and progesterone receptor, but was clearly correlated with tumor size, nuclear anaplasia, and degree of dedifferentiation of the tumor.[62] From these studies, it appeared that a high TLI was associated with an increased probability of disease recurrence, and several studies have shown this to be independent of stage.[61]

Other approaches designed to improve detection of labeled nuclei have used 5-bromodeoxyuridine (BUDR) instead of tritiated thymidine. The BUDR that has been incorporated into DNA is detected by a specific antibody.[31] Even with technical improvements, the TLI does not easily distinguish between normal and malignant cells in a given tissue sample and does not accurately reflect the heterogeneity of the tumor. Combination of the BUDR or tritiated thymidine-labeling techniques with either flow cytometry or image analysis may allow resolution of the different cell populations present in breast cancers.

Newer approaches for the assessment of proliferation in asynchronous, heterogeneous tumor cell populations have used flow cytometry. Flow cytometry can evaluate both the DNA content of tumor cells- and the percentage of cells in S-phase.[58] This method, however, is limited in its ability to detect minor tumor stemlines, which could affect its value in predicting risk for recurrence and therapeutic response.

Recently, Allison and colleagues have combined flow cytometry distribution and absorption cytometry to resolve the DNA distributions of aneuploid tumor and normal host cells present in a heterogeneous tumor.[3] These investigators used an image analysis system equipped with a computerized scanning stage to identify S-phase cells.

These new approaches for assessing the kinetic indices of a tumor hold significant promise for identifying patients at high risk for recurrence[35] and should be especially helpful in selecting a subset of Stage I patients for whom adjuvant therapy would be beneficial. Such indices may also provide criteria for the selection of specific therapeutic drug combinations in the treatment of recurrent disease.

Monoclonal Antibodies

The advent of monoclonal antibody technology in 1975 was one of the most significant advances in modern biomedical research.[46] Monoclonal antibodies are produced by fusing B-lymphocytes from an animal that has been immunized against the target antigen with a drug-selected murine myeloma cell. The hybrid cell resulting from this fusion can be selected by screening culture supernatants for an antibody of desired specificity and immunoglobulin isotype.

Monoclonal antibodies have a number of potential biomedical uses. Future studies will focus on developing their use for the detection of occult malignancy; for phenotyping cancer cells in a given tumor; for determining the degree of tumor cell dedifferentiation; for the detection of specific receptors and growth factors; for the identification of oncogene and proto-oncogene products; for the detection of circulating tumor antigens; and eventually for targeting cytolytic therapy. While a large number of monoclonal antibodies reactive with breast cancer have been produced, only a small number are reactive with breast epithelium.[81]

Monoclonal antibody B72.3, a murine IgG1, is perhaps the best characterized.[14] This antibody recognizes a greater than 10^6 dalton glycoprotein (TAG-72).[41] TAG-72 also appears to be present on fetal gastrointestinal tissue, suggesting that it is an oncofetal antigen.[80] The monoclonal antibody B72.3, which recognizes TAG-72, was reactive with 96% of breast cancers and did not appear to react with normal tissue. The antibody has been used to confirm the diagnosis of cancer in fine needle aspiration breast biopsies and has been able to detect breast cancer cells in effusions.[55]

Results such as those with B72.3 have resulted in increased efforts to use monoclonal antibodies to localize occult tumor by external body scintigraphy. Encouraging results have been reported by a number of investigators.[21,24,49,78] Even so, the question of specificity will need to be addressed in future trials by the simultaneous use of specific and nonspecific radiolabeled monoclonal antibodies of the same immunoglobulin subclass. In addition, studies will need to be performed to determine the absolute amount of antibody uptake in both tumor and normal tissue.

As noted in a previous section, there has been a long-standing interest in producing monoclonal antibodies specific for steroid hormone receptors. Monoclonal antibodies to the estrogen receptor have the advantage of recognizing the receptor independent of the presence or absence of estradiol in the receptor binding site. To date, several antibodies have yielded promising results when used in a radioimmunoassay (RIA) or enzyme-linked immunoabsorbant assay (ELISA).[18,42,50]

Monoclonal antibodies have a potential application in the specific targeting of tumor therapy. From the standpoint of therapy, a monoclonal antibody could act alone, relying on host cell–mediated cytotoxicity or on other Fc receptor–bearing cells to produce antibody dependent cell-mediated cytotoxicity. In addition, monoclonal antibodies can be coupled to toxins (usually bacterial or plant toxins) or to isotopes, thereby directing these agents to specific cells. Using monoclonal antibodies for this purpose has proved more difficult than anticipated.[22] It has been hard to accomplish selective targeting to tumor tissue and to prevent rapid removal of radioactive iodine from the antibody. The host obviously recognizes these antibodies as foreign protein and develops its own antibodies to the murine monoclonal antibodies.

The future, however, promises important uses for these highly specific reagents.[71] Problems related to the varied expression of tumor-associated antigens and the heterogeneity of targeted tumors could be overcome by using a panel of antibodies that included all specificities required. It is possible that the host immune response to the murine antibody could be circumvented by using only the (Fab)$_2$ fragment, since most host antibodies appear to be directed at the Fc portion of the molecule. Recently, recombinant DNA techniques have been used to create recombinant murine-human chimeric antibody which fuses the human immunoglobulin constant regions with murine variable regions.[79]

Also new on the horizon has been the development of anti-idiotype monoclonal antibodies. In this approach, monoclonal antibody specific for a given tumor-associated antigen is used as an immunogen to produce new monoclonal antibodies selected for their specific reactivity with the tumor antigen binding site (idiotype) on the original antibody. Much work has demonstrated previously that specific anti-idiotypic antibodies are an "internal image" of the antigen. As such, they provide a possible way to actively immunize the host against a tumor.[37,51]

SYSTEMIC ADJUVANT THERAPY

Trials comparing patients receiving postoperative adjuvant chemotherapy to untreated controls have shown a significant increase in disease-free survival and in overall survival in the treated group. This decrease in mortality is perhaps as great as 25% in Stage II breast cancer.[10,11,26,28,29,63,82] The results of trials indicate that combination chemotherapy is better than single agent therapy and that results in women over age 50 are less dramatic than in premenopausal women.[7,15,26,28,89] While these findings represent a major advance in the treatment of breast cancer, much work remains to be done.

First, it will still be necessary to weigh the risks and benefits of therapy employing individual agents and combinations of agents whether the drug is cytotoxic or endocrine-specific. Drug toxicities include infertility, cardiac toxicity (with regimens containing doxorubicin), and induction of new cancers, especially myeloproliferative syndrome and leukemia (with the long-term administration of alkylating agents). On the positive side are indications that this risk is relatively low (1.3%) and that no cases occur after seven years.

Second, a number of questions need to be systematically addressed by future trials. For example, how soon should chemotherapy be started? Is there a place for neo-adjuvant therapy? What combinations of drugs are optimal and on what schedules and what dose intensity? What are the interactions with other therapy, such as endocrine or radiation? Preliminary answers to these questions certainly seem to allay earlier fears that combining chemotherapy with radiation would compromise the ability to give full dose systemic chemotherapy. Administration of radiation, in fact, does not seem to decrease hematologic reserves, but may have some effect on normal tissue sensitivity.

ENDOCRINE THERAPY

The advent of antiestrogen therapy and, more recently, the introduction of the aromatase-inhibitor aminoglutethimide as a reversible substitute therapy for adrenalectomy have brought about new options for clinical trials. Aminoglutethimide acts by blocking a series of hydroxylations responsible for the conversion of cholesterol to adrenal steroids. In addition, there is inhibition of aromatization steps, causing a change in the A-ring and a block of androgen conversion to estrogens. Studies have shown that aminoglutethimide therapy is equivalent to adrenalectomy or hypophysectomy and has the added benefit of being reversible. As a result of the successful use of these agents, recent work has suggested the potential benefit of using luteinizing hormone–releasing hormone analogues to suppress follicular stimulating hormone levels and luteinizing hormone levels.[33,57]

This new medical approach to endocrine ablation has virtually eliminated surgical ablative procedures.

The antiestrogens were shown in the early 1960s to cause regression of breast cancer metastases and to do so with much less toxicity than experienced with other hormonal agents.[30] As a result of these studies, the synthetic triphenylethylene, tamoxifen, has become essentially standard therapy. Tamoxifen appears to function primarily as a cytostatic agent and not a cytocidal drug. If this is the case, it will be necessary to evaluate the role of long-term tamoxifen therapy.[43,83] Tamoxifen may also have a potential role in combination with estrogens to effect synchronization of tumor cells prior to treatment with chemotherapeutic agents. Finally, it has been observed that long-term administration of tamoxifen in animal models can prevent carcinogenic induction of breast cancer.[43] These laboratory studies raise the interesting possibility that women having a high risk of developing breast cancer could benefit from prophylactic administration of tamoxifen. Clinical trials will need to be performed to determine the benefits of such therapy compared to risks of osteoporosis and heart disease secondary to antiestrogen.

APPLICATIONS OF MOLECULAR GENETICS TO BREAST CANCER RESEARCH

A large body of evidence indicates a direct association between specific alterations at the DNA level and neoplastic growth.[4,65,70,88] The evidence that has accumulated over the past five years has identified a number of genes whose structure or level of expression is altered in tumors as compared to normal tissues. These observations are the result of two distinct lines of experimentation. The first of these approaches dates from Peyton Rous's discovery, in 1911, that an avian sarcoma could be transmitted by a filterable agent.[69] The agent was later shown to be one of a family of RNA-containing viruses called retroviruses; many such viruses have since been found to cause tumors in animals.[7,8] In a number of cases, the viral genes responsible for cellular transformation have been identified and characterized at the nucleotide level.[6]

A second approach stemmed from the remarkable observation that DNA isolated from some tumors could transmit the transformed phenotype when introduced into nontransformed recipient cells.[48,76] These two approaches converged somewhat surprisingly with the discovery that the cellular genes responsible for transformation in the DNA-transfection experiments were homologous to previously identified transforming genes of RNA tumor viruses.[20,66]

The RNA genomes of retroviruses are transcribed into DNA by reverse transcription and then integrated into the host genome.[85] Integration of the viral DNA into the DNA of the cell may alter the expression of cellular genes by placing them under control of viral regulatory elements.[34,67] Alternatively, cellular genes may become incorporated into the viral genome and subsequently transmitted to other cells by viral infection.[5]

The transforming genes of RNA tumor viruses (termed "oncogenes") are clearly derived from cellular counterparts ("proto-oncogenes"), although the exact mechanisms whereby these cellular genes were captured by retroviruses remain unclear. At present, more than a dozen retroviral oncogenes are known; in many instances, their cellular counterparts have also been implicated in tumor genesis.[76] The proteins encoded by these genes are presumed to play critical roles in normal cell growth and differentiation; in several instances, their roles are known or suspected. For example, some proto-oncogenes encode growth factors or growth factor receptors, while others encode GTP-binding proteins that may function in signal transduction.[9,39,40,86,87]

Altered Gene Expression in Breast Cancer

Amplified DNA sequences have been found in some mammalian cancers; these amplified sequences may include proto-oncogenes. For example, a gene related to c-*myc* (N-*myc*) has been shown to be amplified in several tumors.[1,12,52,72] The presence of amplified proto-oncogenes is significant because of their association with cellular proliferation.

In a recent study, 89 untreated primary neuroblastomas were assayed for amplification of the N-*myc* gene.[74] The degree of N-*myc* amplification in these patients was found to be directly related to stage and prognosis. Similarly, amplification of the c-*myc* gene was found in 32% of 121 patients with primary breast cancer.[23] In other studies, expression of the P21 protein encoded by genes of the *ras* family was found to be significantly elevated in primary breast cancer patients with involvement of more than three axillary nodes.[54]

While the present data do not establish a causal link between gene amplification and malignancy, the identification of specific patterns of gene amplification and expression could provide a means of identifying subsets of breast cancer patients with poor prognosis. This would be especially useful in identifying patients with Stage I disease who might benefit from adjuvant chemotherapy. Such information would also be very useful in developing new therapeutic strategies for Stage II women with a high probability of therapeutic failure. An alternative strategy, for example, might be the use of high dose chemotherapy with autologous marrow transplant.

Molecular Genetic Approach to Understanding Drug Resistance

Breast cancer is one of the adult solid tumors in which almost all patients (60% to 70%) who develop metastatic disease can initially be treated effectively with chemotherapy. Nevertheless, in time these previously responsive breast tumors develop multiple drug resistance.[53] Recent studies suggest that cells exhibiting resistance to multiple drugs undergo similar physiologic changes, and recently, several laboratories have demonstrated a new membrane glycoprotein in resistant cells that binds to a variety of chemotherapeutic agents.[44] Other agents such as calcium channel blockers also bind to this glycoprotein and in so doing are able to reverse cell resistance.[47] The gene that encodes this membrane glycoprotein, *mdr'*, has been cloned and has been shown to be over-expressed in drug-resistant cells.[73] Multiple drug resistance can be transferred to sensitive cells by the introduction of the *mdr'* gene. These discoveries suggest several potentially fruitful approaches to the prevention or circumvention of resistance.

SUMMARY

As physicians treating breast cancer, we must constantly remind ourselves that this is a cancer of many subsets, if not, in fact, many diseases. Some of these subsets will fail rapidly, while some will respond more or less to different therapies. Thus, the direction of future study is to identify those subsets with a high probability of early metastatic spread, to determine the degree of heterogeneity within a given tumor, and to identify therapeutic resistance(s) present in primary or metastatic tumor. The new laboratory technologies of molecular immunology and molecular genetics promise exciting advances. Much more will be learned about the molecular derangements that underlie the malignant phenotype, and new treatment options with greater therapeutic specificity will certainly evolve from these laboratory efforts.

REFERENCES

1. Alitalo K, Schwab M: Oncogene amplification in tumor cells. Adv Cancer Res 47:235–281, 1986.
2. Allegra JC, Lippman ME, Simon R, et al.: Association between steroid hormone receptor status and disease-free interval in breast cancer. Cancer Treat Rep 63:1271–1277, 1979.
3. Allison DC, Chakerian M, Ridolpho PF, et al.: Combined flow and absorption DNA measurements of (^{3}H) thymidine-labeled tumor cells. I. Studies of MCA-11 cells grown as tumors *in vitro* and as exponential cultures *in vitro*. Cell Tissue Kinetics (in press).

4. Ames BN: Identifying environmental chemicals causing mutations and cancer. Science 204:587–593, 1979.
5. Baltimore D, Rosenberg N, Witte ON: Transformation of immature lymphoid cells by Abelson murine leukemia virus. Immunol Rev 48:3–22, 1979.
6. Bishop JM, Varmus HE: Functions and origins of retroviral transforming genes, in *Molecular Biology of Tumor Viruses: RNA Tumor Viruses Ed 2*. Cold Spring Harbor, NY, Cold Spring Harbor Press, Vol 1, pp 999–1108, Vol 2, pp 249–356, 1987.
7. Bishop JM: Cellular oncogenes and retroviruses. Ann Rev Biochem 52:301–354, 1983.
8. Bishop JM: The molecular genetics of cancer. Science 235:305–311, 1987.
9. Bishop JM: Viral oncogenes. Cell 42:23–38, 1985.
10. Bonadonna G, Valagussa P: Adjuvant chemoendocrine therapy in breast cancer. J Clin Onco 4:451–454, 1986.
11. Bonadonna G, Valagussa P, Rossi A, et al.: Ten-year experience with CMF-based adjuvant chemotherapy in resectable breast cancer. Breast Cancer Res Treat 5:95–115, 1985.
12. Brodeur G, Seeger RC, Schwab M, et al.: Amplification of N-*myc* in untreated human neuroblastomas correlates with advanced disease stage. Science 224:1121–1124, 1984.
13. Clark GM, McGuire WL, Hubay CA, et al.: Progesterone receptors as a prognostic factor in stage II breast cancer. N Engl J Med 309:1343–1347, 1983.
14. Colcher D, Horan H and P, Nuti M, et al.: A spectrum of monoclonal antibodies reactive with mammary tumor cells. Proc Natl Acad Sci USA 78:3199–3203, 1981.
15. Cooper RG: Combination chemotherapy in hormone resistant breast cancer. Proc Am Assoc Cancer Res 10:15 (abstract), 1969.
16. Cummings FJ, Gray R, Davis TE, et al.: Tamoxifen versus placebo: Double blind adjuvant trial in elderly women with stage II breast cancer. NCI Monographs 1:119–123, 1986.
17. DeSombre ER, Carbone PP, Jensen EV, et al.: Special report: Steroid receptors in breast cancer. N Engl J Med 301:1011–1012, 1979.
18. DeSombre ER, Thorpe SM, Rose C, et al.: Prognostic usefulness of estrogen receptor immunocytochemical assays for human breast cancer. Cancer Res 46(Suppl):4256s–4264s, 1986.
19. DeSombre ER: Steroid receptors in breast cancer, in McDivett RW, Oberman HA, Ozzello L, Kaufman N (eds): *The Breast*. Baltimore, Williams & Wilkins, 1984, pp 149–174.
20. Der CJ. Krontivis TG, Cooper GM: Transforming genes of human bladder and lung carcinoma cell lines are homologous to the *ras* genes of Harvey and Kirsten sarcoma viruses. Proc Natl Acad Sci USA 79:3637–3640, 1982.
21. Epenetos AA, Britton KE, Mather S, et al.: Targeting of iodine-123-labelled tumour-associated monoclonal antibodies to ovarian, breast and gastrointestinal tumors. Lancet 2:999–1003, 1982.

22. Epenetos AA, Snook D, Durbin H, et al.: Limitations of radiolabeled monoclonal antibodies for localization of human neoplasms. Cancer Res 46:3183–3191, 1986.
23. Escot C, Theillet C, Lidereau R, et al.: Genetic alteration of the c-*myc* proto-oncogene (MYC) in human primary breast carcinoma. Proc Natl Acad Sci USA 83:4834–4838, 1986.
24. Farrands JPA, Perkins HC, Pimm MV, et al.: Radioimmunodetection of human colorectal cancer by an anti-tumour monoclonal antibody. Lancet 2:397–400, 1972.
25. Fisher B, Redmond C, Brown A, et al.: Influence of tumor estrogen and progesterone receptor levels on the response to tamoxifen and chemotherapy in primary breast cancer. J Clin Oncol 1:227–241, 1983.
26. Fisher B, Redmond C, Fisher ER, et al.: Systemic adjuvant therapy in treatment of primary operable breast cancer: National Surgical Adjuvant Breast and Bowel Project experience. NCI Monographs 1:35–43, 1986.
27. Fisher B, Redmond C, Fisher ER, et al.: Ten-year results of a randomized clinical trial comparing radical mastectomy and total mastectomy with or without radiation. N Engl J Med 312:674–681, 1985.
28. Fisher B, Redmond C, Fisher ER: A summary of findings from NSABP trials of adjuvant therapy for breast cancer, in Salmon SE, Jones SE (eds): *Adjuvant Therapy of Cancer IV*. New York, Grune & Stratton, 1984.
29. Fisher B, Redmond C: Breast cancer studies on the National Surgical Adjuvant Breast and Bowel Project (NSABP), in Salmon SE, Jones SE (eds), *Adjuvant Therapy of Cancer*. New York, North-Holland, 1979, pp 215–226.
30. Furr BJA, Jordan VC: The pharmacology and clinical uses of tamoxifen. Pharmacol Ther 25:127–205, 1984.
31. Gratzner HG: Monoclonal antibody to 5-bromo- and 5-iododeoxyuridine: A new reagent for detection of DNA replication. Science 218:474–475, 1982.
32. Greene GL, Sobel NB, King WJ, et al.: Immunochemical studies of estrogen receptors. J Steroid Biochem 20:51–58, 1984.
33. Harvey HA, Lipton A, Max DT, et al.: Medical castration produced by the GnRH analogue leuprolide to treat metastatic breast cancer. J Clin Oncol 3:1068–1072, 1985.
34. Hayward WS, Neel BJ, Astrin SM: Activation of a cellular *onc* gene by promoter insertion in ALV-induced lymphoid leukosis. Nature 209:475–479, 1981.
35. Hedley DW, Rugg CA, Alun BP, et al.: Influence of cellular DNA content on disease-free survival of stage II breast cancer patients. Cancer Res 44:5395–5398, 1984.
36. Henderson IC, Canelios GP: Cancer of the breast: The past decade. N Engl J Med 302:17–30, 78–90, 1980.
37. Herlyn D, Ross AH, Koprowski H: Anti-idiotypic antibodies bear the internal image of a human tumor antigen. Science 232:100–102, 1986.
38. Heubner A, Beck T, Grill H-J, et al.: Comparison of immunocyto-

chemical estrogen receptor assay, estrogen receptor enzyme immunoassay and radioligand-labeled estrogen receptor assay in human breast cancer and uterine tissue. Cancer Res (Suppl) 46:4291s–4295s, 1986.

39. Hunter T, Cooper JA: Protein-lyrosine kinesis. Annu Rev Biochem 54:897–930, 1985.

40. Hurley JB, Simon MI, Teplow DB, et al.: Homologies between signal transducing G proteins and *ras* gene products. Science 226:860–862, 1984.

41. Johnson V, Schlom J, Paterson AJ, et al.: Analysis of a human tumor associated glycoprotein (TAG-72) identified by monoclonal antibody B72.3. Cancer Res 46:850–857, 1986.

42. Jordan VC, Jacobson HI. Keenan EJ: Determination of estrogen receptor in breast cancer using monoclonal antibody technology: Results of a multicenter study in the United States. Cancer Res (Suppl) 46:4237s–4240s, 1986.

43. Jordan VC: Laboratory studies to develop general principles for the adjuvant treatment of breast cancer with antiestrogens: Problems and potential for future clinical applications. Breast Cancer Res Treat 3(Suppl 1):73–86, 1983.

44. Kartner N, Shales M, Riordan JR, et al.: Daunorubicin-resistant Chinese hamster ovary cells expressing multidrug resistance and a cell-surface P-glycoprotein. Cancer Res 43:4413–4419, 1983.

45. Knight WA III, Livingston RB, Gregory EJ, et al.: Estrogen receptor as an independent prognostic factor for early recurrence in breast cancer. Cancer Res 37:4669–4671, 1977.

46. Kohler M, Milstein C: Continuous cultures of fused cells secreting antibody of predefined specificity. Nature 256:494–497, 1975.

47. Kohs WD, Steinkampf RW, Harlick MJ, et al.: Resistance to anthrapyrazoles and anthracyclines in multidrug-resistant p388 murine leukemia cells: reversal by calcium blockers and calmodulin antagonists. Cancer Res 46:4352–4356, 1986.

48. Krontiris T, Cooper GM: Transforming activity of human tumor DNAs. Proc Natl Acad Sci USA 78:1181–1184, 1981.

49. Larson SM, Brown JP, Wright PH, et al.: Imaging of melanoma with I-131-labelled monoclonal antibodies. J Nuc Med 24:123–129, 1983.

50. Lecleroq G, Bojar H, Goussard J, et al.: Abbott monoclonal enzyme immunoassay measurement of estrogen receptors in human breast cancer: A European multicenter study. Cancer Res (Suppl) 46:4232s–4236s, 1986.

51. Lee VK, Harriott TG, Kuchroo VK, et al.: Monoclonal anti-idiotypic antibodies related to a murine oncofetal bladder tumor antigen induce specific cell-mediated tumor immunity. Proc Natl Acad Sci USA 82:6286–6290, 1986.

52. Lee WH, Murphree AL, Benedict WF: Expression and amplification of the N-*myc* gene in primary retinoblastoma. Nature 309:458–460, 1984.

53. Ling V: Drug and hormone resistance, in Bruchovsky N, Goldie JH (eds), *Neoplasia*. Florida, CRC Press, 1982.

54. Lundy J, Grimson R, Mishuki Y, et al.: Elevated *ras* oncogene expres-

sion correlates with lymph node metastases in breast cancer patients. J Clin Med 4:1321–1325, 1986.

55. Lundy J, Lozowski M, Mishriki Y: Monoclonal antibody B72.3 as a diagnostic adjunct in fine needle aspirates of breast masses. Ann Surg 203:399–402, 1986.

56. Mason BH, Holdoway IM, Mullins PR, et al.: Progesterone and estrogen receptors as prognostic variables in breast cancer. Cancer Res 43:2985–2990, 1983.

57. Matnard PV, Nicholson RI: Effects of high doses of a new series of luteinizing hormone-releasing hormone analogues in intact female rats. Br J Cancer 39:274–379, 1979.

58. McDivitt RW, Stone KR, Meyer JS: A method for dissociation of viable human breast cancer cells that produces flow cytometric kinetic information similar to that obtained by thymidine labeling. Cancer Res 44:2628–2633, 1984.

59. McGuire WL, Clark GM, Dressler LG, et al.: Role of steroid hormone receptors as prognostic factors in primary breast cancer. NCI Monographs 1:19–23, 1986.

60. McGuire WL, Horwitz KB, Pearson OH, et al.: Current status of estrogen and progesterone receptors in breast cancer. Cancer 39:2934–2947, 1977.

61. Meyer JS, Friedman E, McCrate MM, et al.: Prediction of early course of breast carcinoma by thymidine labeling. Cancer 51:1879–1886, 1983.

62. Meyer JS: Cell kinetics in selection and stratification of patients for adjuvant therapy of breast carcinoma. NCI Monographs 1:25-28, 1986.

63. Nissen-Meyer R, Kjellgren K, Mansson B: Adjuvant chemotherapy in breast cancer. Recent Results Cancer Res 96:142–148, 1982.

64. Nolva Dex Adjuvant Trial Organisation: Controlled trial of tamoxifen as single adjuvant in management of early breast cancer. Lancet 1:836–840, 1985.

65. Nowell PC, Croce CM: Chromosomes, genes and cancer. Am J Pathol 125:8–15, 1986.

66. Parada LF, Tabin CJ, Shih C, et al.: Human EJ bladder carcinoma oncogene is homologue of Harvey sarcoma virus *ras* gene. Nature 297:474–478, 1982.

67. Payne GS, Bishop JM, Varmus HE: Multiple arrangements of viral DNA and an activated host oncogene (c-*myc*) in bursal lymphomas. Nature 295:209–217, 1982.

68. Press MF, Greene GL: Methods in laboratory investigation. An immunocytochemical method for demonstrating estrogen receptor in human uterus using monoclonal antibodies to human estrophilin. Lab Invest 50:480–486, 1984.

69. Rous P: A sarcoma of the fowl transmissible by an agent separable from the tumor cells. J Exp Med 13:397–411, 1911.

70. Rowley JD: Biological implications of consistent chromosome rearrangements in leukemia and lymphoma. Cancer Res 44:3159–3168, 1984.

71. Schlom J: Basic principles and applications of monoclonal antibodies

in the management of carcinomas: The Richard and Hindu Rosenthal Foundation Award Lecture. Cancer Res 46:3225–3238, 1986.

72. Schwab M, Ellison J, Busch M, et al.: Enhanced expression of the human gene N-*myc* consequent to amplification of DNA may contribute to malignant progression of neuroblastoma. Proc Natl Acad Sci USA 81:4940–4944, 1984.

73. Scotto KW, Biedler JL, Melera PW: Amplification and expression of genes associated with multidrug resistance in mammalian cells. Science 232:751–755, 1986.

74. Seeger RC, Brodeur GM, Sather H, et al.: Association of multiple copies of the N-*myc* oncogene with rapid progression of neuroblastomas. N Engl J Med 313:1111–1116, 1985.

75. Shapiro S, Venet W, Strax P, et al.: Ten to fourteen year effects of breast cancer screening on mortality. JNCI 69:349–353, 1982.

76. Shih C, Padhy LC, Murray M, et al.: Transforming genes of carcinomas and neuroblastomas introduced into mouse fibroblasts. Nature 290:281–284, 1981.

77. Silvertrini R, Diadone MG, Gasparini G: Cell kinetics as a persistent prognostic marker in node-negative breast cancer.   Cancer 56:1982–1987, 1985.

78. Stya M, Wahl RL, Natale RB, et al.: Radioimmunoimaging of human small cell lung carcinoma xenografts in nude mice receiving several monoclonal antibodies. NCI Monographs 3:19–23, 1987.

79. Sun LK, Curtis P, Rakowics-Szulczynska E, et al.: Chimeric antibody with human constant regions and mouse variable regions directed against carcinoma-associated antigen 17–1A. Proc Natl Acad Sci USA 84:214–218, 1987.

80. Thor A, Ohuchi N, Schlom J: Distribution of oncofetal antigen tumor-associated glycoprotein-72 defined by monoclonal antibody B72.3. Cancer Res 16:3118–3124, 1986.

81. Thor A, Weeks MO, Schlom J: Monoclonal antibodies and breast cancer. Semin Oncol 13:393–401, 1986.

82. Tormer DC, Taylor SG, Gray R, et al.: Postmenopausal node-positive comparison of observation with CMFP and CMFP + tamoxifen adjuvant therapy. Recent Results Cancer Res 96:110–115, 1984.

83. Tormer DC, Jordan VC: Long-term tamoxifen adjuvant therapy in node-positive breast cancer: A metabolic and pilot clinical study. Breast Cancer Res Treat 4:297–302, 1984.

84. Tubiana M, Pejovic MH, Chavandra N, et al.: The long-term prognostic significance of the thymidine labeling index in breast cancer. Int J Cancer 33:441–445, 1984.

85. Varmus HE: Form and function of retroviral proviruses.   Science 216:812–820, 1982.

86. Waterfield MD, Scruce GJ, Whittle N, et al.: Platelet-derived growth factor is structurally related to the putative transforming protein, p28*sis*, of Simian sarcoma virus. Nature 304:35–39, 1983.

87. Weinberg RA: The action of oncogenes in the cytoplasm and nucleus. Science 230:770–776, 1985.

88. Yunis JJ: The chromosomal basis of human neoplasia. Science 221:227–235, 1983.
89. Zelen M, Gelman R: Assessment of adjuvant trials in breast cancer. NCI Monographs 1:11–17, 1986.

SECTION FOUR

Psychosocial Issues and Wellness

20. *Multidisciplinary Breast Care Center: Experience at The University of Michigan*

PATRICIA SARAN
MARY ANNE BORD

A woman with a newly found breast lump is usually scared, confused by information from friends and the media, and wants accurate diagnosis and appropriate treatment as quickly as possible. All major medical centers have the personnel and facilities to care for patients with breast disease, but these resources may be physically and functionally separate, so that diagnosis and treatment are oftentimes consuming and costly. In an attempt to resolve this dilemma, the University of Michigan Medical Center (UMMC) established a multidisciplinary breast care center, which has been operating for three years. From our experience with other multidisciplinary clinics, for example, clinics for melanoma, lymphoma, renal transplantation, and burn medicine, we expected that the important factors would be organization and support staff, flow of reports and information, and communication with patients and referring physicians. Specifically, flow of information within the medical center and to referring physicians is mandatory for coordinated treatment, continuity of care, and good relations at the community level.

The literature alludes to the challenge of addressing the above mentioned operational issues when a clinical program cuts across departmental lines.[1,2,3] Additionally, the critical importance of professional skills and commitment of each group member, as well as good communication and mutual trust between team members, have been cited as imperative. These elements result in information sharing, team members willingly learning from each other, and a coordinated service with the patient remaining the main focus. In this chapter, we will describe the UMMC Breast Care Center (BCC), with emphasis on organizational and operational issues.

OBJECTIVES

Most patients with a breast lump will have benign disease. Therefore, the BCC is not just a cancer center. Patients seeking evaluation of a breast lump subsequently diagnosed as malignant should have convenient access to further evaluation by appropriate oncology services. This approach, available within the same center, provides the patient with a greater sense of continuity and security. Thus, the objectives of the UMMC Breast Care Center are:

Rapid evaluation of high-risk patients
"One-stop" approach to management of breast disease
Access to complete information about breast disease and its treatment
Top quality patient care
Cost-effective breast care
Screening for breast cancer
Standardized management protocols
Generation of clinical research
Professional and public education

ORGANIZATION TO MEET OBJECTIVES

The BCC has, as its very core, a multidisciplinary approach to care. Disciplines included are general surgery, medical oncology, radiation oncology, radiology, pathology, plastic surgery, nursing, and social work. Physician coverage for BCC clinic is provided by general surgery, medical oncology, and radiation oncology. All these services see patients with newly diagnosed breast cancer. Treated patients returning for follow-up visits are seen by the service that provided the most recent treatment. Patients with benign disease are seen by the surgical staff.

Nurse coordination is essential in meeting the center objectives, especially in facilitating patient flow and satisfaction. Nurses manage triage, initial assessments, patient and family teaching, follow-up tests and appointments, problem resolution, referral to medical center and community resources, clinic coordination, and direction of clerical support. In addition, they maintain data about the center and act as a first contact resource for other centers managing breast disease.

Secretarial and clerical staff provide the support services necessary for the clinical staff to meet patient needs. The clerk is the patient's initial contact with the BCC and acts as a traffic director: Tests and procedures are scheduled, specimens and X-rays are routed to appropriate departments, and results are obtained so the clinical staff can provide patients with information in a timely fashion. The clerk also arranges for necessary hospital admissions and schedules surgical procedures. The secretary is responsible for transcribing clinic notes, sending letters to referring physicians, arranging meetings, distributing minutes, and typing and distributing other materials related to the center.

The Department of Radiology has committed a block of time on clinic day to perform mammograms and aspirations exclusively for BCC patients. This includes review of prior mammograms and any additional radiographs that may be necessary. The Department of Pathology provides same-day readings of any slides brought with the patient or specimens gathered during clinic. Interpretations and readings are called to the BCC clinic and are also available for discussion at the noon multidisciplinary conference. To facilitate planning, each department receives, prior to clinic, a list of scheduled BCC patients and a brief summary of the reason for the visit.

In addition to the medical and support services outlined above, the oncology social worker contributes to the multidisciplinary team approach. A social worker is available for consultation on both an inpatient and outpatient basis. In addition, support group and peer counselor programs have been initiated through the Social Work Department and include a member from nursing staff.

The BCC is not a freestanding entity, but rather a service that is housed within The University of Michigan Medical Center. There are several advantages to this arrangement: Examination rooms, mammography, consultation, and conference rooms are all located in close physical proximity. Record keeping and flow of information between departments and to the community are managed by existing institutional systems. Because all the specialty diagnostic and treatment modalities are available at the university, patients benefit from these services without having to travel to several locations. This ability to provide comprehensive care assures that patients who are seen initially as outpatients can easily move through the system (including inpatient management) and then be seen for follow-up in the same clinic area where diagnosis took place, by the same medical team. In a large medical facility where patients are being treated by a number of disciplines, there is a great potential for miscommunication and inefficiency. Patients may be unsure of who their physician is and where they are in the course of management. The coordination of BCC activities by nurses is central to managing this problem at UMMC.

Multiple opportunities for making significant contributions to research about breast disease exist with the BCC. Information about the management of both benign and malignant conditions is generated by the activities of the BCC and data are gathered through a variety of mechanisms. Intake data sheets, initial patient assessments, notes from interdisciplinary conferences, clinic logs, and patient records are all available for use in research studies generated by the center. In addition, eligible patients are placed in cooperative studies, for example, the Southwest Oncology Group, and institutional protocols. Currently, a computerized data base is being developed for use in examining statistics about the center and its patients. The data base will also serve as a reference for other institutions seeking information about breast disease and its management.

In its first two years (1985-1987), the BCC has had a total of 1,343 patient visits. A breakdown of this figure shows 920 (68.4%) visits were for benign breast conditions. The remaining 423 visits were for cancer diagnosis, treatment, or continuing care. Approximately 25% of these patients arrive with a diagnosis of breast cancer; another 25% receive a diagnosis of breast cancer at the BCC. The remaining 50% of visits were follow-up visits.

A variety of patients come to the BCC for second opinions. Some, who have had a positive biopsy, come for interpretation and discussion of treatment options. Others have had primary treatment, such as mastectomy, and are now seeking advice regarding follow-up and further treatment. In addition to those patients who are diagnosed with cancer, many patients and referring physicians seek second opinions and consultation about benign breast conditions.

One of the goals of the BCC is to provide cost-efficient care to the extent that all disciplines and services are centrally located, so that timely and efficient care is provided. A flat fee for the initial visit, whether a patient sees one service or the entire team, purposely has been kept under $50. The clinic itself does not generate revenue in excess of operational expenses, but participating clinical departments and the institution itself gain revenue generated from surgical procedures, other procedures. and professional fees.

MARKETING THE BREAST CARE CENTER

Marketing has been incorporated into center activities from its very beginning. The BCC represents a new approach to breast care for the UMMC, so different methods of informing the public have been pursued. Two objectives are: 1) to inform the community about the center and the BCC hotline as a self-referral device, and 2) to capture a greater market share in a community with several providers of breast care.

University Hospital is a referral center, so emphasis is placed on keeping referring physicians aware of The University of Michigan "one-stop" approach to breast care. Brochures have been prepared for both professional and public audiences. The BCC logo is present on these brochures and on all correspondence sent from the center. The logo reinforces the sense of an actual "center" despite the shared nature of facility and staff.

The most effective marketing strategies are interviews and lectures by professional staff to public and professional groups. These have made the presence of the center known in a way that demonstrates our personalized approach to care. Our experience with this type of marketing parallels that of other breast centers; that is, there is a measurable increase in both telephone inquiries and referrals after a program has been presented or an interview conducted.

ORGANIZATION OF THE CLINIC

Triage of calls is performed by the clerk. The professional staff provides guidelines for areas that require clinical judgment. (For example, What category of patient should be scheduled for mammography prior to an evaluation visit for a breast mass?) Calls not covered by the guidelines are referred to a registered nurse. The nurses from radiation oncology, hematology/oncology, and general surgery share this responsibility equally.

When Breast Care Center patients come for a second opinion, they are asked to bring mammograms, pathology slides, and any available reports. This enables the team to do a thorough evaluation and render an opinion the same day as the clinic visit. Once the patient arrives at the clinic, any outside films or slides are sent immediately to the appropriate department. As mentioned previously, a commitment has been made by the Departments of Radiology and Pathology to provide interpretations during the patient's visit.

The role of nurses in assessing patients in the Breast Care Center is critical to the coordination of care and smooth flow through the clinic. Decisions about how this could be achieved were made on such considerations as how much data could reasonably be gathered, the purpose for which it would be used, and how it could be quickly and easily recorded. The nursing assessment form that was developed meets the institutional requirements and is consistent with the Nursing Department's standards of practice. In addition, it has been found to be helpful in assuring that all necessary data is gathered on patients in a consistent manner.

In establishing guidelines for patient teaching of breast self-examination (BSE), the nurses considered who was to be taught, what would be included in that teaching, whether to develop teaching materials specific to the BCC, and how to efficiently incorporate teaching into the clinic flow. Materials from the National Cancer Institute (NCI) have provided the framework for our BSE teaching program. "Breast Exams: What You Should Know" (NCI Publication No. 85-2000) is given to each patient taught BSE. The NCI slide/tape production on BSE, "Breast Cancer: We're Making Progress Every Day," has been adapted and made into a videotape that can be shown easily in the clinic, or transported elsewhere for showing.

Patient flow through the clinic begins with a registered nurse escorting the patient to an examination room and performing a basic health and breast status assessment. She also assesses the patient's knowledge and practice of breast self-examination, follows with appropriate teaching, and may do a breast examination. Teaching BSE may be done either before or after

Table 1.   Breast Self-Examination Teaching

1. One-to-one verbal instruction of necessary steps.
2. Demonstration of appropriate palpation technique; nurse guides the patient's fingers as the patient examines her own breasts.
3. Distribution of BSE booklet, "Breast Exams: What You Should Know," to the patient and to any women accompanying the patient.
4. Showing a six-minute video tape of BSE in a room set aside for this purpose.

the patient has been seen by the physician. Elements taught are listed in Table 1.

After completing the written assessment, the registered nurse communicates her findings with the physician, thus eliminating repetitive questioning of the patient. Following the physician's interview and examination, further medical care is tailored to the individual patient. When appropriate, the need to be seen by other disciplines is discussed with the patient. After the patient is seen by individuals from all necessary disciplines, treatment options are reviewed by those involved and are then discussed with the patient.

Provisions for ongoing care are essential, whether the patient is to be treated at The University of Michigan or elsewhere. The physician, nurse, and clerical staff each provide this in a variety of ways:

1. The nurse reviews future appointments, procedures, and treatments and communicates this information to the patient before she leaves the clinic.
2. An outpatient summary letter is dictated by the physician to the referring or primary physician.
3. One nurse is assigned on a rotating basis to follow-up on all the loose ends of a given clinic day, for example, pathology reports, results of mammography. In this way, details are not lost in the system.
4. The BCC clerk keeps a log of any outstanding laboratory or radiology reports or continuing needs. The log is reviewed at the end of the clinic day by the clerk and the follow-up nurse for completeness.
5. The clerk obtains results of any outstanding studies and directs these to the appropriate nurse and physician.
6. Negative results are shared with the patient by a telephone call by the clerk. Recommended return visit appointments are then made (this applies to those patients who did not receive recommendations during the visit).
7. Positive study results are relayed to the nurse and physician. These are then discussed by the appropriate physicians and further care is planned. The physician then calls the patient.
8. Further appointments are scheduled by the clerk, and the patient is informed of these over the telephone and a written appointment slip is mailed.

9. Scheduling of admissions and operative procedures is arranged by the clerical staff, and the nurse coordinator relays all necessary information regarding the date, location, etc., to the patient.

The nurse's role as coordinator for all the above activities cannot be underestimated. The nurse, in fact, keeps patients and staff informed at all points in the process and follows up on all matters of a clinical nature.

Continuity of care is further supported by the identification of primary caregivers for each patient. Data is kept on each patient, including the names of physicians and nurses who initially saw the patient. Subsequent visits are then scheduled so that the "primary" physician and nurse can see the patient in clinic and manage her care. The identification of primary caregivers within the center is an important source of reassurance to the patient and satisfaction for the professional staff.

QUALITY ASSURANCE

Changes in health care delivery have increased the need for quality monitors and risk indicators. As third party payers and patients themselves shop around to get the best for their health care dollars, providers must be able to demonstrate ability to deliver desired services at reasonable cost. Recognizing this, the BCC conducted a patient satisfaction survey. The survey assessed all aspects of visits (direct and indirect care). Results of this survey indicated a very high level of satisfaction with the center as measured by help with health matters (84%), quality of medical care (84%), and recommendation of the BCC to others (97%). In addition, patients commented that rapid interpretation of tests (both UMMC and outside tests), final recommendations within 24 hours, and availability of all medical specialists contributed to decreasing anxiety and stress. These results indicate that the goals identified by the BCC staff (as described earlier) are being met. But more important, the survey showed that these goals are also valued by our patient population.

Quality assurance has been evaluated on an ongoing basis. For example, nursing assessments and teaching documentation are reviewed quarterly for completeness and compliance with center standards of care. Evaluations have resulted in revision of the assessment process and streamlining of BSE education.

MULTIDISCIPLINARY CONFERENCE

Weekly conferences are held after BCC clinic and participants from general surgery, plastic surgery, oncology, radiation oncology, radiology, nursing, social work, and pathology are present. Patient data, diagnostic findings, and treatment options are presented at this noontime meeting.

The conference serves other purposes as well as those that are patient centered. At this conference, research protocols are discussed, treatment and follow-up algorithms are developed, controversies over treatment approaches are debated, and a great deal of teaching is done. An open invitation is extended to residents, medical students, colleagues, and others. Each discipline learns and shares with the others for the benefit of the patient.

Essential to efficient functioning of multidisciplinary groups is an opportunity for the group to communicate regularly regarding their objectives. The BCC conference has been invaluable in defining goals of the center, communicating these to members, providing an opportunity for involved disciplines to establish roles and responsibilities within the center, and determining treatment plans for individual patients. The social worker, nurses, and representatives from medical staff (including heads of divisions and departments) all consistently participate in these conferences. Indeed, the involvement of so many specialists in the management of patients with breast problems has been cited as a primary factor for many of our referrals. The conference tangibly demonstrates the collaborative management of patients with breast disease and the commitment to a multidisciplinary approach at The University of Michigan.

SUMMARY

While all major medical centers have resources to manage breast disease, this management may not be efficient. The University of Michigan has established a multidisciplinary Breast Care Center that provides screening, diagnosis, treatment, and follow-up, all within the same center. The weekly conference provides a forum where all professionals can interact about patient care and other issues of the center. Our experience has shown this approach to be productive, cost-efficient, effective, and satisfying for patients and professional staff.

REFERENCES

1. Burchell RC, Smith HL, Tuttle WC, et al.: Collaborative practice in obstetrics/gynecology. Implications for cost, quality and productivity. Am J Obstet Gynecol 144:621, 1982.
2. Parker M, Hindle RC: Multidisciplinary team, correspondence. NZ Med J 728:2245, 1983.
3. Yarbro JW, Newell GR: Cancer centers—their relationship to the academic community. J Med Educ 51:487, 1976.

21. Women's Experience of Choice: Confronting the Options for Treatment of Breast Cancer

PENNY F. PIERCE

Breast cancer is the disease most feared by a woman. Its devastation insidiously pervades her body, moving cell by cell, silently, without arousing any sense of danger. That is, until the moment she places her hand on her breast and gasps at the discovery of the intruder.

Shock and disbelief are her first experiences; she feels threatened and out of control by the events that rapidly unfold before her—the tests, examinations, second opinions, and finally, a diagnosis of breast cancer. Before she has time to fully accept the diagnosis and its implications, she is asked to make one of the most profound choices of her life. The experience of discovery and the immediate pressure to make choices overlap, clouding her mind and scattering her thoughts. A woman writing of her thoughts during this time referred to Brutus' words in Shakespeare's *Julius Caesar*, "Between the acting of a dreadful thing and the first motion, all the interim is like a phantasma or a hideous dream."[2]

Every woman has momentarily thought, What if . . . ? How would I feel? What would I do? It is not at all clear how much anticipatory preparation goes on in the minds of women before the diagnosis becomes a reality, but for some women, a preliminary choice is made long before one would expect. Among women in high-risk groups, such as those with a strong family history, the knowledge of being at risk, of being watchful over time, has in a sense prepared them for a positive diagnosis, and they have had the luxury of a lengthy introspection.

THE SOLITARY EXPERIENCE

The majority of women, however, are caught unaware and unprepared for the solitary experience which follows. Judgment and choice, attributes of prudent choice, "depend crucially upon the context in which they occur and the cognitive representation of that context."[9] The major contextual experiences that come into play at the time of diagnosis include vulnerability, a profound threat, and pervasive uncertainty. Hearing the diagnosis for the first time elicits a curious reaction in both the cognitive and affective domain of experience. The following anecdote describes one woman's initial reaction to the diagnosis and the effect of that reaction over the first few days.

> I was kind of in shock when she was telling me about it. And I was very very rational and it was like from the instant that the realization hit me I was . . . my body was taken over by a feeling of fear and apprehension. But I guess as a defense mechanism my mind was a little removed from that and I just kept asking all these questions and getting everything straight in my mind. And the next day I was just totally filled with nonspecific fear. Just a high level of anxiety and sick to my stomach, having no rational thoughts whatsoever, being sure that the worst was going to happen. My mind seemed to let me consciously deal with things a little at a time. . . . I was not thinking of the whole thing in the first person.

Reactions to the diagnosis of cancer include fear, shock, numbness, grief, denial, and loss of control, which are believed to occur in response to a threat that is always perceived as maximally serious.[7] Predecision emotional states such as these have been widely described in the social psychological literature, but very little is known about how these emotions affect decision making.

The ways in which threat influences cognition are not clearly understood, though numerous researchers agree that high emotional arousal lowers efficiency in cognitive function and interferes with rational processes.[16] Soon, if not immediately after hearing the diagnosis, the patient is asked to make choices about treatment, but in fact has few emotional resources at that moment to do so. The following account is characteristic of the manner in which options are presented to patients in clinical practice:

> He started presenting them [options] while he was still stitching me up from the biopsy. . . . The first one was the radiation implant, at the site with radium treatments for five weeks or the mastectomy. And as he was telling me this I was crying, and I just thought I hope this isn't the only time he is telling me this because I needed to hear it once again.

Writing of her experience with breast cancer, Rosamond Campion gave a compelling account of her response to the proposal of surgery: "When mastectomy was proposed, I know there was a vestige of a frozen smile on my face, I know I must have made some sort of autonomic response. But the rest of me had charged ahead wildly on a stubborn, secret trip."[2]

These anecdotal accounts of women's experiences, their personal "stubborn, secret trip," demonstrate an awareness of their own diminished resources during the time of diagnosis when they are also asked to make a decision. Psychological reactions to the diagnosis of cancer are widely appreciated, but there is little awareness (or documentation) of the degree to which the cognitive abilities essential to sound judgment are compromised by the affective response to a threat of this magnitude.

THE AVAILABILITY OF CHOICE

The experience of women making these monumental and irrevocable choices is a new phenomenon and one which deserves further attention. In the pages to follow, a glimpse into the decision-making experience of women confronted with a diagnosis of breast cancer and the task of making a treatment decision will be shared. These 41 women agreed to participate in a study designed to describe their decision making at a stressful and desperate time of their lives, following a diagnosis of cancer of the breast.[15] The scholarly purpose of the study was to capture the experience of individuals having a potentially lethal illness which required that they make a choice between at least two viable treatment options. The clinical agenda, however, was quite different. Not only are patients wandering about in unknown territory when confronting these decisions, so are the health professionals who care for them. There has been considerable controversy in the literature concerning the efficacy and long-term success of less radical therapies. Many physicians have been reluctant to offer alternatives other than mastectomy, which had become "the gold standard by which the worth of all procedures was judged."[19] Until recently, the discussion concerning treatment options flowed in a rather familiar and predictable way because there simply were no options. But today, given the viability of available treatment options,[6] patients are offered choices and told by their physician to "go home and think about what you want to do and call me." How does a women with newly diagnosed breast cancer go about making a choice that will perhaps influence not only the quantity but the quality of her life as well?

In 1890, psychologist William James wrote of the "feeling of effort" in making these difficult choices:[10]

> Whether it be the dreary resignation for the sake of austere and naked duty of all sorts of rich mundane delights, or whether it be the heavy resolve that of two mutually exclusive trains of future fact, both sweet and good, with no strictly objective or imperative principle of choice between them, one shall forevermore become impossible, while the other shall become reality, it is a desolate and acrid sort of act, an excursion into a lonesome moral wilderness.

Many years after James poignantly captured the psychology of decision making, the "lonesome moral wilderness" of the decision experience in the health care setting has remained largely unexplored. At the outset of this study, there were no published studies describing the decision experience of patients confronted with stressful choices. Yet each day, patients look to their health care provider for guidance because they do not know how to make the decision, and fear losing their lives, or the quality of their lives if they make a poor choice. On the other side, the provider does not know how to help the patient and also fears contributing to a faulty decision.

Clearly, the literature lacks any useful explication of the decision-making process of individuals confronted with stressful decisions influencing their health, and in some cases, their lives. Despite the quantity of literature about the application of decision theory to practical problems, there currently are neither adequate descriptions nor prescriptions to guide our clinical practice. Research that identifies and describes the decision-making experience of patients is a reasonable first step toward defining decision interventions.

DEFINING THE PROBLEM

To best describe decision making as it occurs in "real life," newly diagnosed women were asked to become subjects and consent to be interviewed at a time of their choosing after diagnosis and before treatment began. In a free-style unstructured format, each was asked to give her account of how she experienced making the choice. A number of characteristics emerged from the analysis, which served to distinguish the subjects' decision-making activity into descriptive styles. These characteristics, summarized in Table 1, include the salience of alternatives, degree of conflict, locus of responsibility, use of information, type of social support, and the decision rule used to make the choice.

Subjects were classified into one of three styles of decision making, based upon their personal representation of the decision problem. In order of complexity and named by the activity of the subject in facing the problem, these styles are termed the Deferrer, the Delayer, and the Deliberator.

THE DEFERRER

A frequent (41%) and simple style of decision maker is called the Deferrer because she selects the alternative recommended by the physician, deferring to his or her expert judgment.

Table 1. Characteristics of Three Decision-Making Styles

Style	Salience of Alternatives	Degree of Conflict	Responsibility	Information	Social Support	Decision Rule
Deferrer (N = 17, 41%)	None	None	Other	Blunter	Expressive	Preference
Delayer (N = 18, 44%)	Considered at least two options	Minimal	Other	Blunter	Expressive	"First-difference"
Deliberator (N = 6, 15%)	Considered and decomposed at least two options	Moderate	Self	Monitor	Instrumental	"Last-difference"

The Salience of Alternatives

Women in the Deferring group appeared to respond to the immediate appeal of one alternative, quickly choosing with no consideration of other alternatives. Janis and Mann term this style "unconflicted adherence" and explain that it refers to a pattern of deferring decisions to significant and powerful others.[12] The decision experience of members of this group was uncomplicated and effortless. Many, in fact, did not even experience having made a choice. As one subject reported, "I didn't have to make a choice. I never considered the mastectomy." This account is typical among the Deferrers and characterizes how they reduced the field of options to one alternative quickly and without further consideration.

Conflict

These women experienced little or no conflict because they seemed to consider only one alternative. Framing the problem in this simple way allowed the woman to quickly choose an alternative that met whatever basic requirements she had without becoming bogged down in an extensive deliberation. It is only in the Delayer and Deliberator group, where the salience of a competing alternative comes forth, that the woman begins to express conflict and engages in any deliberative activity or search for information.

Locus of Responsibility

An important aspect of patient-physician relationship emerges in this style of decision making. The physician, as expert, serves to provide information confirming the preferred option, and the patient assumes a traditional compliant role accepting the recommended option with little hesitation or reservation. Relationships are characterized by a high level of trust on the part of the patient and paternalism by the physician. Deferring subjects tended to be older, with a mean age of 56 years. Some of their ease in making these choices may be accounted for by their long experience with traditional roles of patients and physicians. As one elderly woman explained, "We feel they're the authority, they study this, they work with all the patients. We were in no position except to take their advice. We feel they have the best interest of their patient at heart." Despite the fact that each subject claimed this was her decision, responsibility for the outcome was more often attributed to the physician, to fate, or to God. The following quote also reveals how readily these subjects deferred to the opinions and judgments of others:

> I didn't have to make a choice, actually. He (the physician) told me lumpectomy was an option, so I just right there felt quite comfortable with what he was telling me, and I never even considered having the mastectomy. He

seemed to be so confident about it. So there was no problem with me making the decision.

Use of Information

One consistent characteristic of this style was the subjects' lack of interest in information. They tended, on the whole, to rely on their feelings and intuition rather than facts or details. Interviews with these women contained a great deal of language about the feelings and reactions they were experiencing rather than specific information about the available treatments or their anticipated outcomes. One may question whether education or social class influenced the adoption of this style, but there was no evidence to lead to such a conclusion.

Information had little value to these subjects; in fact, information about the risks or technical aspects of a procedure was viewed as potentially threatening and avoided whenever possible. Individuals who filter out or avoid threatening information are called "blunters,"[14] which is a term adequately descriptive of this style. Deferrers tended to be risk-averse, describing themselves as "conservative," or "chicken." Their goal was to maximize possible gain and minimize potential loss, wanting the easiest, quickest, and least painful alternative so they could get on with their lives. Regardless of the choice, whether it was a mastectomy or lumpectomy, the subject claimed it was the safest method.

Social Support

For women who used this decision style, emotional distress resulted more from the diagnosis of cancer than from having to make a choice. Their need for social support centered on bolstering them through the reactions of shock and disbelief and making the necessary adjustments to their lifestyles during treatment. Expressive (affect-laden) social support was sought from their friends and families and found to be most helpful during this time.[5]

Decision Rule

Deferring to the physician, though characteristic of this style, is only part of the explanation of how their decisions were made with such ease. Another part of the explanation lies in the structuring of the decision problem. From all the evidence in these interviews, it seems that, for these subjects, the predominant salience of one of the alternatives completely dominated the others, leaving only one preferred option. The decision experience among these subjects appeared almost impulsive to a casual observer. There was no deliberation, questioning, or validating information, simply a declaration of a preferred option. The decision rule for this group was based on a simple "liking" or preference for the chosen option.

In summary, deferring subjects tended to be slightly older, and reported making rapid, conflict-free choices with apparent ease. A need for information was not expressed, and in fact, most subjects avoided it. There was, however, a need for a high level of emotional support to deal with the diagnosis of cancer and its treatment, but this support was not used in an instrumental way to make a decision.

THE DELAYER

The Delayer is the most frequent style (44%) and is distinguished from the Deferrer style by evidence that the subject is recognizing and considering more than one salient alternative. In the latter style, subjects were presented with a number of viable options, but there is little indication that they considered any option other than the one that was readily selected. The Delayer, in contrast, structures the decision problem in a way that allows consideration, and hence deliberation, of at least two options. Subjects reported that they "lined the options up" alongside each other; hence, this style represents the first instance of subjects' weighting the alternatives, even though it occurs in a rather simplistic way. These subjects were slightly younger, with an average age of 45, and they tended to have more concerns about the long-term effects of therapy.

Salience of Alternatives

In this style, the decision problem becomes more difficult when the decision maker sees both attractive and unattractive features to each alternative or they are offered alternatives with no single attribute that helps them discriminate among them. The decision experience of these subjects included more conflict and emotional distress than found in the Deferring group.

Deliberation in the Delaying group was random and superficial. Subjects seemed to be more confused by information and did not have the strong preferences of the Deferrer group. Because there was no outstanding alternative that appealed to the decision maker, she literally delayed the decision until she felt comfortable with a particular option or she was forced into making a choice. It was not unusual for women in this group to take up to six weeks before declaring a choice, and in one instance, a woman totally dropped out of treatment — an unfortunate hazard of indecision. The following is a descriptive account of the experience of a woman with Paget's disease who was still undecided the evening before surgery when she was interviewed:

> So there's not any cut and dry answer to it. And I've really been vacillating back and forth which direction to go. Go the safe route, go the sure route, as sure as they can possibly make it when you're dealing with cancer without a tumor. Or do I take a long shot and go through all the radiology. Every day,

first I think I'm gonna go one way and the next day I think, no I'm gonna go the safe way out and have the complete and when I talked with Dr. D. today, he kind of recommends doing the mastectomy. And I don't know whether that's because he feels more at ease doing that, more comfortable doing it that way, but he still offers me the other route. But I have to decide tonight.

Deliberation for this woman shows how two closely aligned alternatives create conflict and uncertainty in the decision maker. Another subject describes the distressing vacillation she experienced between two alternatives:

I can't keep going back and forth. You'd drive yourself nuts, I think. Should I do this, should I do that? And then that did cross my mind too, you know, after he explained everything with the radiation I thought, hey, maybe it would be easier just to have the mastectomy and get it over with. But I don't know, I'm still not crazy about facing surgery and you know, that kind of surgery. And the biopsy is one thing, but the other I just, I'd rather stick with the radiation and go from there.

Dominance of one alternative was possible when the subject received information that allowed one option to become more heavily weighted than another on some valued dimension of the alternative. In the case cited above, the distaste for surgery finally persuaded her to choose radiation therapy despite the fact that she viewed the mastectomy as an expedient alternative.

Conflict

Conflict and confusion emerged as a dominant experience whenever the decision came into focus. Conflict occurred because the subjects were aware of at least one attractive feature of each alternative but it was not strong enough to completely persuade them to choose one option over another. This state of tension motivated the women toward resolution of the decision conflict by finding a way to ignore, minimize, or eliminate the unattractive alternative. The personal values of these women appear to explain their decision behavior. Subjects tended to order the dimensions in some fashion and base their decision upon the first difference they could detect among them. For example, for a woman with high values for both the breast and expediency of treatment, conflict arose because she did not want a mastectomy, but also had a desire to have the treatment over with quickly and conveniently. A six-week course of radiation therapy seemed undesirable until she fully considered her strong attraction toward keeping her breast. Vacillation between the values of body integrity and expediency of treatment continued until she concluded that six weeks of inconvenience was an acceptable cost to keep her breast for a lifetime.

Another source of conflict and resulting psychological distress resulted from an awareness of the complexity of the decision problem. Janis and Mann have suggested that "the closer together the alternatives, and the more variables the person acquires about them, the more information the person seeks out before he is ready to make a decision."[12] A simple strategy to reduce this tension is to seek information which would serve to differentiate or separate the alternatives and allow one to become more salient. Yet, these subjects did not seek out information but, rather, expressed a desire for someone to tell them the "best" thing to do.

Locus of Responsibility

Delaying subjects preferred that guidance concerning the decision come from an authority figure such as the physician or trusted family member. They wanted to be told the "right" thing to do and were fearful of making a mistake. Though they wanted to make the decision for themselves, they also wanted someone else to be responsible for the consequences.

Use of Information

Information was sought only superficially if at all. Sources of information were most frequently a friend or relative, or someone who had been through the experience. Information was not used extensively, and if they read at all, they preferred reading popular women's magazines.

Social Support

The character of social support was similar to subjects in the Deferring group. A need for consolation and catharsis about having cancer was dominant. As a group, they did not seek social support to help with the decision.

Decision Rule

The decision rule seemed to emerge from an evaluation of each dimension until the first acceptable difference was recognized among competing values. This "first-difference" rule governed the activity of decision making of Delaying subjects.

In summary, the Delayer is slightly more complicated than the Deferrer because women using this style considered, if only briefly, more than one option. They experienced minimal conflict and vacillation as they weighed the attractive and unattractive features of each option. Identification and valuing of dimensions of each option was a more explicit activity than in the previous style. Subjects were more aware and able to communicate their decision-making process, though their affective response was one of confusion and avoidance.

THE DELIBERATOR

The Deliberator is the most complex, though least frequent (15%) representation of the decision problem. It is a complicated style that is difficult for the patient and demanding for the physician who cares for her. Individuals who employed this approach expressed a personal responsibility for making a quality decision and took charge in a manner that appeared more deliberative and purposeful than those using either of the previously discussed styles. The Deliberator resembles the vigilant decision maker described in earlier works by Janis and Mann as one who engages in a deliberative information search to reduce conflict.[12] The vigilant decision maker is mobilized to initiate social contact and seek advice and information from anyone regarded as potentially knowledgeable.[11]

Salience of Alternatives

These women soon became aware of a number of treatment alternatives as well as the controversy surrounding the treatment of breast cancer with conservative therapies. Unlike the other groups, however, these women decomposed each alternative into subsets, which then initiated an elaborate information gathering strategy. There was no immediate solution of the decision problem; rather, they devised a plan or strategy to go about making their decision. Part of the strategy involved identifying and valuing the dimensions of the alternatives with similar and competing values they wished to consider, gathering specific and technical information, and validating their findings with expert consultants. Alternatives were considered independently of each other, in contrast with the Delayer group, where alternatives lacked clear distinctions. By the end of this laborious process, subjects were aware of differences between the alternatives and were conscious of having made trade-offs among them.

Another factor that distinguished Deliberators was the degree to which they considered the risks of each option. They did not take the term "equivalent safety" at face value when considering the option of lumpectomy and radiation therapy against the option of mastectomy. Specific concerns about radiation and long-term effects of conservative treatment were thoroughly pursued. These women were the only ones in the study who questioned risk factors and included the notions of probability and uncertainty in their analysis.

Conflict

The type of conflict experience by these women also differed from the other styles. With the Delayer group, in particular, conflict occurred between two options, and the process became a delicate balancing act until one became heavier than the other in some way. Within members of this group, conflict occurred around the reliability of information, and the advice of experts and friends as well as the particular aspects of the alternatives. The qualitative experience of conflict is best explained by the following excerpt:

> I guess I started by thinking, well it was very confusing and I know that's part of decision making. You go through this period of time when it's very confusing, and you're mixed up, and who are you going to trust, and there's one more piece of information you need to get, and you're going to wait until you get that piece of information. How do you know when you have enough, and how do you know who to trust, and how do you know who the experts are, and all that kind of thing.

Though these women experienced considerable conflict, they seemed able to tolerate it with greater ease than the others, as if they understood that conflict was an inherent part of the process. Women in this group described their experience as an emotional roller coaster, up on days when the information was encouraging and down on days when confusion and fatigue overwhelmed them. Yet, once a strategy was in place, subjects experienced a renewed sense of purpose and mobilized themselves to seek information. In contrast to the other styles, these women were more emotionally distressed over having to make the decision — a quality decision — than they were about the diagnosis of cancer. Using their strategy, the process unfolded into an elaborate information search designed to answer questions until the woman believed that one alternative satisfied a sufficient number of conditions, which she had defined. Adequacy and completeness of the process depended on accurate technical information, and an extensive amount of information to confirm or deny other sources. Information was a necessity for these women. They read scientific reports and primary journal articles, consulted more than one physician, and in several instances, sought consultation at well-known cancer centers.

Locus of Responsibility

Deliberative subjects assumed responsibility for both the process and the outcome of their decision, but they delegated partial responsibility to others for specific tasks. For example, they assigned responsibility for providing honest information about the severity and extent of their cancer to the physician. They required honesty and compassion from their friends, whom they used to talk through their decision-making process.

Physician-patient relationships became more collaborative in this group at the direction of the patient. Many subjects raised the issue of trust and how they would determine criteria by which both the alternatives and the physicians would be judged. Though the idea of physician selection is a relatively new concept, particularly among women, this group engaged in "shopping" behavior, seeking physicians who respected their need for autonomy. One problem confronted by these women, however, was that they rarely had sufficient information upon which to judge the competence of their physicians. Women's rights advocates have noted, for example, that "most women are more demanding and selective of the qualifications of their hairdressers than they are the person to whom they entrust their bodies and/or psyches for health care."[17]

Many physicians found the Deliberator to be threatening and demanding because of her need to question and validate. It was not uncommon, for example, to find these patients had read scientific reports unfamiliar to their physician. These patients were not alarmed to find that their physician had not read the studies, but were dismayed by his defensiveness and at times angry response when she asked penetrating and informed questions. The patient's need, though frequently misinterpreted, was for someone knowledgeable to interpret the technical information and provide a validation of its implications for her particular case.

The relationship required by the Deliberator is best described as a partnership, one in which the patient brings her preferences and values and the physician contributes his or her expertise, experience, and judgment. Shingleton and Shingleton write of the relationship required by the Deliberator that "the physician must enter into a partnership with the patient based on mutual trust and understanding. Failure to recognize and to establish this relationship of trust by the physician denies the patient his dignity as a person and treats him as a thing. This status leads the patient into an unknowing and unresponsible role, causing increasing isolation and loneliness."[18] Physicians who failed to provide this support, or minimized the concerns of these women, soon lost their trust and respect.

Information

Information played a crucial role in reducing conflict among the alternatives, while enhancing a sense of personal control. These women became distressed when they could not get information, or could not reconcile discrepant information. For them, being supported with the provision of appropriate information was essential to their well-being during this time. Miller uses the term "monitors" to describe individuals who seek and use information in this way to prepare themselves for a stressful event.[14]

Social Support

Subjects in this group were the youngest, with an average age of 40, and they required much more instrumental as well as emotional social support. They depended on others to seek out information and refer them to knowledgeable resources. Emotional support was required to sustain them during the process, which took considerable time and energy. They quickly established a network of friends who recommended books to read or experts to visit, or introduced survivors to share their experiences. A typical action is characterized by open and full disclosure of the diagnosis, best described in the following account:

> I talked to everyone I knew. The minute I had mentioned it at work, people found several women on our Board of Directors had also had breast cancer. So because of the controversy going on right now, it was really helpful to me to talk to several different people. I talked in all to three surgeons, an oncologist, and a radiologist. And, the more I talked to people, the more indication I got that mastectomy was not necessarily the way I had to go.

Though this group represents the minority of patients, they demanded the greatest resources from their physicians, families, and friends, which were used in a utilitarian way to aid in gathering information. Repeated visits, longer visits, and interim phone calls were used to answer questions and validate new information as she discovered it.

Decision Rule

The Deliberator develops the most complex representation of the decision problem due to the extent to which she has decomposed the problem into smaller and smaller segments. Unlike the Delayer group, who stopped their evaluation at the "first-difference" point, Deliberators used a "last-difference" rule, reflecting the end product of an extensive and deliberative process.

The cost to the individuals adopting this style was prolonged anxiety, exhaustion, and the expense of seeking the advice of experts. Yet, at the end, most were at peace with the decision and were confident they had done everything possible to minimize the uncertainty that surrounds the treatment alternatives. These women did not speak of satisfaction with their choices as did the previous groups. Rather, they used the term "confidence" to describe their experience of both their choice and the process. Confidence for them was identified as a decrease in conflict, information satiation, and perceived consensus among trusted experts.

Confidence is intimately related to the quality and thoroughness of the decision-making process. Numerous iterations input new information long before these women reached the point at which they were comfortable. Many of them had to go against popular or professional opinion to get the treatment they preferred. Confidence for these women, in particular, came only at the end of an extensive exploration of views and opinions from expert sources. In the final analysis, however, as the next illustration shows, the confidence with their choice came from within:

> I think you had to be, I wouldn't say the word "tough," I think you have to have a lot of belief in yourself and strength in your convictions. For me, it's very hard, I could never have done it even ten years ago. To go against authority, to go against the "educated establishment , I just wouldn't have had the guts, I wouldn't have been able to do it. It's the things I read and the men and women

who have joined groups who say there are options, there are different ways of doing things. Let's look at them and try. And that gave me the strength to say, "You can't rush me, you can't make me do this." You can't scare me to death. And they try, in a very loving way, with their arms around you.

In summary, Deliberators were younger women who experienced greater conflict about the alternatives, engaged in extensive deliberation, and used information to discriminate among alternatives. In addition, Deliberators defined a strategy for making the choice and often engaged in negotiation or bargaining with their physicians. Their decision process involved the identification and weighing of the alternatives and they consciously made trade-offs among them. They reported confidence in their process but remained aware of uncertainty and anticipated future regret regarding their choice.

HAZARDS OF THE THREE DECISION-MAKING STYLES

The major clinical value of the study rests upon an identification of the decision-making styles in a way that is useful in practice to define the information needs, type of support, and style of relationship with the physician. Much more work needs to be done concerning both the identification of information deficits and the assessment of the type of information that will be useful to the patient in making treatment choices. We better understand from this study the relationships between the variables that play a crucial role in making important choices. We have seen, for example, that the amount of information is influenced by the degree of conflict the decision maker experiences in considering alternatives and that the complexity of the decision-making style is determined by the perceived salience of alternatives.

These findings suggest that interventions based on providing information to patients first attempt to identify those subjects who require information to reduce stress as well as those who become more anxious with such interventions. Maslow [13] clearly observed the human need to know as well as the fear of knowing:

> It seems quite clear that the need to know, if we are to understand it well, must be integrated with fear of knowing, with anxiety, with needs for safety and security. We wind up with a dialectical back and forth relationship which is simultaneously a struggle between fear and courage. All those psychological and social factors that increase fear will cut our impulse to know; all factors that permit courage, freedom and boldness will thereby also free our need to know.

Further work needs to be directed toward assessing individual needs for information in stressful decision-making situations. Understanding an individual's decision style is one step in that direction. Classification of the decision-making styles described in this chapter is an attempt to reduce a very complicated process into a framework that may be useful for clinical practice. The value of these descriptive styles lies in its utility in identifying the needs of the patient and prescribe a helping role that matches the style of the decision maker. It would be tempting to place a higher value on one of the decision making styles and offer it as a model of the way patients "should" make decisions. But no such statement is possible from this study — there are no "good" or "bad" styles, but there are potential hazards of each style that must be addressed.

The Deferrer

The Deferrer, for example, has the advantage of making quick choices with little or no conflict. They are spared the laborious task of seeking information, and agonizing through a long period of uncertainty. But, because they have selected an option without obvious consideration of the whole array of options, it is possible that the first quick choice that appeared to meet the needs of the moment may not serve her well over time.

Decisions which subjects report "feel right," are more likely to be based on her emotions and attitudes at the time rather than a deliberative evaluation of the pros and cons of each choice. One of the potential hazards for those who rely on affective feeling states is that they do not integrate a cognitive appraisal of other nonpreferred alternatives.

Another disadvantage for these decision makers is that they have not been involved in the decision and stand the risk of being surprised at the outcome of events. A potential problem for decision makers who confer the responsibility onto others is confirmed by Vertinsky[20] who cautions, "In delegating powers of decision to the professional, the patient often, without intending to do so, delegates to the physician the right to define his objectives." The potential for having very discrepant values between patient and physician is quite strong given the importance of the breast to a woman's sense of identity. As Herbert explains, "Consent is by reliance on the physicians' integrity and good judgment, rather than consent based on adequate presentation of all the information."[8] Self-blame, resentment, or anger may arise at a later time, when the outcome becomes reality and the patient does not remember being told of untoward possibilities. Herbert explains further that "informed consent becomes a legal issue when a patient has had an adverse outcome and the question arises as to whether the doctor adequately considered the possibility of the adverse outcome and adequately communicated that possibility to the patient."[8]

Interventions for the Deferrer

Useful interventions for the Deferrer include providing emotional support in dealing with the diagnosis, offering only specific information required to make an informed choice, and helping them verbalize their preferences. The question of how much information constitutes "informed consent" is everpresent in the minds of physicians when offering patients a choice among equivalent, though controversial, therapies. Of the new informed consent laws concerning treatment of breast cancer, Annas writes, "The question is whether patients were given adequate information at the time they made their decision for surgery. No one asks a patient to settle a scientific dispute, only to decide which of a number of apparently effective treatments she wants."[1] Extensive and detailed information is not useful to these decision makers and only serves to distract them from dealing with the diagnosis, which is their major concern. Yet, they need permission to ask questions, and to express their desires for a particular option. Support for these individuals may be required at a later time as they begin to deal with the consequences of their choice and to reconcile the reality of the outcome with their expectations.

The Delayer

Delayers, in contrast, vacillated among options but only until they were aware of a "first-difference" among them. It is not known what the decision might have been had the subject been persuaded to continue the process. Premature closure of the decision process eliminates the possibility that the decision maker may have found a more satisfactory option. These decision makers tend to get "stuck" between two options and can be easily persuaded to accept a course of treatment simply to get out of the conflict. Their anxiety and confusion makes them vulnerable to the urgings of their families, friends, or physician. Again, this group needs high emotional support, but there are also specific interventions which may be useful.

Interventions for the Delayer

First, they need to know that their experience is a normal part of making a stressful decision and that they should avoid declaring a choice until they are satisfied that it meets the majority of their requirements. Because they tend to want others to assume the responsibility for defining the "best" solution, they need to be reassured that they are in the best position to determine an optimal solution. What these decision makers lack is structure to the process; they tend to proceed aimlessly until they fatigue of the process. A useful intervention is to provide information to increase the salience of different options by pointing out the differences – by actually giving them a format of what should be considered and, at the same time, eliciting their preferences.

Because these patients are frequently highly distressed, physicians are reluctant to give any further information that may prove to be upsetting. Yet, providing appropriate information to patients in decision conflict has potential benefits:

> Clinicians often are concerned that providing patients with detailed information about their disease may create despair. It is useful to know that helping patients become well informed does not create depression but actually assists patients in sustaining hopeful attitudes. Benefits associated with becoming knowledgeable and actively participating in one's care substantially outweigh the theoretical disadvantages of receiving potentially frightening information.[3]

The Deliberator

The greatest hazard for the Deliberator is that through the laborious process of gathering and confirming information, she will simply become exhausted and overwhelmed. Information is absolutely essential to the well-being of the Deliberator; in fact, she becomes most distressed when she cannot get accurate information from reliable sources. Many physicians are unaware of their patients' decisional dilemma because they only see them at diagnosis and treatment. Deliberators need involvement from their physicians in the interim as well; they need facts, instrumental and emotional support, and permission to take the time they require to make a quality decision.

SUMMARY

Burgeoning medical technology has made more alternatives available and has rapidly changed the nature and character of the informed consent dialogue between patient and physician. Understandably, conflict about what treatment alternative to choose, the anticipation of untoward consequences, and feeling quite alone in the decision-making experience is distressing to patients who are asked to participate in making important health care choices.

Decisional conflict is an emerging clinical phenomena that we are not currently prepared to address. Compassion and support are often inadequate in helping with the real problem — the patient does not know what to do and is terrified by the demands of having to make an irrevocable decision. It is time that more attention be directed toward the needs of patients experiencing decisional conflict. As this study has shown, only a minority of patients have difficulty making therapeutic decisions about their health. But for those who do, the psychological distress resulting from decision conflict is profound. These patients require counsel, information, and a structured decision intervention to make a choice that will have an impact on the remainder of their lives. As Crile has long argued in deciding the treatment for breast cancer, "Since there is no scientific evidence proving one treatment better than others, the patient should choose, since it is she who has to live with the consequences."[4] Surely it is the patient's choice, and few would argue that she does not have the moral and ethical right to determine such an important course of her life. Yet, without a clear understanding of the patient's experience of choice, and ways to guide her, she is left to wander about in the territory James calls the lonesome moral wilderness.

REFERENCES

1. Annas GJ: Breast cancer: the treatment of choice. Hastings Center Report, April 27, 1980.
2. Campion R: *The Invisible Worm*. New York, Macmillan, 1972.
3. Cassileth BR, Zupkis, RV, Sutton-Smith, K, et al.: Information and participation preferences among cancer patients. Ann Inter Med 92: 832, 1980.
4. Crile G: *What Women Should Know About the Breast Cancer Controversy*. New York, Macmillan, 1973.
5. Dean A, Lin N: The stress-buffering role of social support. J Nerv Ment Dis 165:4030, 1977.
6. Fisher B, Redmond C, Fisher ER, et al.: Ten-year results of a randomized clinical trial comparing radical mastectomy and total mastectomy with or without radiation. N Engl J Med 213:674, 1985.
7. Haefner DP, Kirscht JP: Motivational and behavioral effects of modifying health beliefs. Public Health Rep 85:478, 1970.
8. Herbert V: Informed consent — a legal evaluation. Cancer 46:1042, 1980.
9. Hogarth RM: Beyond discrete biases: Functional and dysfunctional aspects of the judgmental heuristics. Psychol Bull 90:197, 1980.
10. James W: *The Principles of Psychology*. (1890). Reprinted by the University of Chicago Press, 1952.
11. Janis IL: *Stress and Frustration*. New York, Harcourt Brace Jovanovich, 1971.
12. Janis IL, Mann L: *Decision Making: A Psychological Analysis of Conflict, Choice and Commitment*. New York, The Free Press, 1977.
13. Maslow AH: *Toward a Psychology of Being*. New York, Van Nostrand Reinhold, 1968.
14. Miller SM: When is a little information a dangerous thing? Coping with stressful events by monitoring vs. blunting, in Levine S, Ursin H (eds.): *Coping and Health*. Proceedings of a NATO Conference, 1979.
15. Pierce PF: *Decision Making of Women with Early Stage Breast Cancer:*

A Qualitative Study of Treatment Choices, thesis. University of Michigan, Ann Arbor, 1985.
16. Sarason IG: Anxiety and self preoccupation, in Sarason IG, Spielberger CD (eds.): *Stress and Anxiety*, Vol. 2, New York, Wiley, 1975.
17. Schain WS: Patient's rights in decision making: The case for personalization versus paternalism in health care. Cancer 46:1035, 1980.
18. Shingleton WW, Shingleton AB: Ethical considerations in the treatment of breast cancer. Cancer 46:1031, 1980.
19. Veath JM: Historical aspects of tylectomy and radiation therapy in the treatment of cancer of the breast. Front Radiat Ther Oncol 17:1, 1983.
20. Vertinsky IB, Thompson WA, Vyeno D: Measuring consumer desire for participation in clinical decision making. Health Serv Res, Summer: 121, 1974.

22. Coping with Breast Cancer: Psychological Interventions and Skills

DAVID K. WELLISCH

Hope is both the earliest and the most indispensable virtue. If life is to be sustained, hope must remain, even where confidence is wounded, trust impaired.

Erik Erikson

In writing a chapter on enhancing coping with breast cancer and its treatments, the main issue becomes preservation of quality of psychological life in the face of the dual intrusions of disease and treatment.

By necessity, this chapter must contain two major sections. In the first, the general issue of diagnosis of psychologic problems will be discussed. This will include several issues, such as the types of psychological problems often presented to clinicians treating these patients; factors typical of patients at greater risk for development of disabling psychological symptoms or syndromes; and the issue of normal and expected grief reactions to breast cancer and its treatments versus complicated or pathological grief reactions.

The second section will address the indications for and specific types of psychological interventions. These will include behavioral, psychotherapeutic, and psychopharmacologic interventions.

DIAGNOSIS

Major Categories of Psychological Problems in Breast Cancer

In a large scale review of the current issues in regard to psychological concomitants of breast cancer, four major issues emerge as pivotal.[24] These include: 1) reactive emotional states to illness and treatment, especially depression and anxiety; 2) nausea and vomiting in anticipation of chemotherapy, which is often conceptualized as a classically conditioned syndrome; 3) neuropsychiatric syndromes, which can result from a variety of underlying conditions such as cerebral metastases, carcinomatous neuro-pathies, and metabolic disturbances especially associated with breast cancer such as hypercalcemia; and 4) factors typical of patients at greater risk for developing disabling psychological symptoms. This includes personality dis-orders, which complicate or obstruct medical management.

Reactive Depression

Reactive states of depression and anxiety are almost certainly the most frequent emotional sequelae to diagnosis and treatment of breast cancer. It is difficult to determine the incidence of reactive depression and anxiety to breast cancer and its treatments for a variety of reasons. First, the available studies do not necessarily utilize common diagnostic criteria, and second, available studies do not all assess patients at similar points in their illness or treatment courses. Six studies did follow patients over time and arrived at similar findings on the incidence of "mood disorders" (both depression and anxiety).[43] These studies showed between 15% and 25% of the patients to be sufficiently depressed to warrant psychiatric treatment.[27,40-42,59,72] It is important to note that all of these studies evaluated the emotional outcomes of patients treated surgically by mastectomy; these studies were performed several years ago. It is possible that adequate follow-up studies of patients treated with breast-conserving techniques might show different and poten-tially lower frequencies of depression after treatment.

Focusing on the diagnosis of depression in breast cancer patients presents two major problems. First, the usually accepted "hard" vegetative signs of depression such as appetite disturbance, diminishment of libido, inertia, and severe inability to concentrate may be easily confused with either the disease, or chemotherapy treatment, or both. Thus, identifying the pure symptoms of depression can be quite difficult in such patients. Second, it is not clear what the course of depression is in relation to breast cancer. It might be assumed that psychological trauma and depression might be high-est at the time of diagnosis and operation. Studies show this may not, in fact, be true. For example, in one study where women were followed for one year postmastectomy, the frequency of depression was noted to be much the same at the end of the year as it was at the time of mastectomy.[40] However, it is safe to assume that the intensity of support received by these patients at one year postoperatively was significantly less than that received at diagnosis and operation. Thus, the intensity of the depressive symptoms might actually be greater for the patients at one year postmastectomy, while the frequency is the same. Another study assessed three groups of breast cancer patients cross-sectionally, focusing on phase of disease. They com-pared patients in three phases of disease, including the diagnostic, recur-rent, and terminal phases. Overall, the patients in the recurrent phases showed the highest percentage of overall emotional distress, especially in terms of depression and anxiety, suicidal ideation, social isolation, and mate role disturbance.[59]

It has been suggested that the key symptoms of depression to consider in breast cancer patients might be the more purely psychological ones, including: 1) loss of interest, 2) feelings of worthlessness, 3) diminished ability to think or concentrate, and 4) recurrent thoughts of suicide and death.[51] They are also the criteria for major depression in the Diagnostic and Statistical Manual of Mental Disorders (DSM III).[2] In my experience, it is necessary to look carefully for the presence of extreme irritability and also for sleep disturbance characterized by early morning awakenings.

Anticipatory Nausea and Vomiting

The prevalence of this clinical syndrome is difficult to ascertain for many of the same reasons as is depression. In a systematic review of ten studies, in which a total of 880 patients were evaluated, approximately 329, or 37%, of the patients could be identified as experiencing anticipatory nausea and vomiting.[8]

The prediction of who will develop this syndrome is multifaceted. At least eight different variables have been identified as predictors, including:

1) emetic potential of the chemotherapy regimen or agent (high vs low),[46]
2) multidrug as opposed to single drug regimen,[45]
3) high vs low numbers of previous chemotherapy treatments,[47]
4) strong sensations of taste or smell during chemotherapy,[37]
5) high levels of anxiety,[5]
6) below age 60 vs above age 60, with younger ages having greater susceptibility,[13]
7) an inhibitive vs facilitative (active problem solving) coping style,[1]
8) high levels of frequency, severity, and duration of posttreatment nausea and vomiting.[58]

It has been suggested that the three main variables to consider are emetic potential of the regimen or drug, the strength of the conditioning experience, and the individual's ability to cope with stress. These factors may not be equivalent in influence, with the relative strength of each varying from patient to patient.[8] The most well-supported hypothesis developed to explain this syndrome suggests that anticipatory nausea and vomiting may be a classically conditioned response.[54] This would argue for an association between the pharmacologic side effects of chemotherapy (usually after several courses) and the various stimuli present in the treatment context. These can involve tastes, sights, smells, or even thoughts.

Why is this particularly important or relevant? The issue of decreased quality of life is important but clearly secondary to the issue of patient noncompliance with treatment. Two studies of breast cancer patients' compliance with chemotherapy showed noncompliance rates of 8% and 18% respectively.[17,64] It might be argued that these figures are excellent in terms of noncompliance with other types of medical regimens or treatments. However, noncompliance with chemotherapy for breast cancer can be directly correlated to reduction of survival. Thus, effective management of a syndrome such as anticipatory nausea and vomiting begins to have implications for treatment compliance and therefore ultimate survival.

Neuropsychiatric Syndromes

A key consideration when the breast cancer patient demonstrates changes in mood, thought, or behavior should be the possibility of the existence of an organically based mental disorder. Such disorders can have a wide variety of causes, which mostly fall into two broad classes: disease-related and treatment-related.

Disease-Related. Perhaps most frequent in this category is delirium. Delirium can include:

1. Difficulty in sustaining attention.
2. Disorientation and memory impairment.
3. Perceptual distortion ranging from simple misperceptions to frank hallucinations.
4. Abrupt changes in psychomotoric activity (increased or decreased).
5. Insomnia or daytime drowsiness.[19]

Exact estimates of delirium are yet another area of difficulty. It has been estimated that up to 33% of hospitalized patients have serious cognitive dysfunction, which is often misdiagnosed as a behavioral problem, with delirium as the cause.[30,32]

Goldberg and Tull list three classes of symptom areas that create at least an index of suspicion of underlying organic causes creating neuropsychiatric symptom presentations (Table 1).[19]

Obviously, many of these can and will have psychological reasons for their presence. This list and section only argues for the consideration of organic causes.

There are several potential causes of organic mental disorders in breast cancer patients. These can include: 1) metabolic, such as abnormal levels of calcium, BUN, glucose, cortisol metabolism, or potassium; 2) neoplastic, such as central nervous system metastases; or 3) infectious, such as central nervous system infections. One example is hypercalcemia, with its frequent presentation in breast cancer patients. A study of cancer patients with hypercalcemia showed 58% to exhibit psychiatric symptoms, including

Table 1. Symptom Areas with Possible Organic Cause

Class I Mood	Class II Thought	Class III Personality/Behavior
Depressive symptoms	Memory problems	Poor/questionable judgment
Inappropriate euphoria	Disorientation	Inappropriate behavior
Sudden and extreme fluctuations	Naming problems	Withdrawal
Marked anxiety	General confusion	Uncooperative behavior with no apparent reason
Irritability	Changes in awareness	Aggressiveness or hostility, suspiciousness

depression, anxiety, paranoia, and delirium.[69] A frequent concomitant of metastatic breast cancer is liver failure. This can lead to fluctuating confusion, emotional lability, and restlessness.[56]

A frequent complication of breast cancer is cerebral metastases. Changes in personality have long been known to accompany frontal lobe tumors.[63] In a review of 68 cases with cerebral metastases, 30% had behavioral or mental changes as the presenting symptom.[52]

Treatment-Related. Chemotherapeutic agents have been implicated in contributing to cognitive impairment. In a large scale review of the literature, the cognitive and emotional sequelae of chemotherapy have been broken down into three general categories: 1) organic brain syndromes characterized by memory problems and confusion, 2) depression, and 3) agitation.[50] Several drugs often used in the treatment of breast cancer patients have been implicated in contributing to psychological symptoms. These include: 1) methotrexate,[3] and 2) a combination of cyclophosphamide, methotrexate, and vincristine.[65]

Although these effects have been noted in the literature and also by this writer clinically, these studies and clinical observations are not "clean" in the sense that cognitive impairment can come from coexisting sources besides the chemotherapy, including the disease itself, as previously discussed, and concurrent medications, including steroids, pain medications, antiemetics, and sleep medications.[62]

Factors Typical of Breast Cancer Patients at Greater Risk for Development of Disabling Psychological Symptoms

Several studies have addressed this issue. The result has been the generation of a very large number of factors that profile the patient at greater emotional risk. These studies show the poor adjuster to be generally characterized by previous psychiatric treatment,[68] depression at time of diagnosis,[57,68,72] anticipated or actual lack of support,[4,40,68] and lack of employment.[4,40,43] Other studies have shown that women whose self-esteem has been damaged from failed or lost love/sexual relationships are at heightened risk of psychological morbidity, especially when their treatment is mastectomy.[14,27]

The most comprehensive study to date to delineate the factors of the cancer patient at high risk emotionally is that of Project Omega, conducted at the Massachusetts General Hospital from 1968 to 72.[67] This project was not devoted entirely to patients with breast cancer, although these patients comprised the largest subgroup of the study (35% of sample). In this study, patients were assessed psychosocially, and a psychological intervention protocol was performed to reduce distress. The researchers characterized the patients who profited most from these interventions versus those who profited least on six dimensions, which included:

1) *Personality*: the less well-adjusted patients were more depressive, more pessimistic, more dependent on external structures or people, and less self-reliant
2) *Concerns at screening*: less adjusted patients had more work or financial concerns, more family concerns, more future-oriented concerns, and more self-esteem concerns
3) *Psychological symptoms at follow-up*: less adjusted patients had more symptoms each time
4) *Perception of support from family and doctors*: less adjusted patients felt support was inadequate
5) *Attitude toward recovery*: less adjusted patients were more pessimistic about recovery
6) *Coping at each follow-up*: less adjusted patients showed a poorer resolution of problems with each follow-up

As is evident, some of these categories, such as attitude toward recovery or perception of support from family and doctors, revolve around core personality factors or styles of the patient. The more depressive, ruminative, angry, and challenging patient may be harder to support, may obtain less support, and complain more, with a closed loop phenomenon being created. Some of these personality styles are described in a classic paper entitled "Taking Care of the Hateful Patient." These include: 1) "dependent clingers" who evoke aversion in their physicians, 2) "entitled demanders" who evoke a wish to counterattack in their physicians, 3) "manipulative help rejecters" who evoke feelings of helplessness and depression in their physicians, and 4) "self-destructive deniers" who evoke feelings of malice in their physicians.[25] I have seen all four of these styles in the breast cancer patient population. The key psychosocial variable with such doctor-patient relationships seems less the patient's ability to cope with her disease and treatment and more the physician's ability to understand and cope with these patients' personality dynamics. Such patients require extraordinary effort and time to maintain the doctor-patient relationship as well as the effective medical care of the patient.

Normal or Expected vs Complicated or Pathological Grief Reactions to Breast Cancer

Breast cancer and its treatments present the potential of two major reasons for grief reactions. First, the patient is presented with a threat to her survival and must come to grips with the potential of a terminal outcome even if it is not actually present. Second, alteration or removal of the breast is a loss. This can be true for lumpectomy as well as mastectomy. Given these issues, the patient can be expected to undergo a course of grief, which can be normal or pathological. Such clinical courses, in my experience, can be similar or identical to the loss of a significant other as described in the classic literature on grief reactions.[6,11,12]

Normal Grief

The normal grief reaction is traditionally divided into three phases: shock, preoccupation with the deceased, and resolution. For the breast cancer patient, the first phase, shock, often begins with the suspicion of the cancer and can often end with the mastectomy or, in the case of lumpectomy with definitive radiation, at the end of the course of radiation. Feelings of being dazed, helpless, immobilized, or numb are not at all unusual. In phase two, the experience of numbness can give way initially to feelings of euphoria over surviving the operation or radiation. Very frequently, somewhat later, painful feelings of sadness over the loss of the senses of body image integrity and immortality develop. It is at this point that the clinician would expect to see tearfulness, anger, guilt, and depressive symptoms. It has been shown that as many as 45% of a bereaved group meet the criteria for a major depression at some time within the first year of the loss. There is evidence in at least one prospective follow-up study of breast cancer patients who underwent mastectomy that the majority may experience such feelings for up to a year postoperatively.[40] In phase three, the main theme is resolution and readjustment to life in the absence of a sense of total body image integrity and security of survival. As has been remarked about this phase, "You don't really get over it, you get used to it."[60] This is as applicable for the woman who has lost her breast as for the woman who has lost her husband.

Complicated Grief

Several issues may serve to hamper the adaptive resolution of grief for the breast cancer patient. Those directly related to the patient may include an early traumatic loss in childhood.[5] The physician is well advised to note the patient's family history of breast cancer. If a mother, aunt, or grandmother developed breast cancer and died, this may promote a reexperiencing of unresolved grief and also a sense of helpless panic in the patient at present. Patients with obsessive personality styles who cannot articulate feelings are at greater risk.[34] A history of previous depression is a risk factor.[34] The patient who presents with multiple life crises at the time of diagnosis is at much greater risk.[49]

Another area necessary to evaluate in assessing risk or presence of unresolved grief in the breast cancer patient is her social and family matrix. Three factors have emerged that can be understood as having pathological impact in this realm: 1) lack of encouragement to the patient to freely express her feelings, 2) lack of ability to talk with her spouse or partner, and 3) lack of practical help if and when needed.[39]

Complicated grief can be expected to have two forms, including delayed grief and distorted grief. Both, in my clinical experience, are relevant to breast cancer patients.

Delayed grief is difficult to assess because slight delays in grief when breast cancer is diagnosed or treated are not uncommon. However, absence of grief or very extended delay (i.e., none in first year after diagnosis) would indicate powerful and dysfunctional defenses against inner emotional pain. Such patients often get reinforcement of such repressed or suppressed styles by their social circle or family. The potential outcomes of delayed grief include sudden experiences of acute grief at anniversaries of the date of diagnosis or treatment, or at the time of other minor losses, generalized emotional numbing, symptoms of major depression without acknowledgement of sadness, and, especially, somatization. These somatic symptoms can be the best clue to an otherwise masked depression which has as its cause the unresolved grief reaction.[7] It has been noted in standard grief therapy that viewing the body of the deceased is instrumental in resolving delayed grief. It may follow, therefore, that the breast cancer patient who resists viewing her surgical site or treatment site is experiencing delayed grief and that such viewing is a necessary step in her emotional progression toward recovery.

Distorted grief is the second variant of complicated grief. Here the manifestations of the grief process become distorted. Of the five signs of this type of grief variant, first described by Lindemann in his classic paper, the breast cancer patient who has distorted grief is prone to four.[34] These include: 1) persistent compulsive overactivity without a sense of loss (this is a hypomanic defense against depressive feelings, which can come after breast surgery and can manifest in many ways, one of which may be a driven, urgent, compulsive need to "help" other breast cancer patients); 2) conversion symptoms; 3) social isolation, withdrawal, or alienation; or 4) a major depressive episode. A variant of the compulsive overactivity may be compulsive use of substances. One study, which matched bereaved individuals with an age-matched control group, found the bereaved to use more cigarettes, alcohol, and tranquilizers.[48]

It is sometimes quite difficult for the physician caring for the breast cancer patient to discern where appropriate, functional, and healthy bereavement leaves off and depression begins. A general rule is that acute and later subacute grief are not problematic as long as the patient's personal, occupational, intrafamilial, and social functioning continue, even if on a minimal basis at times. It is more the absence of appropriate and expected grief and the presence of a somatic, hypomanic, or vegetatively depressive response that defines the patient's status as moving from normal grief to complicated grief. This will almost certainly eventuate into a major depressive episode and then chronic depression if left untreated or unattended. Another key difference between the breast cancer patient with appropriate grief and the patient with complicated grief or serious depression is her sense of self. The patient with appropriate grief tends to feel bad, sad, and frightened. She does not feel ruined or worthless. The patient on the other end of this spectrum can feel she is ruined by her disease or treatment and that her person is now worthless. This sense of annihilation of the self becomes a crucial for the distinction between these two states in clinical evaluation.[71]

INTERVENTIONS

This second section will deal with psychological interventions for breast cancer patients. The intent of all of these is primarily twofold: namely, symptom reduction and enhancement of coping with the stresses of diagnosis, treatment, and the subtle but pervasive stress of the "Damocles Syndrome." This syndrome refers to the realities of being a long-term survivor of cancer, without the ability to know when or if recurrence will become a reality.[31] A third and less immediate purpose of psychosocial interventions for breast cancer may seem paradoxical. It is to capitalize on the psychologic crisis and to actually enhance the quality of emotional life through psychological help, a possibility that may best exist when individuals and families are in this kind of crisis.

This section will address three general areas of psychological interventions, in terms of indications for, types, and expected outcomes, including behavioral, psychotherapeutic, and psychopharmacologic interventions.

Behavioral Techniques

Four behavioral techniques have been reported with some frequency in the literature dealing with psychological problems of adult cancer patients — hypnosis, progressive muscle relaxation training, systematic desensitization, and biofeedback. The studies reported in the literature are usually not specifically addressed to breast cancer patients; however, these results and techniques are as applicable for this group as any other disease site.

Hypnosis

Hypnosis is a technique of suggestion and direction used to induce a state of relaxation in the patient and also to create a state of distraction from triggering stimuli. Early, nonsystematic research was done on pediatric and adult cancer patients, with clinical evidence indicating hypnosis could reduce nausea, vomiting, and pain associated with chemotherapy.[8] Later a more experimentally rigorous test of hypnosis with adult cancer patients was done. Results indicated hypnosis produced a reduction in nausea ratings prior to and during chemotherapy, and a complete elimination of anticipatory vomiting.[53] Of clinical interest is the fact that two research groups reported 25% refusal rates of patients approached to participate in hypnosis studies. This reflects the folklore and fear still attached to this procedure.[29,53]

Progressive Muscle Relaxation

Progressive muscle relaxation (PMR) with cancer patients is usually a form of the original technique developed by Jacobson in which the patient learns to tense and then relax various muscle groups in the body. Patients are taught to tense a particular muscle group (i.e., hands, arms, forehead, upper back, shoulders, etc.) until they experience tension, say the word "relax", then focus on the tension released from a particular muscle group. The entire procedure from head to toes takes from 10 to 20 minutes.[44] In a series of well-designed studies on a total of 67 cancer patients, results showed impressive reductions in physiological arousal (pulse rate and blood pressure), nausea, anxiety, depression, and anger during and immediately after chemotherapy. More important, patients in these experimental groups reported significantly less nausea at home in the 36 hours following chemo-therapy.[9,10,38] These studies, combined with others using PMR plus guided relaxation imagery, point to PMR's effectiveness in reducing nausea and emesis associated with chemotherapy.[8]

Biofeedback Combined with Relaxation Training

Biofeedback enables the patient to hear or see visceral, skeletal-motor, or other physiological reactions, usually inaccessible to detection, through use of transducing instrumentation. The motivated patient attempts to repro-duce and maximize the signal indicating the desired response and sustain a pattern of reproducing this signal through control over his or her physiolog-ical responses.[28] This approach plus PMR has been used to a limited extent with cancer patients to reduce physiological arousal, anxiety, and nausea before and after chemotherapy.[8]

Systematic Desensitization

The goal of this procedure is to countercondition a relaxation response to stimuli in an environment (such as an oncology office or clinic), where anxiety has become the conditioned response. In its most basic form, sys-tematic desensitization consists of teaching patients relaxation skills such as PMR, guided relaxation imagery, and breathing exercises and then re-exposing them in a progressive fashion into the anxiety-provoking environ-ment. This was utilized in a study where patients undergoing chemotherapy were randomly assigned to either: 1) systematic desensitization, 2) support-ive counseling, or 3) no treatment control. The patients treated with system-atic desensitization did significantly better than both other groups in reduc-tion of frequency, severity, and duration of anticipatory nausea and vomiting.[44]

The behavioral interventions for cancer patients offer several important advantages: ease of patient acceptance (the patient does not struggle with the issue of defining himself or herself as having "emotional problems" in participating); ease of learning and succeeding, with most patients quickly learning and benefiting from these techniques; ease of adaptability to clini-cal context, where staff and patient can use these techniques in the outpa-tient clinic, hospital room, or at home; and enhanced sense of control on the part of the patient, where the patient can use these techniques at will, wherever or whenever they choose.

The behavioral techniques cannot readily access deeper emotional issues, nor are they designed to facilitate changes in interpersonal relationships.

Psychotherapeutic Techniques

Three general modes of psychotherapy have been used with breast cancer patients, including individual therapy, group therapy, and family therapy.

Individual Therapy

Individual therapy with breast cancer patients can make use of many different theoretical bases and techniques. At a basic level, it consists of the therapist meeting with the patient individually, which allows the patient to ventilate feelings that might not otherwise be ventilated. Three of the primary purposes for such individual therapy are: 1) reducing the patient's sense of emotional isolation, 2) strengthening the patient's defenses, thus enhancing coping, and 3) normalizing the patient's feelings in regard to the stresses of her illness and treatments.

Individual therapy with the breast cancer patient might differ from individual therapy with a non-cancer patient in that: 1) The therapist is likely to be more active, supportive, and self-revealing. It would be counterproductive for the therapist to maintain the more silent or reflective stance often used in conventional psychodynamic or psychoanalytic therapy, and 2) The therapist is less likely to interpret or reduce the breast cancer patient's defenses in order to reach more unconscious issues. The patient's defenses are left intact and strengthened in order to facilitate improved coping. The literature on evaluation of individual counseling of breast cancer patients is not as well-developed as is the behavioral literature previously discussed. Studies have demonstrated beneficial effects, such as reduced negative affects and improved participation in activities. It is unclear, however, whether they actually come from the counseling itself, better information, or early referral.[23,41,43]

There are several clinical indications for and benefits from individual therapy. The indications would include the patient who has sexual problems potentially difficult to discuss in other therapy settings, the patient who is mildly anxious or dysphoric, the patient who needs individual attention and support that cannot be easily obtained in a group, and the patient who has a personality disorder that intrudes into and complicates medical management. Individual therapy with the breast cancer patient can range in duration from brief crisis intervention to therapy lasting the duration of the patient's illness, and even well into the time after the disease is cured.

Group Therapy

Group therapy with cancer patients can take several forms. It can be conducted with patients alone or with patients and family members together. It can focus on purely psychological/emotional issues or be a combination of lecture material followed by focus on emotional issues. The time in the course of her disease and treatment the breast cancer patient attends a group can have a significant bearing on the utility of the group for her. It has been noted that groups are somewhat less helpful for patients undergoing adjuvant treatment.[22,66] For patients with recurrent or even advanced breast cancer, however, the value of the group experience has been clearly noted.[16,36,61] The similarity of issues for patients with advanced disease, especially social isolation, may make this modality more attractive at this phase. For the newly diagnosed or currently-in-treatment patient, symptom control and the need for more individualized attention may make group a less attractive modality.

Indications for group therapy for breast cancer patients would center more on the desire to reduce isolation and the feeling that "I am the only one who has it" and less on the reduction of dysphoric emotional symptoms. The ability to communicate openly about issues related to having cancer and to be secure that the patient will be empathically understood is a distinct advantage of the group modality.

The duration of the group may range from a set number of sessions (such as ten in the American Cancer Society "Make Today Count" program) to an open-ended involvement that may last several months or even years.

Family/Couple Therapy

Family therapy can involve meetings with the entire family unit or subunits of the family. Couples therapy, by definition involves the marital or cohabiting dyad. This can be a high impact therapy, with a small number of sessions resulting in dramatic shifts in family communication and support. The key goals of family or couple therapy with breast cancer patients would include: 1) enabling the family to talk directly and openly about the breast cancer, 2) enabling the family to discuss and plan for terminality if necessary, 3) development for support of all family members, not just the patient, and 4) enabling the couple to break through emotional and sexual impasses that can develop secondary to breast cancer.[70] An important issue in the family therapy of breast cancer patients can be the maintenance of the mother-daughter relationship. In a recent study of families where the mother had breast cancer, 15% of the mother-daughter relationships deteriorated after the patient's diagnosis.[33]

Several indications exist for family/couple therapy of the breast cancer patient. These include poor communication about the patient's diagnosis and treatment, lack of a supportive emotional interaction in the family, the appearance of acting-out in the children closely correlated with the mother's breast cancer, and the revelation of sexual dysfunction in the couple closely correlated to the patient's breast cancer.

Psychopharmacologic Agents

This section will deal with two issues. First, the patterns of use of psychopharmacologic agents with cancer patients will be reviewed. Second, the clinical utilization of three groups of psychopharmacologic agents will be discussed: 1) antidepressants, 2) antipsychotic agents (major tranquilizers), and 3) benzodiazepines (minor tranquilizers).

General Patterns of Use

In one study of psychotropic drugs prescribed to patients in five oncology centers over a six-month period, the following utilization patterns emerged: 1) the largest percentage (44%) of prescriptions for psychotropics were for sleep, 2) the next largest percentage (25%) of prescriptions was for emesis control, 3) prescriptions written specifically for general psychological distress account for 17% of the total, and 4) prescriptions written for psychological distress specifically related to procedures was the smallest percentage (12%). Of particular note was the fact that antidepressants accounted for barely 1% of the prescriptions in this survey.[15]

In a second survey on psychotropic drug use in a terminal cancer population, the following utilization patterns emerged: 1) antidepressants were used with 3% of the population, 2) benzodiazepines were used with 16% of the population (56% of benzodiazepines were flurazepam, probably specifically for sleep), and 3) neuroleptics were used for 7% of the population, almost always prochlorperazine, probably specifically as an antiemetic.[21]

Clinical Utilization

Antidepressants.   Goldberg and Cullen, in an excellent recent review, focus on several clinical issues in utilization of antidepressants with cancer patients. These include clinical indications for use, choice of drug, sedation, anticholinergic effects, cardiovascular effects, and dosage and route (strategy of use).[20]

Clinical indicators for use are sometimes ambiguous in their opinion and as previously discussed by this writer, given the interaction of somatic and psychologic symptoms in cancer. They advise evaluating for the more purely psychologic symptoms as target symptoms for utilizing antidepressants. Antidepressants can be expected to augment analgesia and thus reduce pain.[35] In my experience, they can also reduce an obsessional and limited focus on pain and somatic difficulties.

Choice of medication varies from patient to patient, depending on side effects, potential drug interactions, and routes of administration.[68] Holland recommends antidepressant choice based on desired effect and presenting symptoms. These include: 1) restlessness and insomnia: amitriptyline

(Elavil), nortriptyline (Pamelor), and doxepin (Sinequan), 2) psychomotor retardation, withdrawal, apathy, and also lower potential of anticholinergic side effects: imipramine (Tofranil), and desipramine (Norpramin).[70] Holland and Goldberg and Cullen caution that systematic trials of antidepressants with cancer patients have not yet been done, and these observations and recommendations are based on clinical observation at present.[20,26]

Sedation may be desirable for the patient with insomnia but may be a very undesirable effect in an already fatigued patient. Use of a less sedating antidepressant or administering this only at bedtime may be helpful for this problem.[20] In my clinical experience, administering the medication at bedtime often is helpful in dealing with the frequently dual problems of sleeplessness or agitated sleep and depression.

Anticholinergic effects secondary to use of antidepressants is a standard and expected problem. For the breast cancer patient, this may compound other problems such as dry mouth already in existence secondary to methotrexate, and constipation secondary to narcotics in the patient with advanced disease. In addition, anticholinergic effects can be an underlying cause of delirium.[20]

Cardiovascular effects, especially orthostatic hypotension, are common with antidepressants in all patients and especially with cancer patients.[18] In addition, these drugs also potentially contribute to cardiac conduction difficulties. These factors argue for close monitoring of blood pressure and electrocardiographic status.

Goldberg and Cullen advocate the wise strategy of starting with a low dose and building up slowly in increments to reach therapeutic levels of antidepressants with cancer patients. They believe, as I do, that cancer patients can benefit from and respond to much lower doses of antidepressants than traditional psychiatric patients with major depressions, the reason being that most cancer patients requiring these drugs have not had a history of major depression and are essentially affectively normal, but are suffering from an extreme exogenous stress reaction. This may have become severe or somewhat chronic by the time it reaches the physician's attention.

A key clinical caveat in the use of antidepressants to treat depression in cancer is that they are not a satisfactory replacement for human contact. In short, the drug is not enough. When antidepressants are reasonable and necessary, the additional need exists for psychotherapy, or at the very least a supportive group milieu. Even in the older breast cancer patient where a combination of involutional depression and the external impact of disease and treatment may interact profoundly, utilization of medication and psychotherapy has proved essential.

Antipsychotics.   Goldberg and Cullen point up three potential uses of antipsychotics in cancer patients, which include: 1) emesis control, 2) control of psychomotor agitation associated with delirium, and 3) control of organically induced psychotic symptoms.[68] A fourth category might also include the patient with constant anxiety verging on panic, where decompensation is a threat.

Emesis control with phenothiazines has been previously described.[15,21] This is not without complications. I have seen several instances of severe neurologic side effects with such drugs that have been mistaken for panic or anxiety attacks. Especially implicated has been metoclopramide (Reglan), which can cause significant akathisia.

Antipsychotics have been noted clinically to have beneficial effects in management of organically based delirium and also organic psychosis. Goldberg and Cullen note their efficacy over benzodiazepines, in the absence of double-blind documentation, because of less risk of oversedation and less risk of emergence of a secondary (reactive) psychotic process.[20] They advocate a strategy, also used by our group at UCLA, of rapid neuroleptization by the administration of either haloperidol (Haldol) or thiothixene (Navane). These drugs are reported to have lower potential of anticholinergic activity than the phenothiazines.[20]

Of major significance with breast cancer patients is the fact that all antipsychotic agents create higher prolactin levels. This might tip the balance toward benzodiazepines with breast cancer patients except in two circumstances. One would be in the acutely delirious patient in danger of harming herself or others. The other might be in the patient with advanced disease who is beyond treatment for her disease, but who suffers from panic so severe that she is at the doorstep of clinical decompensation.

Benzodiazepines.   To quote Goldberg and Cullen: "Disabling anxiety, on its part can claim no redeeming attributes."[20]

This group of psychotropic drugs is the most widely used next to the antiemetics. Uses include sleep enhancement, reduction in muscle spasm, and reduction in anxiety. Perhaps the best strategy for this group of drugs in the breast cancer patient is to use them to help enhance coping in the patient facing situational crises in the illness.

Two major problems can exist in use of benzodiazepines with breast cancer patients. First, if the presenting anxiety has as an underlying basis organic delirium, benzodiazepines can worsen or precipitate this state. Second, benzodiazepines can accumulate, an important issue for older patients or for those with liver impairment.[55] The solution to this might be use of shorter acting benzodiazepines such as lorazepam (Ativan) or oxazepam (Serax), which do not depend on the liver for metabolism.[20]

Benzodiazepines do not differ from antidepressants in their shortcomings in solving the problem of the breast cancer patient. The combination of the human plus the pharmacologic element in dealing with the anxiety-based problems of the breast cancer patient is a clinical sine qua non.

A particularly special clinical utilization of benzodiazepines for breast cancer patients may be in helping them more effectively cope with chemotherapy. Given that anxiety is a critical element in anticipatory nausea and vomiting, addition of short-term use of benzodiazepines for the particularly anxious, phobic patient may be particularly helpful. At present, a study is underway at Childrens' Hospital in Los Angeles to investigate the clinical utility of relaxation techniques plus benzodiazepines vs relaxation techniques alone for management of anticipatory nausea and vomiting in chemotherapy treatment (Jay S, unpublished data 1986).

REFERENCES

1. Altmaier EM, Ross W, et al.: A pilot investigation of the psychologic functioning of patients with anticipatory vomiting. Cancer 49:201, 1982.
2. American Psychiatric Association: *Diagnostic and Statistical Manual of Mental Disorders (DSM III)* 3rd ed. Washington, DC: American Psychiatric Assoc., 1980.
3. Bjorgen JE, Gold LHA: Computed tomographic appearance of methotrexate induced necrotizing leukoencephalopathy. Radiology 122:377, 1977.
4. Bloom JR: Social support, accommodation to stress and adjustment to breast cancer. Soc Sci Med 16:1329, 1982.
5. Bowlby J: Processes of mourning. Int J Psychoanal 42:317, 1961.
6. Bowlby J: Pathological mourning and childhood mourning. J Am Psychoanal Assoc 11:50, 1961.
7. Brown JT, Stoudemire GA: Normal and pathological grief. JAMA 250:378, 1983.
8. Burish TG, Carey MP: Conditioned responses to cancer chemotherapy: etiology and treatment, in Fox BH, Newberry BH (eds): *Impact of Psychoendocrine Systems in Cancer and Immunity*. Toronto, CJ Hogrefe, 1984, p148.
9. Burish TG, Lyles JN: Effectiveness of relaxation training in reducing adverse reactions to cancer chemotherapy. J Behav Med 4:65, 1981.
10. Burish TG, Lyles JN: Effectiveness of relaxation training in reducing the aversiveness of chemotherapy in the treatment of cancer. Behav Ther Exp Psychiatry 10:357, 1979.
11. Clayton P, Desmarais L, et al.: A study of normal bereavement. Am J Psychiatry. 125:168, 1968.
12. Clayton PJ, Herjonic M, et al.: Mourning and depression: Their similarities and differences. Can J Psychiatry 19:309, 1974.
13. Cohen RE, Sheehan A, et al.: The prediction of post-treatment and anticipatory nausea and vomiting associated with antineoplastic chemotherapy. Paper presented at the meeting of the Society for Behavioral Medicine, Chicago, 1982.
14. Denton S, Baum M: Can we predict which women will fail to cope with mastectomy? Clin Oncol 8:375, 1981.

15. Derogatis LR, Feldstein M, et al.: A survey of psychotropic drug prescriptions in an oncology population. Cancer 44:1919, 1979.
16. Ferlic M, Goldman A, et al.: Group counselling in adult patients with advanced cancer. Cancer 43:760, 1979.
17. Glass A, Wieand S, et al.: Acute toxicity during adjuvant chemotherapy for breast cancer: The National Surgical Adjuvant Breast and Bowel Project (NSABP) experience from 1717 patients receiving single and multiple agents. Cancer Treat Reports 65:363, 1981.
18. Glassman AH, Johnson LL, et al.: The use of imipramine in depressed patients with congestive heart failure. JAMA 250:1977, 1983.
19. Goldberg R, Tull RM: Medical disorders masquerading as psychiatric symptoms, in Goldberg R, Tull RM (eds): *The Psychosocial Dimensions of Cancer.* New York, The Free Press, 1983, p83.
20. Goldberg RJ, Cullen L: Use of psychotropics in cancer patients. Psychosomatics, 27:687, 1986.
21. Goldberg RJ, Mor V: A survey of psychotropic use in terminal cancer patients. Psychosomatics 26:745, 1985.
22. Golonka LM: The use of group counseling with breast cancer patients receiving chemotherapy. Diss Abst Intl 37:6232, 1977.
23. Gordon WA, Freidenbergs I: Efficacy of psychosocial intervention with cancer patients. J Consult Clin Psychol 48:743, 1980.
24. Greer S, Silberfarb PM: Psychological concomitants of cancer: Current state of research. Psychol Med 12:563, 1982.
25. Groves JE: Taking care of the hateful patient. N Engl J Med 298:883, 1978.
26. Holland J: Use of psychotropics in cancer patients. Oncol Times, 4:12, 1982.
27. Hughes J: Emotional reactions to the diagnosis and treatment of early breast cancer. J Psychosom Res 26:277, 1982.
28. Hunt HF: Behavior therapy for adults, in Freedman DX, Dyrud JE (eds): *American Handbook of Psychiatry* Vol V. New York, Basic Books, 1975, p308.
29. Kellerman J, Zeltzer L, et al.: Hypnotic reduction of distress associated with adolescent cancer and treatment. Part II: Nausea and emesis. Unpublished manuscript, Univ of So. Calif., 1982.
30. Knights EB, Folstein MS: Unsuspected emotional and cognitive disturbance in medical patients. Ann Intern Med 87:723, 1977.
31. Koocher GP, O'Malley JE: *The Damocles Syndrome: Psychosocial Consequences of Surviving Childhood Cancer.* New York, McGraw-Hill, 1981.
32. Levine PM, Silberfarb PM, et al.: Mental disorders in cancer patients. A study of 100 psychiatric referrals. Cancer 42:1385, 1978.
33. Lichtman RR, Taylor SE, et al.: Relations with children after breast cancer: The mother-daughter relationship at risk. J Psychosoc Oncol, in press, 1986.
34. Lindemann E: Symptomatology and management of acute grief. Am J Psychiatry 101:141, 1944.
35. Lindsay PG, Wyckoff M: The depression-pain syndrome and its response to anti-depressants. Psychosomatics 22:751, 1981.

36. Linn MW, Linn BS: Effects of counselling for late stage cancer patients. Cancer 49:1048, 1982.
37. Love RR, Nerenz DR, et al.: The development of anticipatory nausea during chemotherapy. Proc Am Assoc Cancer Res, Am Soc Clin Oncol, in press, 1986.
38. Lyles JN, Burish TG, et al.: Efficacy of relaxation training and guided imagery in reducing the aversiveness of chemotherapy. J Consult Clin Psychol 50:509, 1982.
39. Maddison D, Walker WL: Factors affecting the outcome of conjugal bereavement. Br J Psychiatry 113:1057, 1967.
40. Maguire GP, Lee EG, Bevington DJ, et al.: Psychiatric problems in the first year after mastectomy. Br Med J 1:963, 1978.
41. Maguire P, Tait A, et al.: Effect of counselling on the psychiatric morbidity associated with mastectomy. Brit Med J 2:1454, 1980.
42. Morris T, Greer HS, White P: Psychological and social adjustment to mastectomy: A two year follow-up study. Cancer 40:2381, 1977.
43. Morris T: Psychosocial aspects of breast cancer: A review. Eur J Cancer Clin Oncol 19:1725, 1983.
44. Morrow GR, Morrell C: Behavioral treatment for the anticipatory nausea and vomiting induced by cancer chemotherapy. N Engl J Med 307:1476, 1982.
45. Morrow GR: Prevalence and correlates of anticipatory nausea and vomiting in chemotherapy patients. J Nat Cancer Inst 68:585, 1982.
46. Nerenz DR, Leventhal H, et al.: Factors contributing to emotional distress during cancer chemotherapy. Cancer 50:1020, 1982.
47. Nesse RM, Carli T, et al.: Pretreatment nausea in cancer chemotherapy: A conditioned response? Psychosom Med 42:33, 1980.
48. Parkes CM, Brown RJ: Health after bereavement. Psychosom Med 34:449, 1972.
49. Parkes CM: Determination of outcome following bereavement. Proc R Soc Med 64:279, 1971.
50. Peterson LG, Popkin MK: Neuropsychiatric effects of chemotherapeutic agents for cancer. Psychosomatics 21:141, 1980.
51. Petty F, Noyes R: Depression secondary to cancer. Biol Psych 16:1203, 1981.
52. Posner JB: Neurologic complications of systemic cancer. Med Clin North Am 55:625, 1971.
53. Redd WH, Andresen GV, et al.: Hypnotic control of anticipatory emesis in patients receiving cancer chemotherapy. J Consult Clin Psychol 50:14, 1982.
54. Redd WH, Andresen GV: Conditioned aversion in cancer patients. Behav Ther 4:3, 1981.
55. Salzman C, Shader RI, et al.: Long vs short acting benzodiazepines in the elderly. Arch Gen Psychiatr 40:293, 1983.
56. Schafer DF, Jones EA: Hepatic encephalopathy and the γ-aminobutyric-acid neurotransmitter system. Lancet 18, 1982.
57. Schonfield J: Psychological factors related to delayed return to an earlier

life style in successfully treated cancer patients. J Psychosom Res 16:41, 1972.

58. Scogna DM, Smalley RV: Chemotherapy induced nausea and vomiting. Am J Nurs 79:1562, 1979.

59. Silberfarb PM, Maurer LH, Crouthamel CS: Psychosocial aspects of neoplastic disease: I. Functional status of breast cancer patients during different treatment regimens. Am J Psych 137:450, 1980.

60. Silverman PR: The widow as caregiver in a program of preventative intervention with other widows, in Killelie CG (ed): *Support Systems and Mutual Help*. New York, Grune & Stratton, 1976, p233.

61. Spiegel D, Bloom JR, et al.: Group support for patients with metastatic cancer. Arch Gen Psychiatr 38:527, 1981.

62. Stewart DJ, Benjamin RS: Cancer chemotherapeutic agents, in Levenson AJ (ed): *Neuropsychiatric Side Effects of Drugs in the Elderly*. New York: Raven Press, 1979, p191.

63. Strauss I, Keschner M: Mental symptoms in cases of tumor of the frontal lobe. Arch Neurol Psychiatry 33:986, 1935.

64. Taylor SE, Lichtman RR, et al.: Compliance with chemotherapy among breast cancer patients. Health Psychol 3:553, 1984.

65. Taylor SG, Desoi SA, et al.: Phase II trial of a combination of cyclophosphamide, vincristine, and methotrexate in advanced colorectal cancer. Cancer Treat Rep 64:25, 1978.

66. Vachon MLS, Lyall WAL, et al.: The effectiveness of psychosocial support during post-surgical treatment of breast cancer. Int J Psychiatr Med 11:365, 1982.

67. Weisman AD, Worder JW, et al.: Psychosocial screening and intervention with cancer patients. Res Rep, 1980.

68. Weisman AD: Early diagnosis of vulnerability in cancer patients. Am J Med Sci 271:187, 1976.

69. Weizman A, Eldar M, et al.: Hypercalcemia-induced psychopathology in malignant diseases. Br J Psychiatr 135:363, 1979.

70. Wellisch DK, Jamison DR, et al.: Psychosocial aspects of mastectomy: The man's perspective. Am J Psychiatr 135:543, 1978.

71. Wellisch DK, Schain WS, et al.: Psychosocial correlates of immediate versus delayed reconstruction of the breast. Plast Reconstr Surg 76:713, 1985.

72. Worden JW, Weisman AD: The fallacy in postmastectomy depression. Am J Med Sci 273:169, 1977.

23. Rehabilitation

MARY M. WAKEFIELD

The treatment of breast cancer has changed dramatically in recent years. Clinical trials have suggested that according to the extent of the disease, results from lumpectomy and radiation therapy equal those of modified radical and radical mastectomy. As stated by Pollard et al., the best treatment for cancer of the breast is unclear, but the treatment of choice should depend on the resulting quality of life.[6]

When comparing rehabilitation outcomes after the different operations for breast cancer, one sees that radical mastectomy results in severe postural changes, frequent decrease in range of motion and strength in the shoulder, and often chronic lymphedema. With the advent of less drastic operations, gross disfiguration due to pectoral muscle loss and scar contracture is diminishing. No more does the flexed posture and protracted shoulder blade need to interfere with movement.

Some things, however, have not changed. In 1976 Pollard et al. determined that early physiotherapy following all forms of treatment for carcinoma of the breast is a most important factor in achieving better shoulder movement.[6] With respect to the need for early mobility, I have not found documentation of wound dehiscence when early supervised activity is initiated postoperatively, and I concur with his beliefs about the necessity to initiate early physical therapy. Sachs et al. mentioned that the physician relates more easily to an in-hospital approach to postoperative patient care.[8] As hospitalization for this patient population is about five days, it is vital that physical therapy be initiated immediately after operation.

POSTOPERATIVE COMPLAINTS

Patients exhibit a variety of complaints following mastectomy. Loss of skin mobility on the chest wall is of primary concern. Formation of adhesive fibers resulting from dissection of the skin flaps and fascia helps in setting the stage for shoulder joint dysfunction. A cycle of pain, muscle spasm, and loss of range of motion can be established.[9] Another significant cause of shoulder dysfunction is trauma to the long thoracic nerve during axillary dissection. Paralysis of the serratus anterior muscle can occur and impair activities such as reaching.

Patients who overcompensate with posture for the lost weight of the breast, or who are very tense, may develop chronic spasm of the trapezius or rhomboid muscle groups. Early intervention and instruction in relaxation and posture methods can break this cycle of pain and spasm.

Specific complaints of pain can usually be sorted into the following categories: sharp, intermittent chest wall pain caused by cutaneous nerve regeneration or nerve entrapment in adhesions; aching, sharp pain in the anterior chest caused by spasm of the pectoralis major muscle; upper arm pain caused by referred discomfort from the trapezius, rotator cuff, or cervical spine; posterior upper arm pain or paresthesias associated with cutaneous nerve regeneration; and lower arm or antecubital pain, which may signal cellulitis. The latter usually must be treated with antibiotics.[9]

PHYSICAL THERAPY INTERVENTION

At The University of Michigan, four major areas were identified where physical therapy intervention is needed for persons who have had operations for breast cancer: posture, range of motion, strength, and management of lymphedema.

Posture

Patients need to be made aware in advance of potential postural changes that may occur after mastectomy. Although surgical procedures have become less disfiguring, patients can still develop asymmetry depending on the extent of their operation. As with any surgical scar, protective splinting, leaning toward the side of discomfort, and trunk flexion may occur. Even with drains in place in the early postoperative period, it is important that the patient be made aware of accentuated poor posture and be instructed in its correction. Instruction in exercise includes chin tuck with back erect, scapular retraction, and shoulder elevation. During ambulation, natural arm swing is encouraged. When carrying objects, ideally both upper extremities should be used. Unless otherwise advised by the surgeon, however, no more than five pounds should be carried on the involved side for a period up to eight weeks postoperatively. Since the upper and lower trunk are closely related, a lumbar pillow may be of value for sitting activities, in addition to arranging supportive chair and table heights that allow good trunk support when the patient is using her involved upper extremity. Finally, therapists should instruct the patient in overall good posture habits.[10]

Range of Motion

In a prospective study, Wingate has shown that patients undergoing postoperative physical therapy have achieved better range of motion and return to their preoperative state sooner than patients who receive no therapy.[11] She reported that, at three months following operation, those patients having had physical therapy immediately after the operation still retained an advantage over patients who had not undergone physical therapy.

When physical therapists begin the postoperative exercise program, patient instruction often must occur while drains are still in place. While the drains are in, 90 degrees of shoulder flexion and abduction are allowed on the involved side. After removal of the surgical drains, full range of motion of the shoulder should be attainable within two to four weeks after mastectomy. We feel this length of time allows for full range of motion and prevents the soreness sometimes seen with overaggressive exercising. Careful instruction in postoperative exercise is given in order to avoid movement substitutions.

Examples of exercises given include: 1) upper extremity wall climbing for shoulder flexion and abduction; 2) hands behind the neck and head erect with elbows winging out and in slowly; and 3) reaching behind the neck toward the small of the back, then reversing this to reach from the small of the back toward the shoulder blade, as when drying one's back with a towel. In addition, patients are encouraged to perform their activities of daily living in order to attain the goal of full mobility. Figures 1–4 illustrate postoperative range of motion exercises. Wingate lists ten activities covering many of the possible functional movements for the involved shoulder (Table 1).

At times, the healing of the scar can interfere with full upper extremity mobility. Extensive adhesions may develop with pectoral fascia dissection. As soon as sutures are removed, mobilization of the skin on the involved chest wall can be initiated. Use of gentle but firm massage over the scar and surrounding surface can prevent adhesions at the scar–soft tissue interface. By desensitizing the scar, movement of the surrounding tissue and upper extremity can be assisted.[9]

Group activities also help these patients to accomplish their mobility goals. Activities such as dance classes, organized programs through the YWCA, and water exercise classes have shown favorable results. The physical accomplishments of freedom of movement, tension release, and control of pain are enhanced by the psychological and social support of a peer group.[2,4,5] Bonds can be established between individuals who have undergone the experience of mastectomy, and theses women can share the coping mechanisms they have used to deal with changes in their body image and loss of a body part in addition to regaining mobility.

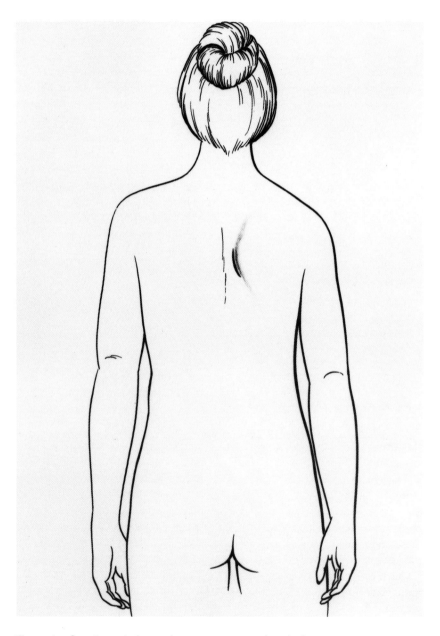

Figure 1.   Serratus anterior weakness causes scapular winging.

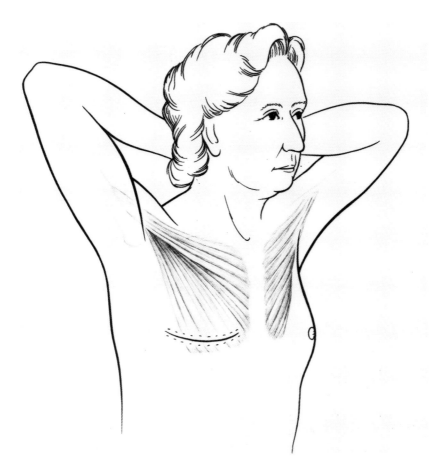

Figure 2.   Pectoral stretching.

Strength

When working with the breast cancer patient, physical therapists need to address specific muscle strengthening as well as overall conditioning. In addition to immediate postoperative physical therapy, breast cancer patients can benefit from an exercise program throughout the postoperative phase, even during radiation and chemotherapy treatments, with modifications made as necessary.[12]

The specific muscles of concern following mastectomy are the pectoralis major, latissimus dorsi, and the serratus anterior. Though changing surgical technique has allowed preservation of these muscles, disuse and decreased mobility still necessitate exercise instruction. Examples of specific strengthening exercises include wall push-offs, advancing to modifications of the

Table 1.   Evaluation of the Affected Shoulder

Using the arm on your operated side are you able to:

1. Brush and comb your hair?
2. Get a T-shirt, blouse that does not unbutton, or tight-necked sweater over your head?
3. Put on a pair of pants or pantyhose and pull them up?
4. Close a back-fastening bra?
5. Completely zip up a dress with a back-fastening zipper?
6. Wash the upper part of your back, i.e., shoulder blade area, on the same side as the operation?
7. Wash the upper part of your back, i.e., shoulder blade area, on the opposite side from the operation?
8. Reach into a cupboard over your head?
9. Make a double bed?
10. Carry a grocery bag containing three 1-lb cans, a 3-lb roast, a 3-lb bag of apples, and one or two other items so that the bag weighs approximately 10 lb?

Reprinted from *Physical Therapy 65:896,* 1985 with the permission of the American Physical Therapy Association.

push-up, for serratus anterior strengthening and the use of progressive weights for latissimus dorsi strengthening (Figure 5).

In terms of general conditioning exercise, i.e., swimming, walking, and biking, frequency and duration must continually be reassessed with respect to the choice of treatment modality after surgical therapy. Both patients who lead fairly sedentary lives and those used to exercising must be educated and screened before beginning a prescribed program. Activity recommended should be based on the collective assessment of those involved in the patient's care.[12] Basically, these should include the oncology nurse clinician, dietitian, and physical therapist in consultation with the appropriate physician, e.g., the medical oncologist, radiation oncologist, or the surgeon. The importance of continuing the exercise program at home is stressed, and a series of exercises requiring no equipment and stressing the three key areas of proper posture, mobility, and strengthening is prescribed.

Lymphedema

Lymphedema, when encountered, continues to be difficult to treat. Specific measures found useful for decreasing the associated swelling include squeezing a soft ball, arm elevation, and gentle but firm massage of the upper extremity in a distal to proximal direction. Gilchrist has described a method of breaking down lymph pools in the subcutaneous fat.[3] He suggests applying repeated pressure with the thumbs up and down the length of the ulna, including the back of the hand. He feels that if this pressure treatment is performed early, appreciable edema will not develop. Gilchrist

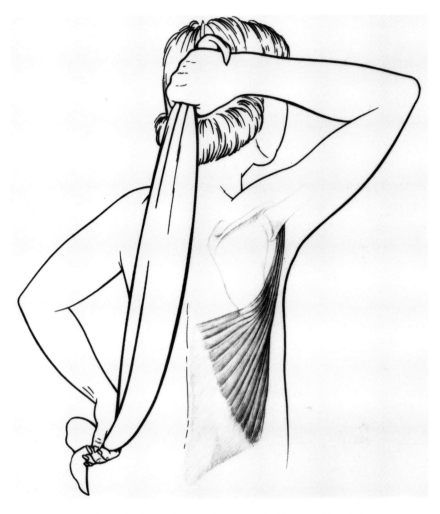

Figure 3.   Latissimus dorsi stretching and movement of the shoulder girdle.

goes on to state that since there will not be a prolonged period of lymph stasis, fibrosis will not develop and pressure treatments may be needed less frequently.

When formal pressure treatments are needed, a device known as a sequential lymphedema pump has been found to be more effective for control of the chronic swelling of lymphedematous tissue than the standard constant pressure pump.[1,7] The sleeve on the lymphedema pump is made up of several overlapping compartments that apply pressure sequentially. Application of the sleeve allows distal to proximal milking of the extremity.

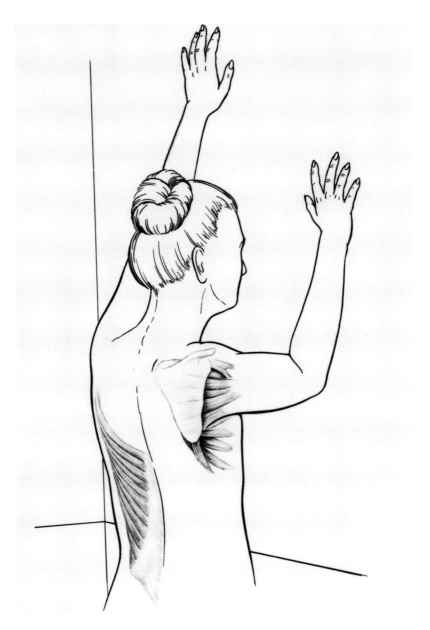

Figure 4. Latissimus dorsi stretching with external shoulder rotation, flexion, and abduction.

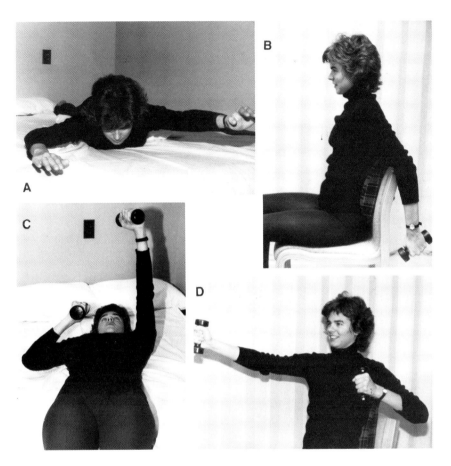

Figure 5. Muscle strengthening exercises. *(a)* Hand weights used for upper extremity strengthening; *(b)* upper extremity strengthening with trunk supported in supine position; *(c)* shoulder girdle strengthening in prone position; and *(d)* good posture is promoted with lumbar pillow during upper extremity strengthening exercise.

As the first compartment fills and then empties, the following compartment does the same and likewise up the sleeve. Since each compartment is filled for a short period of time, higher pressures than conventionally utilized in the constant pressure pump are employed. For upper extremity swelling, pressures as high as 120 mm Hg are used, compared with the 30–60 mm Hg used with constant pressure. Depending on the severity of the lymphedema, an initial protocol could be 24 hours of continuous use of the pump with higher pressure used during waking hours, followed by 4- to 6-hour sessions with 30-minute breaks until further reduction is seen.

When desired reduction in the extremity size is obtained, fitting for a pressure sleeve and gauntlet is necessary to maintain a soft limb. There are a variety of pressure garments available at this time. The most comfortable appear to be those without a seam in a three-dimensional weave. For long-term reduction in a swollen upper extremity, a sleeve and gauntlet must be worn.

SUMMARY

Mastectomy results in the loss of a body part and a dramatic change in one's body image. By promoting good posture, mobility, and strength, the physical therapist has the opportunity to help these patients adapt in an active way to this physical change. Along with psychological and social support by health professionals, as well as family involvement and peer contact, these patients need to physically take control of their lives for their postoperative activity and overall well-being.

REFERENCES

1. Browse NL: The diagnosis and management of primary lymphedema. J Vasc Surg 3:181–184, 1986.
2. Dietz JH: Cancer of the breast, in Dietz JH (ed.): *Rehabilitation Oncology*. New York, John Wiley & Sons, 1981, pp 82–101.
3. Gilchrist RK: The postmastectomy massive arm: Usually preventable catastrophe. Am J Surg 122:363–364, 1971.
4. Healey LE: Role of rehabilitation medicine in the care of the patient with breast cancer. Cancer 28:1666–1671, 1971.
5. Molinaro J, Kleinfeld M, Lebed S: Physical therapy and dance in the surgical management of breast cancer. Phys Ther 66:967–969, 1986.
6. Pollard R, Callum KG, Bates T, et al.: Shoulder movement following mastectomy. Clin Oncol 2:343–349, 1976.
7. Richmand DM, O'Donnell TF Jr, Zelikovski A: Sequential pneumatic compression for lymphedema, a controlled trial. Arch Surg 120:1116–1119, 1985.
8. Sachs HS, Davis JM, Spagnola M, et al.: Comparative results of postmastectomy rehabilitation in a specialized and a community hospital. Cancer 48:1251–1255, 1981.
9. Stumm D: Rehabilitation of the breast cancer patient. Clin Management 2:20–22, 1982.
10. Wilhite OD: Pre and postoperative rehabilitation exercises for the mastectomy patient. Home Health Care Nurse Jan/Feb:34–39, 1984.
11. Wingate L: Efficacy of physical therapy for patients who have undergone mastectomies. Phys Ther 65:896–900, 1985.
12. Winningham ML, MacVicar MG, Burk CA: Exercises for cancer patients: Guidelines and precautions. Phys Sports Med 14:125–134, 1986.

24. Diet and Exercise in the Management of the Breast Cancer Patient

CARL E. ORRINGER
GORDON A. SAXE

Interest in the therapeutic potential of diet and exercise has grown considerably in recent years. The approach is now accepted as an important ingredient in successful cardiac rehabilitation and may also have merit as an adjunct to the treatment of cancer, especially carcinoma of the breast. In this chapter, we will discuss the potential of a program based on dietary modification and tailored exercise in the treatment of breast cancer.

DIET AND CANCER OUTCOME: THE RATIONALE FOR DIETARY INTERVENTION

The past decade has witnessed an explosion of interest and research in the area of diet, nutrition, and cancer. Epidemiological studies have demonstrated that diet is associated with the incidence and mortality of many human cancers. Laboratory investigations have indicated that dietary factors may play a major role in the pathogenesis of cancer, both in the initiation stage of carcinogenesis, and in the later promotional stage.

As a result of such findings, organizations including the National Academy of Sciences, the National Cancer Institute, and the American Cancer Society have proposed cancer prevention dietary guidelines. Recommended dietary changes include a reduction in total calories, fat, and alcohol, and increased consumption of whole grains, fruits, and vegetables. Particularly recommended are daily servings of foods rich in vitamins A and C (such as dark green and deep yellow vegetables) as well as cruciferous vegetables (the cabbage family).[28]

Scientific interest in the preventive potential of diet has given rise to an important question: Can dietary modification, following these guidelines, improve outcome in existing cancers? This question has been addressed in animal, epidemiological, and metabolic studies.

Table 1. Tumor-Inhibiting Micronutrients in Animal Studies

Micronutrient	Organ
Vitamin A	Cervix,[9] Prostate,[23] Forestomach[9]
Vitamin E	Colon,[11] Skin[36]
Retinoids	Respiratory tract,[30] Bladder,[39] Skin,[5]
Selenium	Breast,[9,21,35,43] Liver,[2,12,18,19] Skin[10]

Animal Studies

Among the earliest of the animal studies were those of Tannenbaum.[40] He found that both caloric and fat restriction individually inhibited the development and growth of induced, as well as spontaneous, mammary tumors in mice. More recently, Davidson and Carroll[13] demonstrated that feeding a fat-free diet inhibited dimethylbenzanthracene (DMBA) carcinogenesis in Sprague-Dawley rats. This diet led to tumor regression in half of the rats, but tumors could be induced to regrow by reinstituting the high-fat diet.

Development of animal tumors at sites besides breast has also been inhibited through modulation of dietary macronutrient levels. Colon tumor development in rats has been inhibited by fat restriction, resulting in both fewer tumors and reduced metastasis to the abdominal cavity, lungs, and liver.[29] Pancreatic tumors have been inhibited in hamsters by a low-fat diet,[4] and in rats by caloric restriction,[31] and amino acid modulation.[38] Tumor development in animals has also been inhibited in a variety of organ systems through the administration of micronutrients (Table 1).

Epidemiological Studies

Epidemiological studies have associated obesity and dietary fat intake with recurrence and survival in breast cancer. Several investigators have found that obese breast cancer patients have a greater chance of early recurrence and shorter survival than do nonobese patients.[1,6,7,15,41,50,51] Differences in survival between treated Japanese and American breast cancer patients have been observed and have been attributed to the lower fat content of the Japanese diet, compared with the American diet.[33,48] This may be due either to differences in the biology of premenopausal and postmenopausal disease, or to the fact that fat consumption decreases with age among Japanese women.[22]

More recently, Marshall and colleagues found in a historical prospective study of breast cancer that, when controlling for disease stage and patient age, the risk of death increased 1.4-fold for each 1000 grams in monthly fat intake. The relationship was found to be even more pronounced for women with distant disease, in whom survival time did not vary according to age.[17]

In contrast to the above studies, Willett found, in a case-control study of American nurses, no significant difference in breast cancer incidence between women in the lowest quintile of fat consumption (mean fat intake of 33% of calories) and the highest quintile (44% of calories).[46] While this study calls into question the potential benefits of modest fat reduction on breast cancer incidence, these findings have been challenged on the grounds that its principal dietary assessment instrument may have biased results toward the null hypothesis (M Buzzard, personal communication). Whether or not this criticism is valid, this study does not address the question of whether severe, as opposed to moderate, fat restriction might either reduce incidence or increase disease-free or overall survival in breast cancer.

To our knowledge, there is only one epidemiological study showing a correlation of diet with survival at a site other than breast. Saxe and co-workers conducted a historical prospective study of 110 pancreatic cancer patients advised to follow a low-fat diet based on whole grains, fresh vegetables, legumes, and fruit. In 25 patients in this group who were able to comply with the recommended diet, there was increased one-year survival (56% vs 10%, P = .01) in comparison with pancreatic cancer patients from the SEER (Surveillance Epidemiology and End Results) national data base.[34]

Metabolic Studies

The hypothesis that diet affects the course of and survival from malignancy, especially in postmenopausal and advanced stage breast cancer, is supported by metabolic studies of: 1) the role of estrogen receptors (tumor hormone binding globulin or albumin) in the promotion of estrogen receptor–positive breast cancer, and 2) the influence of dietary fat, calories, and obesity on the production of endogenous estrogens.

The effectiveness of hormonal therapies, such as oophorectomy, adrenalectomy, and aminoglutethimide in breast cancer is dependent upon the level of estrogen receptors.[32] Tamoxifen, which appears to operate by binding estrogen receptors, thereby preventing receptor binding of endogenous estrogens, has a demonstrated disease-free and overall survival advantage in estrogen receptor–positive, but not in estrogen receptor–negative disease.[14]

The central biological role of estrogen receptors appears to be due to their responsiveness to endogenous estrogens. Cho-Chung has postulated that tumor cell membrane estrogen receptors, when bound by estrogen, translocate to the nucleus, where the estrogen is released. Estrogen then binds DNA, stimulating cell replication and tumor growth.[8] Estrogen binding (and hypothetically, nuclear translocation) of receptors is a function of the level of endogenous estrogens. This may be due to either of two mechanisms. Endogenous estrogens may saturate the available estrogen receptors, or they may induce mammary ductal cells to produce more estrogen receptor proteins.[3,16,24,44]

Not all endogenous estrogens appear to be biologically active, however.

While case-control studies have shown no differences in serum levels of androgens, progesterone or its urinary metabolite pregnandiol, prolactin, or the three major estrogens (estrone, estradiol, and estriol) not bound to sex hormone–binding globulin or albumin in breast cancer cases.[42] Because they are unbound, these estrogens are free to bind receptor sites and stimulate mammary tumor growth.

The principal source of endogenous estrogen production in postmenopausal women is the aromatization of androstenedione to estrone.[49] Since the primary site for this reaction is adipose tissue,[25] the fat and calorie content of the diet influences estrogen levels. While it is not clear whether this reaction results in increased levels of unbound estrogens, it has been established that British women (a high-risk group for breast cancer) produce more unbound estrogen than lower risk Japanese women.[27]

Thus, it appears that estrogen receptor binding of unbound estrogen stimulates tumor growth, that the rate of binding is dependent upon the level of unbound estrogen, and that the level of unbound estrogen may be influenced by dietary factors, obesity, or a combination of the two.

Clinically Controlled Trials of Dietary Intervention

Taken together, animal, epidemiological, and metabolic studies support the hypothesis that breast cancer may be responsive to dietary change. Each of these approaches, however, has limitations that necessitate cautious interpretation. For example, while animal studies have linked both macronutrient and micronutrient modulation to tumor inhibition at various sites, it is always questionable whether animal results can be extrapolated to humans. Epidemiological studies have detected height and weight associations with outcome in human breast cancer, but are weakened by imprecise dietary assessment methods and by the requirement that cause and effect be inferred. Metabolic studies of endocrine mechanisms lend biological credence to the dietary hypothesis, but it is difficult to discern precise causal relationships. Clearly, unbiased evaluation of the dietary hypothesis requires a clinically controlled study of dietary intervention.

In a recent review, Wynder[49] concluded that:

> These and other findings suggest that it may be appropriate to perform a randomized prospective clinical trial on the efficacy of a low-fat diet as adjuvant therapy in postmenopausal breast cancer. . . . An important stipulation for such a trial is that it be limited to postmenopausal patients with lymph node involvement; this subgroup is often most resistant to chemotherapy and is also most likely to respond to dietary adjuvant therapy.

Although the data in support of a trial of a low-fat diet are stronger for postmenopausal breast cancer, the inclusion of premenopausal women may also be worthy of consideration for several reasons. First, dietary modification may provide a survival advantage and means for disease control in premenopausal disease. While premenopausal breast cancer may not be as responsive to diet-induced modulation of estrogen levels as postmenopausal disease, it may be sensitive to other effects of dietary change. For example, fat restriction, either singularly or in tandem with increased levels of putatively protective nutrients, e.g., beta-carotene, vitamin C, indoles, and omega-3 fatty acids, which are also a regular part of a balanced low-fat diet, may regulate neoplastic growth through a variety of pathways: through alteration of prostaglandin metabolism, by enhancement of immune surveillance or natural killer cell activity, or by protecting against free radical processes and lipid peroxidation of cell membranes.[37]

Another important reason for including premenopausal patients is that dietary modification might have major effects on other aspects of health and quality of life. For example, one of the more distressing side effects of adjuvant CMF (cyclophosphamide, methotrexate, 5-fluorouracil), a chemotherapeutic regimen commonly employed in advanced premenopausal breast cancer, is inexplicable weight gain. This may add to the negative self-image that many women are already experiencing after the cosmetic changes caused by surgical and radiation treatments. A low-fat, low-calorie diet might help to relieve this problem. In addition, as diet change would require the active involvement of patients, the institution of dietary changes might be of psychological benefit in that it could help the patient to regain a sense of control over the course of her illness.

EXERCISE AND CANCER

Years ago the idea of recommending regular physical activity to patients with coronary artery disease was considered dangerous and inappropriate. In 1987, the use of exercise therapy as part of a structured program of cardiac rehabilitation is considered standard care. Patients with neoplastic diseases are subjected today to newer and more aggressive treatment modalities designed to eradicate or slow the progression of the malignant process. These patients, however, like patients with cardiac disease in the past, have not been afforded the potential for improved health that regular physical exercise may provide.

Physical therapy has been increasingly used since the early 1970s in the rehabilitation of patients treated surgically for breast cancer.[20] In the past, when radical mastectomy with or without extensive radiation therapy was commonly performed, dysfunction of the involved musculoskeletal system and marked lymphedema provided major rehabilitative difficulties for those patients. With the increasing use of more limited surgical procedures and improved techniques of delivering radiation therapy, physicians may now help their patients to minimize musculoskeletal functional loss.

Chemotherapy is being increasingly used as adjunctive therapy for breast cancer. Some of the common side effects of chemotherapy, including nausea, vomiting, diarrhea, anorexia, and anemia, may hamper the patient's ability and motivation to participate in a physical training program. In addition, those patients whose medical regimens involve corticosteroids may be predisposed to additional complications, including diabetes, osteoporosis, hypertension, and hyperlipidemia.

The role of cardiovascular exercise in the treatment of patients with breast cancer has been only minimally examined in the medical literature. Winningham and MacVicar studied 16 subjects and divided them into three groups: 1) six healthy exercising women, 2) six exercising patients with diagnosed Stage II breast cancer for which they were receiving chemotherapy during the study, and 3) four nonexercising cancer patients. These patients underwent symptom-limited, graded exercise tests before and after the study to evaluate maximal oxygen consumption and the Profile of Mood States (POMS) survey to assess tension-anxiety, depression-dejection, anger-hostility, vigor-fatigue, and confusion-bewilderment before and after the study. Patients were trained three times a week using a bicycle ergometer at 60% to 85% of their maximal heart rate for 20 to 30 minutes per session. Cancer patients improved their work capacity by 20.7% when compared to controls (-1.8%), and achieved an improvement of fitness comparable to that of healthy patients (17.4%). On the POMS test, the cancer patients demonstrated significant score reduction on the tension-anxiety and confusion-bewilderment scales.[47]

The same two authors conducted a survey of 254 cancer patients who were identified as regular exercisers. Forty-four percent of these patients reported difficulty maintaining their exercise programs, and half of these stated that their major problem was easy fatigability. Two thirds of the study patients were able to maintain some sort of exercise throughout their treatment regimen, even though they did not recieve specific guidance about exercise. Eighty-five percent of the respondents felt that exercise counseling was a significant unmet need for patients with cancer.[26]

Exercise and Immune Function

It is still not clear whether regular cardiovascular endurance exercise has a beneficial, detrimental, or no significant effect on the immune function of patients with cancer. Watson and associates studied a group of 46 healthy individuals and subjected them to a 15-week cardiovascular endurance training program in which they exercised for 45 to 60 minutes five days a week at an exercise intensity between 70% to 85% of their maximal oxygen consumption. The study demonstrated that such physical training in these normal subjects results in: 1) significantly increased T-cell mitogenesis, reflecting the ability of T-cells to respond, grow, and divide when stimulated by nonspecific mitogens, 2) significantly increased numbers of mature

T-lymphocytes as measured by the formation of E-rosettes (lymphocytes to which at least three sheep red blood cells become attached during incubation), and 3) significantly suppressed natural killer cell activity, which may be due to enhanced maturation of natural killer cells into more mature T cells.[45] It is apparent that effects of such immune modulation on patients with breast cancer and other malignancies may be a consideration if cardiovascular exercise is to be recommended as adjunctive therapy for these patients.

THE UNIVERSITY OF MICHIGAN APPROACH

Because of the mutual interest in the total care of our patients with breast cancer, a program to enhance total body fitness and nutritional status is under development by the Breast Care Center and MedSport. MedSport has two divisions, Sports Medicine for the diagnosis, treatment, and rehabilitation of sports injuries, and Cardiac Programs, the scope of which has progressively expanded to encompass other medical conditions in which diet and exercise would be expected to be beneficial.

Patients who enter the Breast Care Center health enhancement program initially undergo a medical evaluation, including a history and a physical examination. Particular attention is paid to the staging of the disease and the type of therapy that has been carried out. Baseline blood studies are obtained, including a complete blood count, lipid profile, and biochemical screen. Percent body fat is estimated using skin fold thickness.

Exercise Recommendations

Postmenopausal patients or those over 40 years of age are asked to perform a symptom-limited, graded exercise test, performed to determine the patient's current level of cardiovascular fitness and for the development of an exercise prescription. We recommend that this test not be performed within 48 hours of the previous dose of intravenous chemotherapy, or if the patient has experienced significant recent vomiting or diarrhea as a result of oral chemotherapy.

Healthy individuals coming for an exercise program are generally given the coefficient of $x = .65$ to $.85$ in the Karvonen formula:

Exercise heart rate = Resting heart rate + x(peak exercise heart rate – resting heart rate)

We recommend that breast cancer patients should be exercised initially at lower levels, using a coefficient of $x = .30$ to $.60$. These patients, many of whom tend to fatigue easily secondary to physical deconditioning, recent operative therapy, or medication, find such recommendations to be non-threatening and acceptable. Premenopausal patients under 40 years are given exercise recommendations based on estimated maximal heart rate, and treadmill testing is not required.

We advocate the performance of weight lifting and, in selected cases, the use of exercise machines for enhancement of muscle tone and strength. Light weights are recommended so that the patient can perform 8 to 15 repetitions of the activity over the full range of the muscle's motion. Various flexibility activities are also recommended to improve this aspect of fitness.

We integrate cardiovascular endurance, muscle tone and strength, and flexibility exercises into our total body fitness approach to training. This method proceeds as follows:

Stage 1. Warm-up activities performed on a treadmill, a bicycle ergometer, or a track for 5 to 10 minutes.

Stage 2. Flexibility and range of motion exercises and isometric stretching for 4 to 6 minutes.

Stage 3. Aerobic exercises at target exercise heart rate on a treadmill, bicycle ergometer, and/or track for 10 to 15 minutes.

Stage 4. Muscular activities involving weight lifting and calisthenics performed in a circuit training sequence for 15 to 20 minutes

Stage 5. Aerobic exercises as for Stage 3 for 8 to 10 minutes.

Stage 6. Low-intensity muscular endurance upper body activities performed on a rowing machine or hand crank ergometer for 4 to 6 minutes.

Stage 7. Cool-down activities involving slow walking, flexibility, range of motion, and isometric stretching for 10 to 12 minutes.

Patients are checked during exercise to determine their heart rate response to exercise and are taught how to measure their own heart rate. We recommend that the above activities be performed two to three times a week at our facility, and at least 30 minutes of walking, light cycling, swimming, or other desired activities be performed several additional times a week outside of the program facility.

It is expected that there will be variations in adherence to the program, depending upon the patient's sense of well-being relative to the underlying disease process as well as to the required medical treatment. We do anticipate the usual responses, however, to a regular exercise program, including improved cardiovascular endurance, muscle strength, and flexibility; reduced body fatness; increased bone mineral content and reduced tendency to develop osteoporosis; improved lipid profile; and improved psychological profile.

Dietary Recommendations

Patients with breast cancer entering the program receive sound nutritional advice emphasizing weight reduction to as close to ideal body weight as possible; reduced consumption of total fat, saturated fat, and cholesterol, and especially of fatty meats and high-fat dairy products; increased intake of whole cereal grains, pasta, and legumes; increased consumption of fresh vegetables and fruits; decreased use of highly processed foods containing excessive amounts of artificial flavorings and colorings; avoidance of excessive amounts of salt and sodium-containing foods, as well as sugary foods; and increased fish intake.

Our goals are accomplished through individual and group dietary counseling and patient self-monitoring. In the individual sessions, a registered dietician meets with each patient and analyzes her individual diet, and provides personalized counseling to improve the patient's dietary habits and instructs her in how to monitor her dietary intake. The group counseling involves educational classes on a variety of topics, such as diet and cancer, food label reading, dining out, vegetarian eating, and food additives. We also provide cooking classes in which patients are instructed in a variety of meal preparation techniques, and we have grocery shopping classes, during which we take our patients to a local supermarket and teach them how to make healthier food choices.

At the termination of the program, we repeat the measurements taken at the beginning to assess the effect of the program. We believe that it is likely that those patients who participate regularly will gain improved health as a result of our efforts to enhance their fitness and nutrition. Whether these interventions will provide an improvement in the prognosis of our breast cancer patients remains to be determined.

SUMMARY

We postulate that dietary modification and physical exercise may be of value as adjunctive therapy in the treatment of breast cancer. The basis for this opinion is reviewed in this chapter. The collaborative model provides the setting for examination of the clinical role of such interventions, and will serve as a site for the development of research protocols to address the numerous unanswered questions about this new therapeutic approach.

REFERENCES

1. Abe R, Kumanai N, Kumagai M, et al.: Biological characteristics of breast cancer in obesity. Tohoku J Exp Med 120:351, 1976.
2. Balanski RM, Hadsiolov DH: Influence of sodium selenite on the hepa-

tocarcinogenic action of diethylnitrosamine in rats. CR Acad Bulg Sci 32:697, 1979.

3. Bird CE, Houghton B, Westenbrink W, et al.: Estradiol receptors in human breast carcinomas. Can Med Assoc J 124:1010, 1981.

4. Birt DF, Salmasi S, Pour PM: Enhancement of experimental pancreatic cancer in Syrian golden hamsters by dietary fat. JNCI 67:1327, 1981.

5. Bollag W: Therapy of epithelial tumors with an aromatic retinoic acid analog. Chemotherapy (Basel) 21:236, 1975.

6. Boyd NF, Campbell JE, Gerrmanson T, et al.: Body weight and prognosis in breast cancer. JNCI 67:785, 1981.

7. Burt JRF, Schapira DV: The effect of obesity on recurrence and ER status in breast cancer patients. Proc Am Assoc Clin Oncol c-6, 1983.

8. Cho-Chung YS: Cyclic AMP and tumor growth in vivo, in Kellen JA, Hilf R (eds): *Influences of Hormones in Tumor Development.* Boca Raton, FL, CRC Press, 1979, pp55–93.

9. Chu EW, Malmgran RA: An inhibitory effect of vitamin A on the induction of tumors of forestomach and cervix in the Syrian hamster by carcinogenic polycyclic hydrocarbons. Cancer Res 25:884, 1965.

10. Clayton CC, Baumann CA: Diet and azo-dye tumors: Effect of diet during a period when the dye is not fed. Cancer Res 9:575, 1949.

11. Cook MG, McNamara P: Effect of dietary vitamin E on dimethylhydrazine-induced colonic tumors in mice. Cancer Res 40:1329, 1980.

12. Daoud AH, Griffin AC: Effect of retinoic acid, butylated hydroxytoluene, selenium, and sorbic acid on azo-dye hepatocarcinogenesis. Cancer Lett 9:299, 1980.

13. Davidson MB, Carroll KK: Inhibitory effect of a fat-free diet on mammary carcinogenesis in rats. Nutr Cancer 3:207, 1982.

14. Delozier T, Julien JP, Juret P, et al.: Adjuvant tamoxifen in postmenopausal breast cancer: Preliminary results of a randomized trial. Breast Cancer Res Treat 7:105, 1986.

15. Donegan WI, Hartz AJ, Rimm AA: The association of body weight with recurrent breast cancer. Cancer 41:1590, 1978.

16. Elwood JM, Godolphin W: Oestrogen receptors in breast tumors: Associations with age, menopausal status, and epidemiological and clinical features in 735 patients. Br J Cancer 42:635, 1980.

17. Gregorio DI, Emrich LJ, Graham S, et al.: Dietary fat consumption and survival among women with breast cancer. JNCI 75:37, 1985.

18. Griffin AC, Jacobs MM: Effects of selenium on azo dye hepatocarcinogenesis. Cancer Lett 3:177, 1977.

19. Harr JR, Exon JH, Weswig H, et al.: Relationship of dietary selenium concentration, chemical cancer induction, and tissue concentration of selenium in rats. Clin Toxicol 8:487, 1973.

20. Healy JE: Role of rehabilitative medicine on the care of the patient with breast cancer. Cancer 28:1666, 1971.

21. Ip C: Factors influencing the anticarcinogenic efficacy of selenium in dimethylbenzanthracene-induced mammary tumorigenesis in rats. Cancer Res 41:2683, 1981.

22. Koloncl LN, Hankin JH, Lee J, et al.: Nutrient intakes in relation to cancer incidence in Hawaii. Br J Cancer 44:332, 1981.
23. Lasnitski I: Reversal of methylcholanthrene-induced changes in mouse prostates in vitro by retinoic acid and its analogs. Br J Cancer 34:239, 1976.
24. Lesser ML, Rosen PP, Senie RT, et al.: Estrogen and progesterone receptors in breast carcinoma. Cancer 48:299, 1981.
25. Longcope C, Pratt JH, Schneider SH, et al.: Aromatization of androgens by muscle and adipose tissue in vivo. J Clin Endocrinol Metab 46:146, 1978.
26. MacVicar MG, Winningham ML: Promoting the functional capacity of cancer patients. Cancer Bull, 1986, in press.
27. Moore JW, Clarke GMG, Takatani O, et al.: Distribution of 17-estradiol in the sera of normal British and Japanese women. JNCI 71:749, 1983.
28. National Research Council: *Diet, Nutrition and Cancer*. Washington, DC, National Academy Press, 1982.
29. Nigro ND, Singh DV, Campbell RL, et al.: Effect of dietary beef fat on intestinal tumor formation by azoxymethane in rats. JNCI 54:429, 1975.
30. Port CD, Sporn MB, Kaufman DG: Prevention of lung cancer in hamsters by 13-cis-retinoic acid. Proc Am Assoc Cancer Res 16:21, 1975.
31. Roebuck BD, Yager JG Jr, Longnecker DS, et al.: Promotion by unsaturated fat of azaserine-induced pancreatic carcinogenesis in the rat. Cancer Res 41:3961, 1981.
32. Rose DP: Postmenopausal oestrogen production and its inhibition, in Stoll BA (ed): *Endocrine Relationships in Breast Cancer*. London, Wm Heinemann Medical Books, 1982, pp187–214.
33. Sakamoto G, Sugano H, Hartman WH: Comparative clinicopathological study of breast cancer among Japanese and American females. Jpn J Cancer 25:161, 1979.
34. Saxe GA, Garces N, Carter JP: A study of diet and cancer of the pancreas. Master's thesis, Tulane University, New Orleans, 1985.
35. Schrauzer GN, Ishmael D: Effects of selenium and of arsenic on the genesis of spontaneous mammary tumors in inbred C_3H mice. Ann Clin Lab Sci 4:411, 1974.
36. Shamberger RJ: Relationships of selenium to cancer. I. Inhibitory effect of selenium on carcinogenesis. JNCI 44:931, 1970.
37. Shamberger RJ: Increase of peroxidation in carcinogenesis. JNCI 59:1712, 1977.
38. Sidransky H: Chemical and cellular pathology of experimental acute amino acid deficiency. Methods Achiev Exp Pathol 6:1, 1972.
39. Sporn MB, Squire RA, Brown CC, et al.: 13-cis-retinoic acid: Inhibition of bladder carcinogenesis in the rat. Science 195:487, 1977.
40. Tannenbaum A: The genesis and growth of tumors. III. Effects of a high fat diet. Cancer Res 2:468, 1942.
41. Tartter PI, Papatesstas AE, Ioannovich J, et al.: Cholesterol and obesity as prognostic factors in breast cancer. Cancer 47:2222, 1981.

42. Thomas DB: Hormones and hormone receptors in the etiology of breast cancer. Breast Cancer Res Treat 7[Suppl]:11, 1986.
43. Thompson HJ, Taglaferro AR: Effect of selenium on 7,12-dimethylbenzanthracene-induced mammary tumorigenesis. Fed Proc 39:1117, 1980.
44. Thorpe SM, Rose C, Petersen BV, et al.: Estrogen and progesterone receptor profile patterns in primary breast cancer. Breast Cancer Res Treat 3:103, 1983.
45. Watson RR, Moriguchi S, Jackson JC: Modification of cellular immune functions in humans by endurance exercise training during β-adrenergic blockade with atenolol or propranolol. Med Sci Sports Exerc 18:95, 1986.
46. Willett WC, Stampfer MJ, Colditz GA, et al.: Dietary fat and the risk of breast cancer. N Engl J Med 316:22, 1987.
47. Winningham ML, MacVicar MG: Response of cancer patients on chemotherapy to a supervised exercise program, abstracted. Med Sci Sports Exerc 17:292, 1985.
48. Wynder EL, Kajitani T, Kuno J, et al.: A comparison of survival rates between American and Japanese patients with breast cancer. Surg Gynecol Obstet 117:196, 1963.
49. Wynder EL, Rose DP: Diet and breast cancer. Hospital Practice April, 1984, pp73.
50. Zumoff B, Dasgupta I: Relationship between body weight and the incidence of positive axillary nodes at mastectomy for breast cancer. J Surg Oncol 22:217, 1983.
51. Zumoff B, Gorzynski JG, Katz JL, et al.: Nonobesity at the time of mastectomy is highly predictive of 10-year disease-free survival in women with breast cancer. Anticancer Res 2:59, 1982.

25. Nursing Management of the Patient with Breast Cancer

KATHLEEN A. CALZONE
SHARON J. NOFFSINGER
PATRICIA A. SARAN
DIANE K. SOMMERFIELD

The care of the breast cancer patient provides a unique opportunity for surgical, radiation, and medical oncology nurses to provide comprehensive care collaboratively. Multiple disciplines intervene in the diagnosis and treatment process, sometimes singly and at other times simultaneously. Patients can be overwhelmed, and perhaps lost, with so many professionals involved in their care. Oncology nurses are in a position to facilitate the coordination of care for these patients. While each of the three roles has unique functions, there are many that are common to each area.

One of the responsibilities that is shared by each oncology nurse is screening and detection, the first step in the fight against breast cancer. The active participation of nursing in teaching breast self-examination (BSE) on a one-to-one basis or in public presentations is vital to increasing patient and public awareness and compliance. Besides the BSE technique, teaching includes encouraging questions and expression of fears. In conjunction with BSE, the nurse provides information about mammography, its early detection capabilities, the low risk of radiation used, the recommended frequency, and the physical sensations experienced while having a mammogram. People also need to be aware of advances and new developments in breast cancer research and treatment. This information increases the chance for early detection. At many points in the health care system, the nurse reaches individuals and family members. Public health awareness programs, clubs, or group forums can be utilized (with the nurse serving as organizer, facilitator, or lecturer) to reach larger numbers of people.

The patient with breast cancer will encounter a number of oncology nurses throughout the diagnostic and treatment phases of her illness. No matter which specialty is involved in treating a patient, the goals are the same. This chapter presents an overview of the scope of nursing roles in the care of these patients.

SURGICAL ONCOLOGY NURSING

When there is a suspicion of breast cancer, the patient will first encounter a surgical oncology nurse, who practices in ambulatory care and inpatient settings. The surgical nurse assumes responsibilities that assist in the functioning of the multidisciplinary team. Shared responsibilities may include phone triage of patients, initial history and health assessments, breast self-examination teaching, follow-up regarding test results and recommendations, and contributing to research data collection.

Surgical background and knowledge is important to this patient population, but teaching only the surgical and medical therapies and the biologic processes involved is not sufficient. Information conveyed must also include anticipated sensory feelings, impact on lifestyle, and concrete preparatory instructions. Patients newly diagnosed or suspected of breast cancer require a quiet environment and a confident, competent approach. The nurse's ability to discuss the planned procedures as well as rationale provides an atmosphere of confidence and hope.

The surgical nurse, with her knowledge of the necessary equipment, supplies, handling of the specimen, and appropriate patient care, facilitates a smooth and uncomplicated biopsy (fine needle aspiration, Tru-Cut®, punch). More extensive biopsies (incisional, excisional, wire localization) are done on an outpatient basis. Despite breast biopsy's classification as a minor procedure, all patients having a breast biopsy need information, teaching, and support. The nurse's knowledge is maintained by the periodic observation of surgical procedures and regular, open communication with operating room and recovery room personnel. These activities assist her in devising written materials that reflect current practices.

Providing information as is listed in Table 1 in the clinic setting promotes a feeling of security and confidence in the patient. A number of the teaching points will be readdressed by the operating room/recovery room nursing staff and the surgeon. Repetition is quite often necessary for the patient at a highly stressful time.

Today's economic climate has resulted in admissions the same day as the procedure, shortened hospitalizations, and a longer list of approved outpatient procedures. Preoperative preparation, counseling, and teaching has now become the responsibility of the nurse in ambulatory care. Legislative measures also have influenced and underscored the need for an informed and well-prepared patient. The nurse's contribution cannot be underestimated.

Knowledge about the implications of a major surgical procedure and potential complications is invaluable. During the first postoperative visit,

Table 1. Nurse's Surgical Teaching

Location of surgical suite and family waiting room
Time and date of procedure
Estimated length of procedure
Name of surgeon
NPO status
Medications
   To continue regular medications or not
   Prescription for discomfort
   Anesthesia planned
Appropriate clothing, e.g., firm support bra
Need for responsible adult to provide transportation home
Type of excision, expected tissue loss
Effect of surgical scar on future mammographic readings
Changes in breast self-examination
Suture material material, need for removal or not
Type of dressing, e.g., transparent, pressure, etc.
Bathing following procedure
Activity level and work restrictions
Signs and symptoms of normal healing
Symptoms or problems to report
Contact names and phone numbers
Clinic visit after procedure
Approximate date pathology report available

the nurse assesses the patient for complications, assists in her treatment, and provides approaches to continuing care. Since the surgical nurse is aware of the operative date, and because of short hospital stays, some referrals are made prior to admission. The referral services may include the physical therapist, social worker, Reach to Recovery volunteer, peer counselor, business office, and so on.

The surgical nurse is in a position to share insights and information with all nurses caring for the breast cancer patient. This is accomplished both formally (in-services, conferences, interdisciplinary rounds) and informally. Ongoing dialogue between the inpatient unit nursing staff and the surgical nurse ensures consistent patient education materials, follow-up of patients after discharge, and information sharing. Information regarding an individual's needs or problems may be incorporated in care plans both in the outpatient and inpatient settings. Familiarization with units' routines, policies, resources, and changes in care is valuable.

Nursing rounds on hospitalized patients supply a wealth of information to the surgical nurse and are a source of comfort and continuity. These also provide an opportunity to verify the content and appropriateness of any teaching and referrals. Because of the presence of the surgical nurse during the diagnostic and surgical treatment process, patients often freely share their feelings and observations of care. Information on the emotional support of the breast cancer patient and family, which is abundant in the nursing literature, is constantly incorporated into the practice of the surgical oncology nurse.

The services of the surgical oncology nurse are not limited to the diagnostic and primary treatment phases of breast cancer. A surgical biopsy to determine the presence of metastatic lesions or a second primary requires the understanding and comfort of a knowledgeable nurse. Should a venous access device become necessary, the surgical nurse's familiarity with the various devices and procedures not only augments the medical oncology nurses's teaching, but assists in troubleshooting. Surgery, the oldest treatment modality, and nursing have been complementary through the years, but breast cancer care has now expanded to include other treatment modalities and disciplines. Management of the patient with breast cancer requires a collaborative approach among nursing specialties as well.

RADIATION ONCOLOGY NURSING

The major focus of the radiation oncology nurse's role in the care of patients with breast cancer is patient education and counseling. The nurse in radiation oncology participating in a multidisciplinary breast team first encounters patients during the treatment decision–making phase. Patients frequently are uncertain and have questions about radiation therapy as a treatment option for breast cancer. In addition to dealing with a diagnosis of cancer, which is stressful, patients are having to make a decision about a lesser known treatment modality. A collaborative relationship with social workers has been developed to assist in meeting counseling needs.

Initially, the nurse assesses the extent to which the patient is coping. By the first visit to the radiation oncology department, a patient has had some time to adjust to the diagnosis of breast cancer, make a treatment decision, and often have the necessary operative therapy. Since the use of primary radiation therapy to treat early stage breast cancer is relatively new, few individuals are knowledgeable about this option, and many are skeptical. In addition, patients have often heard comments from "well-intentioned" acquaintances such as: "How do you know that is going to work?" or "You may get burned."

Many patients initially question the use of radiation therapy to treat cancer at a time when the public is being told to limit X-ray exposure. Others may have doubts about their treatment decision and fear recurrence of disease. The radiation oncology nurse encourages patients and family members to ask questions and provides information about treatment. Arrangements are often made for patients to talk with former patients who are articulate and positive about their treatment, which is also very helpful. Concerns about radiation treatment are ongoing; therefore, throughout the treatment course reassurance is provided by the radiation oncology nurse.

Another patient concern is the requirement of daily treatment for five to six weeks. Driving time and travel problems can be disruptive and a source

Table 2. Nurse's Radiation Therapy Teaching

Constant audio and television communication with staff
Position determined at simulation will be used for all treatments
No pain associated with actual treatment (like getting an X-ray)
Linear accelerator produces a loud humming noise when on
Length of entire procedure (approximately 15 to 20 minutes)
Length of actual treatment (one to two minutes)
Verification of treatment area with weekly X-rays
Weekly complete blood counts
Weekly examination by a physician

of additional stress. Nurses assist patients and families by facilitating discussion of travel considerations, offering possible solutions, and making appropriate referrals, such as to the American Cancer Society.

During the consultation appointment, range of motion in the affected arm is assessed so that potential problems are identified prior to simulation. Range of motion exercises are reviewed, and the necessity for daily performance is reinforced and assessed periodically throughout treatment.

A treatment planning session (simulation) is necessary before treatment can begin. The procedure is first explained at the consultation appointment so that anticipatory anxiety is lessened. Teaching simple relaxation techniques and listening to taped music are interventions that are helpful in decreasing any anxiety and discomfort associated with simulation. The types of immobilization devices and simulation procedures can vary from place to place; therefore, each radiation oncology department develops its own description of simulation that the radiation oncology nurse will use in patient teaching. The patient usually begins treatment within two days of simulation. The information in Table 2 is presented to the patient prior to the first treatment.

At the first treatment, the radiation oncology nurse explains the procedure, elicits special concerns, and gives reassurance. This does much to alleviate the anxiety associated with the start of radiation treatments. During the first week, patients are taught about skin care, and potential side effects and their management. Side effects for patients undergoing breast radiation are generally related to skin reactions and fatigue. Weekly physical assessments are done on all patients being treated. Skin changes are expected, but are short-term and easy to manage. The extent of these changes ranges from dryness, mild erythema, peeling (dry desquamation), pruritus, and slight tenderness to moist desquamation and marked erythema. More severe side effects are seen most commonly in skin fold areas, i.e., axilla, inframammary fold, and supraclavicular area (neck edge). Women with larger, pendulous breasts are more likely to experience moist desquamation; when this occurs, dressings such as Vigilon may be used until the area has healed. Skin care teaching is listed in Table 3.

The extent to which patients experience fatigue is quite variable because

Table 3.   Radiation Therapy Skin Care Teaching

Use of mild soap to cleanse treated breast, e.g., Ivory or Neutrogena
Avoid vigorous towel drying
Avoid use of creams, lotions, deodorants, etc., on treated area
Comfort of soft, loose-fitting bra, or no bra during treatment
Dressings for moist desquamation, should it occur
Redness may increase for as much as seven days after treatment ends

of life situation, personality, and distance traveled to and from radiation therapy. Fatigue may begin halfway through a treatment course and persist for a few months following completion. Being informed of this side effect early in the treatment process prevents anxiety, which could develop if this were perceived as a new symptom. Strategies that the nurse recommends for managing fatigue include having family members help with household duties, taking naps, going to bed earlier, and prioritizing, deleting, or deferring activities.

Rare side effects that may occur several months posttreatment include myositis in the pectoral region, arm edema, rib fracture, and pneumonitis. Patients are informed about these effects and how to manage them.

After the boost method is determined, the nurse explains the procedure. Patients being treated with external beam radiation are informed about the greater potential for skin reaction. Those receiving implants require more information about the surgical procedure, including expected sensations, loading procedure, inpatient care, and follow-up. Patients and family members usually require more reassurance about the implanting of radioactive sources, because of the fear of increased exposure to other parts of their body. Discussion of these concerns is facilitated by the radiation oncology nurse.

As therapy is completed, patients are given information about follow-up and continuing self-care. Understanding the follow-up process, and realizing a nurse is available if there are any problems, lessens anxiety associated with separation from a therapeutic atmosphere. The importance of monthly BSE is reinforced and the procedure reviewed. This is particularly important because postradiation changes make BSE more difficult. A major focus of the radiation oncology nurse role at this point is assisting patients to gain confidence in doing BSE.

Radiotherapy is also used for palliation. Patients with metastatic disease may require more nursing care because of increased physical and psychological distress. Relief of physical distress is of prime importance, but accompanying psychosocial stress cannot be minimized or ignored. Nurses assist patients and families in dealing with issues related to more advanced disease. When patients are receiving radiation therapy for pain relief, the nurse's expertise in the use of multiple methods of pain management, including nonmedical therapies, is invaluable in assisting patients until pain relief is achieved.

Education of other nursing personnel is also a component of the radiation oncology nurse's role. Conducting inservice programs and sharing information with other nursing personnel about mutual patients is particularly helpful with this less understood form of treatment. Conducting nursing research is another component of the role and is particularly pertinent because of the comparatively limited number of studies that have been conducted.

As more people have become aware of radiation therapy as primary treatment for breast cancer, more are choosing this modality. Nurses have an important role in caring for patients undergoing radiation therapy for breast cancer. The role of the radiation oncology nurse is emerging as a challenging and important area of nursing specialization that dramatically affects patient care.

MEDICAL ONCOLOGY NURSING

The population encountered in medical oncology nursing comprises patients in all stages of disease. Nursing management includes the care of patients receiving adjuvant therapy, those receiving therapy for metastatic disease, and those enrolled in investigational studies. Treatment forms vary, but include antineoplastic agents, antiestrogen therapy, and a variety of investigational agents, including biologicals. Once therapy is completed (whether the individual remains disease-free requiring follow-up, or progression occurs and the patient requires palliative care), the medical oncology nurse continues as an essential resource for patients.

Clinical research is frequently a component of medical oncology nursing practice. Comprehensive understanding of the purpose of a research protocol and its format and ramifications is essential for patient management. The nurse is an integral part of the health care team whose overall objective is to establish improved treatment alternatives. Nursing contributions to a successful clinical trial are essential. The role integrates patient management and coordination, data collection, and subsequent analysis.

The realm of clinical research also includes the nurse as an independent primary investigator. Areas of research encompass symptom management, psychosocial interventions, and safety standards. Medical oncology nurses practice in the following settings:

- Inpatient hospital units
- Ambulatory care centers
- Private practice offices
- Clinical research centers
- Home care agencies
- Hospices

Collaboration between nursing in these different areas assures continuity and consistency of teaching and care.

Throughout all patient settings and various stages of disease, the medical oncology nurse incorporates high-level assessment skills and develops comprehensive care plans to address the areas of prevention, detection, symptom management, psychosocial issues, and comprehensive care follow-up.

The nurse also maintains a technical domain, which includes the performance of or assistance with medical procedures. Nursing care is required for patients undergoing bone marrow aspirations, lumbar punctures, thoracentesis, paracentesis, and other procedures. A thorough understanding of the procedure is required to adequately assist the physician and to effectively prepare the patient and explain the procedure to her. Administration of antineoplastics and investigational agents is major responsibility, requiring additional nursing education, training, and technical expertise. Other nursing activities involve the administration and monitoring of intravenous hydration, antibiotics, parenteral and enteral nutrition, blood products, and symptom and pain control medications.

The medical oncology nurse's role frequently begins when a patient is to receive neo-adjuvant or adjuvant treatment. At this time (and during all stages of disease), a major nursing focus is the psychological support of the patient and family. The nurse frequently develops intervention strategies to address depression, altered body image, altered lifestyle, sexual concerns, infertility, uncertainty and concern about disease recurrence, fear of death, and grieving. In addition, the medical oncology nurse assists patients and families in accepting the concept or rationale for adjuvant treatment.

When receiving chemotherapy, most patients are treated on an outpatient basis or discharged from the hospital soon after treatment ends. Chemotherapy has both short-term and long-term side effects; consequently, many problems occur at home. Therefore, the patient and family are responsible for managing and reporting both changes of condition and uncontrolled side effects. The nurse explains the treatment program, side effects, and how to manage them. Written resources covering this material are given to patients to provide concrete information at home. Each chemotherapy drug has individual side effects and may affect each patient differently. The issues discussed with the patient are listed in Table 4.

To ensure patient safety and prompt intervention, the patient is taught to call immediately to report the symptoms listed in Table 5. The nurse also supplies information about available services such as peer counselors, support/information groups, and the wig bank, and such organizations as the American Cancer Society and cancer foundations.

If a patient develops metastatic disease, clinical management requires an increasingly broad spectrum of nursing interventions and activities. A major nursing activity is symptom management. Symptoms can result from the disease process or be secondary to treatment programs. The medical

Table 4. Nurse's Chemotherapy Teaching

Increased potential for infection and bleeding
Gastrointestinal symptoms
  Nausea and vomiting
  Diarrhea
  Constipation
  Stomatitis
Alopecia
Skin changes, including
  Acne
  Photosensitivity
  Pruritus
Nerve or muscle changes
Changes in sexual functioning and desire
Reproductive concerns and issues
Emotional changes
Fatigue
Medications, prescription and over the counter
Alcoholic beverages

Table 5. Symptoms Requiring Immediate Contact with Professional Staff

Nausea or vomiting persisting for more than 24 hours
Inability to eat or drink for 24 hours
Diarrhea persisting for more than 24 hours
Significant change in bowel habits over two or three days
Development of mouth sores
Temperature of 101°F or higher
Persistent cough
Burning on urination
Bleeding that persists more than 10 to 20 minutes
Blood in urine or stools (either bright red or black bowel movements)

oncology nurse is responsible for patient and family education, monitoring, documenting, and assisting in the management of all symptoms and problems that arise. One of the most distressing problems encountered is pain. Dispelling myths about drug addiction or drug selection, assuring adequate pain control, and safety are vital. Some of the other symptoms addressed are listed in Table 6.

When metastatic disease progresses, the nurse continues to provide emotional support. The decision to discontinue treatment is a delicate issue, during which time the nurse provides support and information. Assisting the patient and family with increasing limitations is a major responsibility.

Preparing a family to care for a patient in end-stage disease encompasses many areas. The medical oncology nurse assumes the task as educator and coordinator. The patient must have adequate supplies and services at home, including nursing care, dressings, oxygen, dietary supplements, and hospital equipment. The nurse educates the family to manage many of the previ-

Table 6.   Nursing Problems Requiring Management in Metastatic Disease

Fatigue	Shortness of breath
Nausea and vomiting	Skin breakdown
Diarrhea	Decreased mobility
Constipation	Ascites and edema
Nutritional deficit, weight loss	Depression
Dehydration	Mental changes

Table 7.   Issues in End-Stage Care

Family and social impact
Teaching technical skills, such as
    Feeding tubes
    Microvolume infusion pumps
    Permanent right atrial catheters
Hospice/respite care
Grief and loss
Legal implications
Funeral arrangements
Bereavement

ously mentioned symptoms. In addition, other areas need to be addressed (Table 7).

The clinical realm of the oncology nurse is very broad, but the nurse is limited in her ability to manage all patient problems. Consequently, patient triage to other members of the health care team is necessary. Collaboration with the physician, social worker, dietician, physical therapist, and pharmacist is essential. The role of the medial oncology nurse as coordinator and provider of consistent and effective care cannot be overemphasized.

The medical oncology nurse has a unique and challenging role in the management of the patient with breast cancer. She cares for patients at diagnosis, through treatment, follow-up and, too frequently, recurrence and death. The long-term, intense nurse/patient/family relationship that develops results in the opportunity to deliver quality nursing care. Although stressful, this nursing role is a very rewarding and satisfying experience.

CONCLUSION

There are myriad resources to support the nurse in her professional development. The Oncology Nursing Society, National Intravenous Therapy Association, National Hospice Organization, American Cancer Society, and the National Cancer Institute are indispensable in providing a forum for professional education and growth. Networking with colleagues concerning current issues is also a means of growing professionally. Most recently, the development of the Oncology Nursing Certification examination has presented a new challenge to oncology nurses. It assures a consistent knowledge base and offers opportunity for professional recognition of expertise. Educational institutions have also developed graduate programs for master's level specialization in oncology nursing.

Oncology nursing has developed as a specialty area of nursing in response to cancer being a major health problem. Whether the nurse's prime focus is education, clinical practice, administration, or research, she will be concerned with the provision of optimal care to individuals with a diagnosis of cancer and to family members as well. Because of a constantly changing approach to the diagnosis and treatment of breast cancer, nurses must be informed of these changes in order to provide competent and compassionate patient care. Care of the breast cancer patient demands collaborative nursing practice, which promotes quality patient care.

BIBLIOGRAPHY

1. Bouchard-Kurtz R, Speece-Owens N: *Nursing Care of the Cancer Patient.* St. Louis, C.V. Mosby Company, 1981.
2. Burns N: The medical management of cancer and the nurse's role, *Nursing and Cancer.* Philadelphia, W.B. Saunders Company, 1982, pp82–206.
3. Crowley, SA: *Chemotherapy Side Effects Management Handbook.* Ann Arbor, University of Michigan Hospitals, 1984.
4. Friel M: Concepts related to the nursing care of surgical oncology patients, in Vredovoe DL (ed): *Concepts of Oncology Nursing.* Englewood Cliffs, N.J., Prentice-Hall Incorporated, 1981, pp221–269.
5. Greifzu S: Breast cancer: The risks and the options. RN 49:26–32, 1986.
6. Hassey K: Radiation therapy for breast cancer: A historic review. Nursing management for breast cancer. Semin Oncol 1:181–188, 1985.
7. Henke C: Emerging roles in the nurse in oncology. Semin Oncol 7:4–8, 1980.
8. Hubbard S, Donehower M: The nurse in a cancer research setting. Semin Oncol 7:14, 1980.
9. Kobza L: Assessing post-mastectomy care in a community hospital. QRB 9:116–119, 1984.
10. Lichter A: Nonmastectomy treatment of breast cancer. Postgrad Med 79:93–103, 1986.
11. Mast M: Primary care of the mastectomy patient. Nurse Practitioner 9:27–28, 30, 32, 1984.
12. McNally JC, Stair JC, Somerville ET: *Guidelines for Cancer Nursing Practice.* Orlando, Grune & Stratton, 1985.
13. Pfeiffer C, Mulliken J: *Caring for the Patient with Breast Cancer: An Interdisciplinary/Multidisciplinary Approach.* Reston, VA, Reston Publishing Company, 1984.
14. Voss S: Ambulatory surgery scheduling, assuring a smooth patient flow. AORN 43:1009–1012, 1986.

15. Whitehead D: A minor surgical procedure? Nursing Timcs 80:45–46, 1984.
16. Wilson C, Strohl R: Radiation therapy as primary treatment for breast cancer. Oncol Nursing Forum 19:12–15, 1982.
17. Yasko JM: *Care of the Client Receiving External Radiation Therapy.* Reston, VA, Reston Publishing Company, 1982.
18. Yasko JM: *Guidelines for Cancer Care: Symptom Management.* Reston, VA, Reston Publishing Company, 1983.

26. *Social Work with the Breast Cancer Patient*

CLAUDIA W. KRAUS
LEE K. ROSENBLUM

When a woman is given a diagnosis of breast cancer, she enters a transitional crisis that will alter her life in fundamental and enduring ways. From the time that a patient discovers she has breast cancer until long after she completes treatment, she and her family undergo a series of profound changes. They are faced with many decisions, must quickly absorb new information, learn the meaning and implications of unfamiliar medical terminology, and confront social stigma. They are facing a potentially life-threatening disease, perhaps quite early in life. There are many psychological transitions as well. She may reevaluate fundamental assumptions about the future, lifestyle, body image, sexuality, and mortality. Comprehensive care of the breast cancer patient necessarily includes addressing the psychosocial issues that affect the larger context of her life. Although other members of the breast care team may address these concerns, it is the role of the social worker to focus primarily on the issues of psychosocial adjustment, and to intervene therapeutically with the patient. The social worker may be one of the only nonmedical professionals with whom the patient has contact. His or her broad training in psychological assessment, crisis intervention, counseling, and group work, combined with knowledge of community resources and familiarity with the medical setting, enables the social worker to bring a valuable perspective to patient care.

The functions of the breast cancer social worker are, by necessity, diverse. In order to meet the various patient needs, the social worker may arrange transportation, coordinate hospital discharge plans, offer individual and family counseling, consult with teachers and psychotherapists in the community, conduct support groups, refer to community resources, and develop educational programs and materials. The underlying goals that unify these diverse professional activities are twofold: to help the patient maintain psychological and social functioning during a time of stressful transition; and to help her integrate the crisis into her life in a way that will promote healthy, long-term adjustment.

347

Following are two case examples illustrating some of the range of social work involvement with breast cancer patients:

CASE 1   Mrs. G. is an attractive 57-year-old woman diagnosed with breast cancer, who was seen by social work after her mastectomy. She was referred to and seen by Reach to Recovery while in the hospital. During the initial assessment with the social worker, the great importance of her breasts and appearance to her self-esteem were discussed. She raised concerns about how her husband would accept her after the loss of her breast; she was reluctant to talk with her husband about her worries. As they talked further, the social worker was able to help Mrs. G. recognize that these fears weren't based on anything he had said or done, but were a normal part of adjusting to her new body image. The worker helped bring into focus how supportive and accepting Mr. G. was actually being to his wife, and encouraged her to discuss her concerns directly with him. When she was still hesitant, the social worker arranged to meet with both of them to discuss the normal process of resuming intimacy after mastectomy. Because of the patient's questions about breast reconstruction, the social worker arranged for her to meet with a peer counselor who had had breast reconstruction. Mrs. G. found this very helpful. After going home from the hospital, she found the transition easier than she had expected. Some time later she attended a Breast Reconstruction Program and decided to go ahead with the reconstruction. At her one-year follow-up visit, the social worker met with Mrs. G. She reported that things were going well and that there were no problems that needed to be addressed.

CASE 2   Ms. S. is a 35-year-old single parent with daughters three and eight years old. Prior to her diagnosis of breast cancer, she was working at a convenience store that did not provide health insurance. Ms. S. was referred to the social worker at the clinic for assistance in obtaining coverage for the surgical treatment she would need. The social worker was able to help guide Ms. S. through a complex application process for assistance at a time when she was quite stressed. The social worker learned that Ms. S. had little support other than from an unreliable boyfriend. She had no close friends or family. The social worker arranged for Ms. S. to meet with a peer counselor when she was in the hospital for her lumpectomy. She was able to talk with the same peer counselor when she learned she would undergo adjuvant chemotherapy. Ms. S. seemed to be adjusting well to her operation and chemotherapy until eight months into her one-year course of treatment. At that point, she contacted the social worker whom she had remembered from previous contacts, asking for some help. When the social worker met with her, she reported that her boyfriend decided to leave her. Upon further assessment, she related that her eight-year-old daughter was fearful and unwilling to go to school. The social worker learned that Ms. S. had not directly told the children about her medical problems or explained the treatments that made her feel sick once a week. The social worker helped Ms. S. find ways to explain the illness and treatments to the children in ways they could understand and find reassuring. The social worker helped Ms. S. to understand the impact of a mother's illness on children as well as helped her grieve the loss of her boyfriend. In addition, the social worker referred her to the Breast Cancer Support Group, where she would be able to talk with others in similar situations. Ms. S. continued to see the social worker for counseling until the end of her chemotherapy. The social worker referred Ms. S. to a local counseling agency for continuation of her treatment.

As illustrated in those examples, it is the role of the social worker to assess various areas of functioning and to provide resources to strengthen and supplement the patient's own resources. This may include the traditional social work role of providing access to social services such as public assistance or transportation. However, this may also entail counseling the patient to utilize her own psychological resources, which have become paralyzed due to crisis. It may mean helping the patient mobilize her support network, by enhancing communication with a spouse, or involving extended family and friends in her coping strategies. The social worker may also develop resources, such as programs and groups, which address particular needs of the breast cancer patient and her family.

In order to best serve the patient, the social worker should contact her as soon after diagnosis as possible. The period of involvement may continue through hospitalization for surgery, adjuvant treatment, breast reconstruction and ongoing follow-up, if appropriate. Contact is often reinitiated at a time of recurrence and continued treatment. At the University of Michigan Medical Center, a comprehensive support program has been developed which addresses the patient's changing needs through the course of diagnosis, treatment, and follow-up.

STAGES IN ADJUSTMENT

A patient diagnosed with breast cancer faces new experiences and issues with which she must cope. These issues and her reactions change as she goes through her course of treatment. From observation of patients, as well as descriptions of their experiences, we identify six stages in adjustment to breast cancer which parallel steps in the diagnosis and treatment process. There is variation among patients in their adjustment to the illness, and overlap of stages. It is important for the members of the treatment team to be aware of the sequence and timing of this adjustment process, as the patient's needs will vary during the process. Others have described stages in adjustment somewhat differently.[14]

Finding a Suspicious Lump

When a patient discovers a lump that she believes may be cancer, she suddenly faces many of her worst fears and some crucial decisions. For many, the most important issue at this point is the need to clarify whether this lump is breast cancer, and whether her fears are accurate. She must decide whether the lump warrants further attention, and if so, how urgently.

Most patients describe their initial reaction at the discovery as shock and fear, often followed by efforts to reassure themselves. There is no way to alleviate their fears until the visit with the physician. Many patients describe feeling as if they are swept along by their fears, with little control over them.

Confirmation of Diagnosis

When the suspicious lump is found to be cancer, the patient's fears are confirmed, and she must begin to absorb the implications of her diagnosis. Since there is still no way of knowing what the full extent and impact of the disease will be, her primary concern is about suffering or dying. At the same time that the patient is grappling with her feelings, she must make a decision with her physician about treatment. Will she have a mastectomy or lumpectomy and radiation therapy? Can she face the loss of a breast? Or, can she tolerate approximately six weeks of daily radiation treatments? She has a great deal of information and many decisions to consider.

At this stage, patients may feel more anxious than usual, more fearful, moody, depressed, or have difficulty concentrating and performing usual tasks. Many describe feeling that everything seems strange, almost like in a dream. The breast cancer becomes the central focus in her life.

In the Hospital

After the operation, she has completed what is perhaps the most significant change that she will undergo. Although she has undergone the primary treatment for her disease, she must await test results to know whether she is likely to be free of the disease and whether she will have to undergo further treatments. The patient is torn between wanting to get on with adjusting and being unable to do so until she learns what adjustments she must make. There are a number of milestones at this stage: viewing and touching her incision for the first time; having others, especially her spouse or partner, do so; assessing other's reactions to her; and beginning to resume activities of normal life.[5]

The majority of patients are able to cope effectively, and are surprised to find that the operation was easier than anticipated. However, some patients have problematic reactions, with strong fears or anxiety; some experience resurfacing of preexisting problems or issues, especially relating to losses in the past. Patients may be moody and irritable, and find minor problems and delays intolerable.[7]

Going Home

When the patient goes home from the hospital and has received test results, she begins the task of living with cancer. She begins to return to her usual activities of home, family, job, and friends. She knows her treatment plan and can begin to realize the full impact of what has happened. She and her family may be rethinking many of their assumptions about life and reordering their priorities.[15]

The process of returning to familiar surroundings and activities often brings the emotional impact of her situation more fully to awareness. There is less need and ability to use denial as protection. In the hospital, she had more structured support from staff and visitors, as well as subtle encouragement to be strong and be a "good patient."[13] Some of the feelings and reactions that she had in the hospital may be intensified, such as a sense of loss or moodiness. But as the patient passes some of the milestones and resumes prior functioning, she becomes more confident and the feeling of mastery over her experiences grows.

Adjuvant Treatment

When the patient is undergoing adjuvant radiation therapy or chemotherapy, the most important concerns she faces are whether the treatment will be effective and whether side effects will be manageable. The duration of therapy, especially chemotherapy, can extend and impede the process of returning to normal functioning begun in the previous stage.[7,9] Unfortunately, the treatment presents the patient and her family with additional adjustments, such as treatment schedules, hair thinning, nausea, and weakness.

What most patients describe concerning adjuvant treatment is that they have an ongoing, unavoidable reminder of their disease. Depression and discouragement are not uncommon reactions. Problematic reactions that arose earlier may still continue. On the other hand, many of the same patients report feeling hopeful and protected while in treatment. During this period, patients have ongoing contact and support from the treatment team. Their anxiety may increase as the end of treatment approaches.[6]

Long-Term Adjustment

When the patient has finished the planned treatment, she enters the long-term adjustment phase. She must come to terms with whatever losses she has experienced and learn to handle the fear of recurrence. She must integrate her altered view of the world to incorporate the new awareness of her vulnerability brought into focus by her experiences.

As described previously, some patients experience increased anxiety as they come to the end of their treatment and proceed "on their own." This anxiety is likely to be intensified around the anniversaries of treatment events, as well as at follow-up visits. Some patients have difficulty adjusting to the changes in their view of the world — faith in God, their own future well-being, and the value of their lives and activities. Patients may seek explanations or reasons for their cancer. This struggle to understand the disease is a common manifestation of trying to control fear through knowledge.

MODALITIES OF SOCIAL WORK INTERVENTION WITH THE BREAST CANCER PATIENT

There are three aspects of patient functioning which the social worker must assess, the psychological, the relational, and the social. The psychological aspect of functioning is the internal resources of the patient herself, including her ability to adapt to change, to make decisions, to cope with loss, and to come to terms with what has happened. The relational aspect is the quality of communication and support she receives from the people in the inner circle of her life. Much has been written about the value of this support in adjusting to her illness.[1,11,12,15] The third aspect, the larger circle of social support, includes provision of basic needs, such as financial resources, housing, and transportation. Some women have deficits in these aspects of functioning, even during the best of times; during a time of crisis, resources in each of these areas can be overstrained.

During this transition to an altered sense of self and the world, a period sometimes prolonged by adjuvant treatment, the patient and family are particularly open to, and often seek, information to help them grasp and conceptualize what is happening to them. During this time, the social worker has the opportunity to intervene in ways that the patient might not have accepted at other times in her life.

Although the specific issues being dealt with are different at the various stages discussed previously, the social work interventions are somewhat consistent. Much of the work is supportive — reinforcing appropriate coping, clarifying feelings, enhancing communication with the family, providing a realistic perspective, and providing access to information from the medical team, peer counselors, and community programs. By serving as a sounding board to the patient, the worker can clarify ambivalence and help reduce discouragement about the treatment, as well as providing help in the ongoing efforts to learn to live with her new identity: cancer patient. The social worker can also provide crisis intervention, helping deal with grossly dysfunctional reactions.

In order to address the changing concerns arising at different points in the treatment, and specific individual needs, the social worker must use a variety of interventions. The modalities of social work interventions with the breast cancer patient can be classified in four categories: 1) initial assessment, 2) counseling, 3) psychosocial programs, and 4) linking with community resources. Each of these interventions serves specific needs, and is best used during particular phases of the diagnosis, treatment, and follow-up.

Initial Assessment

There are two primary goals in the social worker's initial contact with the patient that are worked on concurrently: identification of problems in the above-mentioned aspects of functioning that may require intervention, and intervention to assist her in adjusting to the disease and its treatment.

In assessing the psychological functioning, the social worker seeks to determine the manner and effectiveness of the patient's coping. By assessing how the patient and family have adjusted to losses and important changes in the past, the social worker can determine what unresolved issues may resurface,[16] and gain perspective on the patient's current functioning. The social worker inquires about others whom the patient has known with cancer, especially breast cancer, in order to understand the patient's frame of reference and expectations. The social worker assesses how well the patient understands her medical situation and the accuracy of her expectations of what lies ahead.

In assessing the relational aspects of functioning, the social worker determines the existence, make-up, and strength of the patient's support network. The social worker evaluates the resilience of her significant relationships, the supportiveness of her spouse or partner. The social worker may address concerns about self-image and the resumption of intimacy. The reactions of children, parents, and others in the family are assessed,[17] as well as what information has been given to them. The social worker identifies friends and others beyond the family on whom the patient can rely for support at times of crisis. Assessment is made of how well the patient is actually utilizing the support system identified — partner, family, and friends.

In assessing the larger circle of social support, attention is directed toward such basic needs as financial resources, employment, housing, transportation, child care, and medical cost coverage.

In the initial contact, in addition to assessing, the social worker intervenes in several ways, seeking to help with identified concerns. The social worker may provide the patient with information in an effort to alleviate fears and concerns. He or she may help the patient clarify questions for the medical team, enhancing her understanding, and decreasing her anxiety. The social worker helps the patient to accept her feelings through supportive discussion of them and provision of perspective about how other patients have felt. Patients are often reassured to learn that what they have been feeling is not unusual and is part of the normal process of adjusting. The social worker is able to discuss problem-solving strategies with the patient, helping her resolve concerns more effectively. For example, when the social worker assesses that the patient is not relating well to her spouse, he or she might discuss ways to enhance communication and encourage closeness. When appropriate, the social worker might discuss helpful ways the patient can explain the illness to her children and address their fears. In addition to the supportive intervention provided at this point, the social worker may be planning useful follow-up measures, such as the involvement of peer counselors, support groups, Reach to Recovery, or longer term counseling.

This initial contact is conducted with the understanding that it may not necessarily expand into ongoing counseling. Certainly, if problems are recognized that warrant ongoing therapy, the social worker would seek to link the patient with an appropriate therapist. The basic nature of this contact is evaluative and supportive. The interview is conducted with clarification of these goals. Some patients feel that they are adjusting well, and keep these interviews quite brief. However, most patients find it useful to talk with a professional familiar with situations like theirs.

Counseling

The social worker is among various professionals offering counseling in the medical setting. Although the psychologist, psychiatrist, and nurse specialist may also be involved, the social worker is in an important position on the medical team. He or she is available during the times of the patient's greatest crisis or need, and is trained to provide psychosocial assessment and counseling. The social worker may have an introduction into the family on the basis of practical problems such as financial or transportation needs. However, the skilled social work clinician will be able to assess the larger psychosocial system, and intervene with more than the simple provision of resources.[4]

In this context, counseling refers to three types of intervention: short-term counseling focused on adjustment to the illness, a specific problem or decision; psychotherapy for underlying problems intensified by the diagnosis or treatment; and crisis intervention. In order to intervene accurately and appropriately in diverse circumstances, the social worker must be familiar with family systems theory, psychodynamics, psychopathology, crisis intervention, and grief and loss issues.

The social worker may meet with a patient/family only once, or the social worker may have the opportunity to work with a family over a number of years, as different concerns or crises arise. This type of continued intervention allows trust to build over time that is atypical in "short-term" work. The social worker in this setting is in a strong position to help a patient/

family who is experiencing problems but resistant to seeking the help of counseling.

The most common type of counseling will be short-term, issue-focused, and aimed toward coping effectively with, and mastery of, their situations.[4] This may include work around such issues as resumption of intimacy after mastectomy, talking to children about the diagnosis, or adjusting to family role changes. As with any serious illness, the diagnosis of breast cancer may intensify preexisting problems in a marriage, with a difficult adolescent, with child abuse, alcoholism, or adjustment to role changes, among others. The social worker must be adroit at assessment and intervention, as there may be only one opportunity for engaging the family or patient. The task is to help the patient recognize the benefit of further help. A social worker may establish a traditional treatment relationship with the patient or make a referral to a mental health agency.

The social worker must be available for crisis intervention with patients who are acting in a way that may be dangerous to themselves or others. The high stress of a cancer diagnosis creates a context in which crisis is likely. In the medical setting, this may include not only the suicidal patient, but the intensely anxious patient, the patient in psychological shock, or the one refusing necessary treatment.

In some cases, the social worker will refer the patient to an outside agency or psychotherapist. Some social workers offer individual, marital, or family therapy in the medical setting. Many patients who would otherwise not pursue needed treatment will accept treatment when it is available in a familiar environment.

When the social worker provides counseling in the medical setting, certain issues need special attention. These include clarification of confidentiality of the counseling relationship; separation of psychotherapeutic needs from medical needs; and definition of the recipients of therapy, perhaps other than the patient. When these issues are appropriately addressed, the social worker can offer excellent treatment in the medical setting.

Psychosocial Programs

At the University of Michigan Medical Center, Social Work, in conjunction with Nursing, has developed an extensive network of psychosocial programs combining support and education at the medical center. The programs currently include peer counseling, weekly support groups, a monthly education series, and a breast reconstruction program. These programs allow the patient to gather and integrate information, which helps her and her family adjust. Some patients remain active in these programs for as long as two to three years posttreatment.

Peer Counseling

Breast cancer patients who have finished treatment and done well inspire hope and optimism in patients who are newly diagnosed or facing a treatment transition. Not only does the veteran patient's mere presence inspire hope, but she can also help demystify the disease and treatment process by sharing her own experiences.

The use of patient-to-patient interaction as a therapeutic intervention in the medical setting is a very delicate matter. In order to assure appropriate and responsible interaction, such contacts should be part of a formalized program with clear guidelines, training, and supervision provided by professionals.

The peer counselor is most helpful at transition times when the patient expresses anxiety about the unknown. At such a time, she is being inundated with medical information and is trying to conceptualize what will happen to her. Talking with someone who went through what she is facing seems to help her approach the situation with more hope. The peer counselors are trained not to give medical advice, but share their own experiences. Following are some of the specific ways peer counselors are used in our program:

Immediately postdiagnosis. The patient is referred to a peer counselor by a social worker as soon as possible after diagnosis. It may be hard for this patient to believe that this intense crisis is temporary. Talking with a peer counselor enables her to learn that "there is life after breast cancer" and provides her with new perspective and hope.

Mastectomy/lumpectomy decision. For some women, making the choice between lumpectomy and mastectomy can be difficult. We have found that it is helpful for these women to talk with two peer counselors, one who underwent lumpectomy and radiation therapy, and another who underwent mastectomy. The process of decision making is facilitated as the patient gains more concrete expectations about the impact of the treatments.

Adjuvant treatment. Many patients have misconceptions about radiation and chemotherapy. The peer counselor who has gone through treatment can demystify it.

Reconstructive surgery. Some women know immediately that they want reconstructive surgery and others take years to come to a decision. In either case, a peer counselor can provide a role model of adjustment and be very useful in helping a patient know what to realistically expect.

In addition to the benefit to the patient, this program is also very valuable for the peer counselor herself. There is a sense of "graduating" from receiving to giving support. Although she has finished treatment and has no evidence of disease, she is still a cancer patient; being a peer counselor allows her to reframe her self-concept as a cancer patient in a positive way.

Support Groups

Because of the diverse needs of these patients, we offer several different group experiences. The groups provide a setting in which a woman can compare her experiences and develop new perspectives. They also provide new information about the disease and coping with it,[2] and are a safe context in which tears as well as humor are accepted. All are facilitated jointly by a nurse and a social worker, enabling integration of the medical and psychosocial issues.

Short-term groups. The patient is offered a ten-session weekly group that combines discussion of experiences and feelings with educational material. This group is for women actively dealing with issues of adjustment, whether immediately postoperatively, during adjuvant treatment, or later. The topics discussed often include family relationships, fear about the future, nutrition and cancer, dealing with stress, and use of mental imagery, etc. Physicians from various departments are also invited to speak on such topics as radiation therapy, chemotherapy, new research, and mammography. The patients find these meetings very helpful, and are often able to ask questions that they have felt intimidated to ask in the clinical setting. In addition, the group may view one of several videotapes produced by social workers at the University of Michigan Medical Center. These videotapes show interviews with patients and their families, and physicians on the psychosocial concerns of breast cancer patients.[3,8]

We provide separate groups for mastectomy and lumpectomy patients because we have found their needs to differ. We have found that the lumpectomy patients required special support as they encountered friends and family who questioned the soundness of their medical decision, accusing them of choosing breast preservation out of vanity. Mastectomy patients may have concerns and anger about the loss of their breast. Although many of the other issues are very similar, we have found that the separate groups work well.

Long-term group. After the weekly group ends, some participants wish to continue group involvement, but on a less frequent basis. A monthly series entitled "Healthy Living After Breast Cancer" is offered. Speakers are drawn from the medical and academic campuses as well as the community. Women who have participated in any of the groups are invited to attend. Some may come for a while, stop for a few months or a year, and then attend again. This group addresses the psychosocial needs of these patients.

Breast Reconstruction Program

Although most patients know that reconstructive surgery is an option, many questions, concerns and misconceptions arise. When a patient's expectations are that reconstruction will erase the emotional and physical wounds of her mastectomy or that her lost breast will be perfectly restored, she will experience disappointment and poor overall adjustment. Because of this, extensive information and careful preparation are crucial.

Many patients wonder whether they should have reconstruction. Some may dread the idea of another hospitalization; some may feel they are too old to be concerned about their appearance. Others may not realize that the operation will be covered by their insurance. These concerns can be addressed with straightforward information. Patients may be curious about what the reconstructed breast will look and feel like, about sensation, and about nipple reconstruction.

In order to meet the needs of patients and their families at this stage, we have developed a special program addressing medical and psychosocial concerns. The Breast Reconstruction Program includes a slide presentation by a plastic surgeon, as well as a panel discussion by women who have had reconstructive surgery. The various types of reconstruction are discussed, and the panel members talk openly about their own experiences. This program increases patients' understanding of the possibilities as well as limitations of reconstructive surgery. It helps women clarify their reasons for wanting the surgery and their expectations about the outcome.

Community Resources

In addition to providing other services, Social Work has a primary function — to link the client with helpful resources. Common resources utilized for breast cancer patients include support programs and groups, financial resources, housing, transportation, sources for wigs and breast prostheses, legal aid, community mental health agencies, and genetic counseling. Access to these resources can strengthen the patient's ability to cope during periods of crisis and enhance long-term adjustment.

As mentioned previously, many patients benefit from the use of support groups in adjusting to breast cancer. In addition to the groups mentioned previously, social workers refer patients to support groups in the larger community.

One of the community resources that is used consistently at the University of Michigan Medical Center is the Reach to Recovery program of the American Cancer Society. Reach to Recovery is a well-established program that provides a visit, usually on a one time basis, by a trained volunteer who has had breast cancer with no recurrence. The volunteer shows the patient exercises to improve arm mobility, brings a temporary prosthesis and lightweight bra, describes other prostheses, and discusses some of her own experiences. Most patients find the visit quite helpful, as it comes at a time when they are eager for information on how others have managed in their situation. The social worker seeks to have as many patients as possible receive these services prior to discharge from the hospital to improve the patient's perspective and outlook early in the adjustment process. On occasion, arrangements have been made for the husband of a volunteer to meet with the husband of the patient if that has been indicated.

The program, initially designed for mastectomy patients, does not at present include lumpectomy volunteers. Some lumpectomy patients are referred to Reach to Recovery; although the situations are different, the exercises and some of the information are useful. There is a program under development to provide a comparable service by lumpectomy volunteers.

There are other programs affiliated with the American Cancer Society that serve breast cancer patients in classes or groups of other cancer patients. "I Can Cope" and "CanSurmount" are guided discussion groups for cancer patients and their families that can be found in many communities. Some patients find these group discussions quite useful and benefit from the topics covered, as well as the group support. Not all patients feel the need for ongoing discussions about coping with cancer; others would not feel comfortable discussing their feelings and problems in a group setting. Both factors are considered by the social worker before making a referral to these groups.

SUMMARY

As described, the social worker assesses several aspects of adjustment: psychological, relational, and support; and intervenes to improve functioning. The social worker can also act as a consultant on the Breast Care Team, to interpret patients' background, situations, and behavior for the rest of the team. This trained perspective can be useful to other medical staff in understanding confusing or illogical behavior and in planning patient care. The social worker can also provide insight into the adjustment process in general and how staff can assist with it in their care of the patient.

We have presented the general sequence of steps breast cancer patients go through in the psychosocial adjustment to breast cancer. As has been discussed, most patients and families adjust fairly well, without overt psychopathology. Yet even these patients are making significant and difficult transitions psychologically, relationally, and socially. The social worker can intervene in various ways to assist the patient.

The medical and surgical care of breast cancer has progressed toward more effective and less invasive treatments. The diagnosis does not imply the risk of mortality, disfigurement, and suffering for patients that it once did. However, it remains a diagnosis with important and profound implications, especially in terms of the psychosocial adjustments it necessitates.

REFERENCES

1. Bloom JR: Social support, accommodation to stress and adjustment to breast cancer. Soc Sci Med 16:1329–1338, 1982.
2. Euster S: Rehabilitation after mastectomy: The group process. Soc Work Health Care 4:3, 1979.

3. Foley SM: *Hobson's Choice: The Experience of Women on Adjuvant Chemotherapy*, videotape. Ann Arbor, University of Michigan Media Library, 1981.

4. Goldberg R, Tull R: *The Psychosocial Dimensions of Cancer.* New York, Macmillan, Inc., 1983.

5. Grandstaff NW: The impact of breast cancer on the family. Front Radiat Ther Oncol 11:146–156, 1976.

6. Holland JC, Rowland J, Lebovits A: Reactions to cancer treatment: Assessment of emotional response to adjuvant radiotherapy as a guide to planned intervention. Psychiatr Clin North Am 2:2, 1979.

7. Hughes J: Emotional reaction to the diagnosis and treatment of early breast cancer. J Psychosom Res 26:2, 1982.

8. Kraus CW: *Perspectives on Breast Cancer Treatment: It's Come a Long Way*, videotape, Ann Arbor, University of Michigan Media Library, 1986.

9. Majes NL, Mendelsohn GA: Effects of cancer on patients' lives: A personalogical approach, in Stone GC, Cohen F, Adler NE (eds.): *Health Psychology.* San Francisco, Jossey-Bass, 1979.

10. Meyerowitz BE, Watkins IK, Sparks FC: Psychosocial implications of adjuvant chemotherapy: A two year follow-up. Cancer 52:1541–1545, 1983.

11. Peters-Golden H: Breast cancer: Varied perception of social support in the illness experience. Soc Sci Med 16:483–491, 1982.

12. Quint JC: The impact of mastectomy. Am J Nurs 63:11, 1963.

13. Rollin B: *First You Cry.* Philadelphia, J.B. Lippincott Co., 1979.

14. Schain W: Psychological impact of the diagnosis of breast cancer on the patient. Front Radiat Ther Onc 11:68–89, 1976.

15. Scott DW, Eisendrath SJ: Dynamics of the recovery process following initial diagnosis of breast cancer. J Psychosoc Oncol 3:4, 1985/86.

16. Simmons CC: The relationship between life change losses and stress levels for females with breast cancer. Oncol Nurs Forum 11:2, 1981.

17. Wellisch DK: Family relationships of the mastectomy patient: Interactions with the spouse and children. Isr J Med Sci 17:993–996, 1981.

27. *Update on the Psychosocial Issues of Breast Cancer Treatments*

WENDY S. SCHAIN

The diagnosis and treatment of breast cancer pose a greater threat to mortality and immortality in more complex ways than was initially assumed. Expanding awareness regarding psychosocial issues in the long-term adaptation of breast cancer patients has shifted the focus from an exclusive preoccupation with survival measures (namely, longevity, disease-free periods, and response rates) to a more comprehensive concern that also addresses the quality of life responses of these women.

For almost 100 years, mastectomy was synonymous with breast cancer surgery, and women and physicians alike accepted, with varying degrees of painful resignation, the necessary mutilation and emotional distress associated with such a procedure. The psychosocial literature in this area has been accumulating for the last 30 years, and describes the nature and frequency of postmastectomy disturbance.[7,25,27,32] While there is some conflict over the magnitude and duration of the ensuing turmoil, "all these studies point to a substantial percentage of women having psychological and social adjustment problems as a result of mastectomy."[31] Many women and their spouses suffer from depression, anxiety, suicidal thoughts, sexual problems, diminished self-image, and family maladjustment. Although exact predictors are uncertain, it seems that every woman who has a mastectomy is potentially at some risk of emotional morbidity.[44]

Given the widespread deleterious effects of radical breast surgery, medical investigators have been committed to finding an alternative therapy that would not compromise survivorship but might indeed preserve body integrity and protect psychological well-being. The alternative treatments now being used and evaluated extensively in this country are a variety of procedures that are subsumed under the generic title of conservative management.[20] This broad classification generally means that the primary operation for the breast cancer is a less radical procedure, and that the conservative procedure may be considered definitive or boosted with radiation therapy. Recent investigations into outcome of these various procedures revealed no significant difference between the two approaches in terms of survival.[15,36,50] Therefore, one must ask "if the two treatment regimens have equal impact on the survival of patients, but one of them leads to a better quality of life, (should not) the decision be in favor of the one resulting in the better quality of life."[30] The major question that surfaces is whether all of the psychological anguish heretofore associated with mastectomy is categorically eliminated when the cherished body part is not surgically amputated. If this is not so, then a number of assumptions about emotional consequences of breast cancer must be reexamined. Factors other than type of treatment clearly have an impact on subsequent adjustment.

Holly Peters-Golden makes a succinct distinction between breast cancer patients whose distress is rooted primarily in their diagnosis of cancer and those patients whose distress is predominantly colored by their having had to lose a breast.[37] As far back as 1979, a surgeon reported on a series of 81 patients treated with breast conservation surgery and concluded that the improvement in quality of life issues for these women and in their fears about their disease was so far superior to the mastectomy patients that it defied belief.[46] Whether this is so for all breast cancer patients whose breast is spared, or for certain subsets of patients, is a major concern which merits serious attention and will be addressed in this paper.

The thrust of this article, therefore, is to provide an update of psychosocial research in breast cancer and to shed some light on what is known, what is currently debatable and conflicted, and what is largely unexplored and critical for future research. The content of this presentation, it is hoped, will provide a data base of quality-of-life issues for women undergoing a variety of breast cancer treatments and allow health care providers to plan optimal therapy and rehabilitation based on both an understanding of the biology of the disease and an awareness of the psychology of the individual woman.

QUALITY OF LIFE

Quality of life is the major issue here and conjures up a variety of different meanings containing a variety of associated factors. Most succinctly, one can define the concept as "those problems, the problems of living that are sometimes called psychological and social, that are common to us all, and its inevitability, the fear of disability and deformity, and the loss of self-sufficiency; as well as the loss of ways to maintain self-esteem and the ability to sustain and fulfill our social roles."[13] Irrespective of the diversity of definitions of this term, consensus would support an interpretation of the concept based either on: (1) very specific aspects of life (or critical domains) compared to (2) a more global description of one's happiness and well-being. For purposes of this chapter, the former definition will be utilized and the majority of attention will be given to three specific areas of response. The three factors that will be used here seem to comprise a significant proportion of the quality-of-life reactions for breast cancer patients. They are ostensibly three independent critical domains and were identified separately by Meyerowitz[29] and Steinberg.[47] Both of these investigators used psychological tests and interviews to factor-analyze those variables that could be described as the major ingredient contained in the more generic term "quality of life." The following three critical domains could be compared across treatment groups and analyzed to distinguish the degree of disruption experienced by a woman in the most important areas of her overall functioning: (1) mood or psychological symptoms; (2) life pattern changes, including social, familial, and work relations, style of dress, sexual interaction, and leisure time pursuits; and (3) worries or fears and uncertainties about the future.

MASTECTOMY

Mastectomy has often been referred to as the surgery that most women fear most and is associated in the literature with a wide range of psychological turmoil. Early studies reported that these women suffered from severe anxiety, depression, and feelings of hopelessness, which lasted for years following initial treatment.[3,38] Studies conducted in the United Kingdom more than 20 years later [27,32] substantiated the earlier findings and added to the understanding of the relationship between loss of the breast and subsequent psychological adjustment problems. Maguire[27] reported disruptive psychological reactions in mastectomy patients he studied, which ranged from between one fourth to one third of the population. Specifically, 25% had mood disturbance and anxiety, which occurred in the form of tension, inability to relax, headaches, sweating, panic attacks, and palpitations. In addition, more than 20% of the breast cancer population had depression, compared to only 12% of the benign biopsy control group from that study. Furthermore, 27% of the mastectomy patients reported problems in their sexual adjustment, the exact nature and magnitude of which were not detailed. Morris,[32] another investigator from the United Kingdom, compared 69 women with breast cancer to 91 women with benign disease and found that almost one half (46%) of the mastectomy group acknowledged psychological distress related to the loss of their breast and subsequent disfigurement resulting from the surgery. At one year after the mastectomy, 24% still experienced upsetting mood reactions, disruptions in their sexual relations, diminished marital satisfaction, and an overall lessening of feelings of well-being.

Disfigurement and Altered Body Image

The issue of disfigurement and an altered body image appears to be a major component of the depression experienced by these women and a significant contributor to the reduced pleasure associated with sexual activity. It is not clear, however, as Bransfield[7] noted, whether an altered body image is an inevitable consequence of mastectomy which elicits sexual disturbances, or whether diminished sexual responsiveness follows mastectomy but is unrelated an altered body image. In an empirical investigation conducted by Taylor[48] on 78 breast cancer outpatients, poorer psychological adjustment was associated with feelings of lopsidedness and disfigurement related to having had a breast amputated rather than to the actual trauma of the surgery itself. Taylor went on to disclose that the negative self-perceptions associated with mastectomy were linked to subsequent changes in sexual and affectional patterns in the marriage. To what extent such a change in marital relations and sexual interaction is due to body image insult is not clear, but the author concluded that psychosocial adjustment problems may have more to do with treatment-related factors than illness-related factors. It appeared that the mastectomy patients' negative views of themselves following their surgery were strongly dictated by changes in their physical appearance, since their perceptions of themselves as attractive and capable women were diminished, irrespective of objective changes in overall level of functioning.

Age and Social Support

Two other major variables that are likely to affect postoperative adjustment are age and involvement of support people such as one's spouse or lover. In a landmark set of consecutive studies by Jamison, who evaluated mastectomy patients,[22] and Wellisch, who assessed those women's husbands,[52] the importance of these two factors was confirmed. Both authors reported that younger women felt they had a poorer postoperative adjustment in general. Specifically, this was because the mastectomy had a strong negative impact on their sexual relations. Approximately one fourth of the study group acknowledged suicidal ideation and felt some of the extreme negative feelings they were having were a result of their having had more positive reactions to sex prior to mastectomy, and consequently, more sense of loss and anxiety following their amputation. Furthermore, these women acknowledged that they thought the loss of a breast would be generally destructive to their husband/wife interaction and particularly damaging to their sexual relations.

In the study by Wellisch,[52] which explored the reactions of the spouse of these mastectomy patients, it was concluded that the involvement of the mate in decision making and in hospital visits could be considered a benchmark for determining marital satisfaction after mastectomy. It could also be used as an index of change in the couple's sexual activity. The author concluded that the better the man felt about the relationship to begin with, the less detrimental he felt the mastectomy was likely to be and the less changes in intimate behaviors he would anticipate. This could be correlated to the frequency of visits to the hospital. Interestingly, while slightly less than one fourth of the husbands had not seen their wives naked after the mastectomy operation, the decision in this matter was not exclusively the choice of the man. The view of the patient herself, regarding her feelings of being defective, not sexually desirable or attractive, influenced whether she was (1) initiating sexual relations, or (2) responsive to her partner's overtures.

In another study, which also used a retrospective questionnaire to study postmastectomy sexual relations, more than half of 47 women admitted to experiencing between three and six changes in their sexual relations in the direction of decreased frequency, decreased satisfaction, or both.[1] While this study was a self-report of women's sexual relations and was not particularly sophisticated in design, it was one of the first to expand the evaluation of changes that can occur in one's sexual repertoire beyond just assessing frequency of intercourse. Specifically, Abt asked respondents to note any changes in kissing, nude behaviors, change in breast stimulation, use of nighttime clothes when making love, and fantasy. Until fairly recently, measurement of sexual consequences following mastectomy had been primarily focused on genital intercourse and the difference in frequency and satisfaction with orgasm. The earlier, more narrowly focused view of sex distorts the magnitude and range of intimate and affectionate behaviors that may change as a result of body-altering surgery or cancer diagnosis. While the exact nature of interaction between marital satisfaction, sexual adaptation, and psychological comfort following mastectomy is not totally clear, the critical connection between affectionate responses and psychological distress in cancer patients has been more than alluded to.[26]

Clifford[8,10] conducted two studies that helped to clarify the nature of the relationship between sexual responses and marital satisfaction following the loss of one's breast. He concluded that the impact on the marital relationship was directly in proportion to the degree of upset experienced by the woman. Specifically, if the mastectomy patient could restrict her upset to a small part of her self-evaluation (namely, her breast area) and not let it spoil her overall estimate of her self-esteem or worthiness, the ramifications for the couple would be tolerable. If, on the other hand, the mastectomy patient experienced herself as damaged in a serious manner as a result of having lost a breast or having cancer, then the quality of the marital relationship would suffer more significantly. For the woman who experiences a major subtractive effect from mastectomy, it is to be expected that a great many facets of her marital and social functioning could be diminished.

Interestingly, Clifford stated that too often one asks what impact the mastectomy has on the woman's marriage, when the more appropriate question might be: What impact does the marriage have on the adjustment to mastectomy? Specifically, in what ways does a supportive, caring partner ease the pain of such a devastating experience, and how does one's mate aid the mastectomy patient in feeling loved, desired, and sexually attractive?

In recent years, a number of authors have documented the salutary effect that social support has on adaptation to patients undergoing stress in general, and breast cancer in particular.[25,37] Social support acts as a buffer against feelings of isolation and loneliness, diminishes one's feeling of victimization, and significantly enhances the individual's sense of feeling valued and loved. While there are discrepant findings in the literature regarding the percentage and intensity of postmastectomy distress, it is well known that the stress of this diagnosis and operation cause considerable upset in almost all aspects of a woman's life and may exert a negative influence long after the physical scars have healed. If the magnitude and duration of postmastectomy distress is as significant as it appears to be from reports in the literature, then one must extract from this information important guidelines to help physicians and other health professionals identify and intervene with these women who are at high risk for emotional morbidity.

The body of knowledge about coping and breast cancer is a separate tome and would take considerable effort and space to formalize, but some general governing principles can be put forth here. First, women whose self-esteem is primarily rooted in physical beauty and traditional values of femininity are likely to be the most devastated by the loss of the breast.[18,19] In addition, younger rather than older women seem to be especially distressed by their breast cancer surgery, particularly if it involves amputation of such a socially prized organ. Factors that probably contribute to this difference are multiple and include: the insult to body integrity, the threat to one's sexuality, and the necessary compromises that cancer treatments dictate. These infractions on quality of life are likely to be experienced more intensely by the younger, possibly single, or childless woman.

Interestingly, there is some suggestion in the literature that psychological factors may not only be different as outcome variables between younger and older women, but they may also account in part for the etiology of this disease.[5,14] The possible link between psychological characteristics and progression or regression of the tumor is more than intimated in the literature also. A major area of interest is in personality types and survivorship, and whether the characteristic "fighting spirit" type individual compared to the passive and stoic patient lives longer. Several studies reported in a chapter by Levy and Schain[24] discuss this area of investigation and explore in detail the connections between age, social support, coping strategies, personality, and incidence and outcome of breast cancer. In this chapter, there is put forth a preliminary statement that indicates emotional passivity may not be the most adaptive response in coping with breast cancer. In fact, the authors state quite candidly "the expression of complaint—the articulation of distress—may not only be psychologically adaptive but may have survival value."[24] Therefore, more vocal and aggressive women fare better. This assumption certainly requires additional follow-up research with significant implications for interventions to be developed. One might begin to think about constructing assertiveness training programs to teach more effective coping strategies to patients, which might conceivably influence the course of their disease.

Pregnancy and Breast Cancer

The issue of age in the breast cancer patient must also be considered in planning treatment programs, both medically and psychologically. The critical issue of pregnancy and breast cancer must be addressed with a seriousness that correlates with the gravity with which it is experienced by the young woman for whom it is a major quality-of-life concern. One must acknowledge that today, unlike a decade ago, more women are delaying pregnancies until their thirties and are being diagnosed with breast cancer considerably before middle age. There is conflicting evidence in this area that confuses both the professional and the patient. On the one hand, there is some suggestion in the literature that early pregnancy and the hormonal aftereffects could have a protective effect on women at high risk for breast cancer.[51] On the other hand, there are reports that intimate pregnancy in a woman who has had breast cancer could be detrimental to her health.[35] Such opposing notions are very unsettling, and the fear that a future pregnancy could aggravate disease in a woman who has breast cancer and desperately wants to become pregnant is a very anxiety-provoking state. In my own clinical practice, I have heard repeatedly from women struggling to resolve this issue, that cancer has provoked a need to constantly deal with losses and limitations resulting from: (1) the actual disease; (2) the consequences of treatments; or (3) the threat of future recurrence.

If a given woman resolves the ambivalence about becoming pregnant and does conceive and carry the baby, a number of additional critical questions have to be addressed. First, if she develops symptoms during the first two trimesters, what kinds of diagnostic tools are available to follow her adequately without injuring the fetus? Second, if there is evidence of recurrence, what should be the fate of the pregnancy? And third, does the fear of a future cancer or a preoccupation with an existing one (as is the case when breast cancer is diagnosed at the end of a pregnancy or very shortly thereafter), interfere with appropriate mothering behavior and bonding with the new baby? The psychological and physical energy that go into taking care of a new baby and also dealing with treatment demands of breast cancer are almost mutually exclusive for some period of time. Controlled clinical trials in this area are out of the question, but survey evaluations of patients who have had a pregnancy subsequent to their breast cancer could enlighten the health profession so that some reasonable index of emotional reactivity during this condition can be identified and quantified. In addition, there is an expressed and as yet unmet need in the community to provide a support system for this small group of women and facilitate their decision making in regard to this matter.

The Postmenopausal Woman

Interestingly, there is a corresponding issue of equal intensity for the postmenopausal woman. A fairly sizeable population, who are either suffering from natural or iatrogenic menopausal symptoms, experience a serious diminution in their quality of life and the aftereffects of cancer treatment even when there is no evidence of disease. Clinical complaints range from the distress imposed from severely disruptive hot flashes and mood swings, to the stated depression and accompanying anger that is associated with painful sexual relations. It is reasonable to assume that some women might be relieved to have an excuse to reduce or eliminate sexual intercourse, but my own clinical experience is that a significant number of these women are terribly saddened by the threatened loss of intimacy and the conditioned aversive response to sex, which often develops in response to the pain associated with penetration. There does not seem to be consensus about the use of postmenopausal hormones as a treatment for this condition, but the majority of opinions seem opposed to the introduction of exogenous hormones to ameliorate this condition.[28] Topical lubricants are not the solution to the severity and magnitude of the problem of senile vaginitis in this population of breast cancer patients. Concerned physicians and mental health professionals must focus on this issue to bring relief to the large numbers of women who suffer markedly from this condition.

RECONSTRUCTION

If a significant proportion of the anguish and emotional morbidity associated with mastectomy is due to the loss of such a socially prized body part (which fosters feelings of disfigurement and depreciated worth), then one might assume that restoration of that body part and replacement of the breast projection might lessen such reactions. This does seem to be the case for a significant number of mastectomy patients. Slightly more than a decade ago, it was believed that only those women who could not adjust to the physical defect created by mastectomy would consider breast reconstruction. It was assumed that these women were less well-adjusted and less able to cope with their altered body image and so would go in search of replacing their lost organ. The other group of more well-adjusted women could accept their disfigurement with appropriate resignation and learn to live with their amputation. In the last nine or ten years, various researchers have not only challenged this assumption but presented clinical case material and empirical findings which refute such a tenet. In one of the earliest investigations into this matter, Clifford[9] concluded that women who went in search of "restitution" for their altered body were exhibiting evidence of positive coping and assertive, effective problem-solving maneuvers, not neurotic reactions. The desire and active effort to change an undesirable physical defect, which is indeed reversible today, is more likely the outgrowth of adaptive coping responses than of maladaptive defensiveness. Another research team that evaluated postmastectomy patients and compared a group who sought reconstruction with their mastectomy counterparts (who did not want this operation) published results that confirmed this fact. The women who sought reconstruction were quite well-adjusted and devoid of any clinically significant psychopathology and maintained a high level of psychosocial functioning.[21] The old view of discontented neurotic women as the only ones who opt for reconstruction has been put to rest.

In reference to which women seek this reparative operation, and what motives that prompt them to do so, the answer is not so settled. There is no universal theme to explain women's choice to undergo more surgery after a mastectomy. However, certain reasons do seem to factor out this subset of mastectomy patients. While the reasons cited by women seeking breast reconstruction represent a wide range of contributing factors, the most prevalent motives appear to be (1) to feel whole again and (2) to get rid of the external prosthesis.[53] These two reactions are intimately connected since it is very difficult to feel truly intact, an external prosthesis is not easily incorporated into one's body image, and the woman is often aware of the irritation and self-consciousness accompanying wearing a false breast. In addition, when one focuses on her "falsie," there is often an underlying connection to the awareness that the breast is missing because of having had cancer. Therefore, the fear about possible recurrence (which is usually hiding only tenuously beneath surface consciousness) may be reactivated. The desire to have an internal prosthesis implanted under the chest wall may indeed be related to a wish to lessen the connection between the external prosthesis, the experienced body alteration, and the underlying anxiety about the dread disease.

Timing of Reconstruction

If the accepted axiom today is that breast reconstruction has a salutary effect on a mastectomy patient's psychological adaptation, the pressing issue is no longer whether this operation should be performed, but when in the course of treatment is the most propitious time to reconstruct the patient? Earlier views about the timing of breast reconstruction were rooted in the belief that a patient could better appreciate the outcome of her reconstructed breast only after she had lived with the defect of mastectomy and truly mourned the loss of her natural breast.[21] A number of surgical oncologists and breast reconstruction surgeons[23,39] put forth the notion that the mastectomy patient would like the cosmetic appearance of her new breast only after she lived without one. Therefore, it was advisable to delay the reparative operation. In addition, there was serious concern about the possible hazards of a reconstructive surgery performed simultaneously with the cancer operation.[45] Dowden[12] helped allay these concerns and appealed to the profession that immediate breast reconstruction would likely benefit a sizeable population of breast cancer patients and not deleteriously affect the group who might experience recurrence. What was necessary, then, was to study the psychological consequences of this type of reconstruction and determine, if it was not medically unsafe, what the psychological advantage and disadvantages might actually be.

Early investigations in this regard concluded that mastectomy patients did not have to live with the deformity of a missing breast to appreciate the benefits of a reconstructed one. Noone,[34] in an early research study investigating this issue, concluded that there was no less satisfaction in the immediate group than in the population who had delayed reconstruction. Teimourian[49] stated the patients' overall level of satisfaction with delayed reconstruction was reported to be about 90%, and Noone's research revealed that 92% of the immediate group was satisfied with the results. In another study, which compared 25 women undergoing immediate reconstruction to 28 who underwent the delayed procedure, the authors concluded "the sooner, the better"[43] was a reasonable recommendation to make regarding breast reconstruction. Specifically, it was revealed that women who underwent immediate breast reconstruction were less depressed, less anxious, less hostile toward their physicians, and absolutely no less satisfied than women who had the delayed procedure. In addition, the women who had their ablative operation and their reconstruction simultaneously reported less overall trauma with their breast cancer operation and expressed less subjective distress over the surgery than the group who had delayed reconstruction. On the other hand, the immediate group did report more physical discomfort, which was probably related to the simultaneous axillary dissection that was performed on them, while the delayed group did not have that to contend with at the time of reconstruction. Early conclusions in this regard tip the scale in favor of immediate breast reconstruction, sparing women some of the agony associated with living with a deformity that undermines their self-esteem, sexuality, and sense of physical integrity. As was discussed by Dowden,[12] since the insertion of an internal prosthesis seems to pose no threat to tumor progression, decisions about immediate breast reconstruction need to be predicated on the woman's anticipated loss associated with the mastectomy disfigurement and the imagined benefit to be derived by avoiding such a depressing state.

Clearly there are subsets of mastectomy patients who are ineligible for this procedure because of medical conditions, and there are also those women who will prefer to delay the reconstruction or who would be emotionally better suited to do so. This latter group comprises women who cannot process all the options presented to them before their initial surgery and need to finish one problem before confronting another. Another group of mastectomy patients who would do well to wait are those who are especially anxious about their disease and for one reason or another fear that they will not get the necessary follow-up for their cancer if they simultaneously have a reconstructive (or cosmetic) operation. In addition, there is a subset of mastectomy patients who are clearly not motivated to replace the breast that is to be removed, but the reasons may be quite diverse. Furthermore, some patients need to have the reconstruction to look forward to as part of an investment in the future and as a reward for getting through the ordeal of mastectomy. Therefore, delayed reconstruction has significant benefit for these women.

On the other hand, some women are excellent candidates psychologically for immediate reconstruction. These include women who are:

1. Extremely invested in their breasts as synonymous with their self-worth.
2. Resistant to mastectomy if intraoperative repair is not considered as an option.
3. Very well-read and know and express that they feel the benefits of such a procedure outweigh identified risks.
4. Assertive in their requests and their life-style and for whom wearing an external prosthesis compromises their activities.
5. Strongly negatively influenced by having seen the mutilating effects of mastectomy in a family member or close friend.
6. Cancer phobic about their existing breast, have had multiple biopsies and a history of breast cancer in themselves or a family member, and want to ease the pain of a prophylactic mastectomy with synchronous reconstruction.[17]

Sexual Responsiveness and Reconstruction

One additional element that requires elaboration here is the view the woman has about her sexuality and how critical her breasts are to her sense of physical attractiveness and sexual desirability. Breast reconstruction has been found to increase sexual responsiveness[49] in a population of mastectomy patients who feel diminished by having lost such an important part of their body and one so intimately connected to feeling sexually attractive. Why this is so is not self-evident or simple as one might assume, and the clinical investigation of this problem has been minimal. However, an interesting laboratory study conducted by Gerard[16] has added considerable understanding to this complex phenomenon. She compared the sexual excitement of mastectomy patients and reconstructed patients by using a photoplethysmograph to document vaginal blood flow as an index of arousal while the women were listening to romantic and erotic tapes. Her findings revealed that reconstructed patients are more easily sexually aroused than their mastectomy counterparts. The clinical interpretation of this finding appears to be related to the anxiety that mastectomy patients feel about their altered body, which gets translated into a negative preoccupation with their physical appearance. This obsessing preoccupation about their body distracts them from being able to concentrate their energies on the lovemaking experience. Instead of being able to tune into the pleasurable aspects of the sexual stimulation and related good feelings, the mastectomy patients were more focused on their body's differences and were not able to relax, let go, and abandon themselves up to the experience of the moment. The women who had been reconstructed, it appeared, could distance themselves from concentrating on the physical aspects of their body (or self-perceived defect) and get into the fantasied or real sexual act. There was a notable difference between the two study groups in regard to the lag time between stimulus and reaction and also in terms of the magnitude of the sexual excitement experienced. The mastectomy patients had more difficulty in getting "turned on."

The above findings have serious implications for health professionals from both the medical and behavioral sciences in terms of understanding the connection between women's sexual behavior and interest in breast reconstruction. Although a number of breast reconstruction patients state they do not have erotic sensations in the reconstructed breast, the link between body parts and sexual responsiveness is more complex than can be explained by anatomic connections. Breast reconstruction does facilitate a reintegration of one's body image and does contribute to feeling whole again.[6] This finding is clarified by an observation made by Nathan and Johanning,[33] who reported that the closer a woman can remain to her presurgical state physically, the less distressed she may feel generally, and the less disrupted she may be specifically in regard to her sexual responses.

In an effort to lend additional understanding to the relationship between intact breast image and sexual responsiveness, Wellisch and Schain[53] constructed a study to evaluate the difference in psychosexual outcome of women who had undergone breast reconstruction and who subsequently elected to have or not to have nipple/areola reconstruction. The nipple-added group (n = 33) compared to the nonnipple-added (n = 26) reported significantly greater satisfaction with breast reconstruction in regard to: (1) overall satisfaction; (2) satisfaction with size; (3) satisfaction with softness of the breast; (4) satisfaction with nude appearance; and (5) satisfaction with the sexual sensitivity of the reconstructed breast. Findings from this study are noteworthy in the respect that the nipple-added group expressed increased satisfaction with sexual responsiveness in the reconstructed breast. The addition of the nipple/areola complex to the reconstructed mound could not in and of itself increase sensory response. This reported reaction must have to do with somatosensory reactions rather than anatomic or physiological connections. The identified outcome, therefore, must be dependent on a complex set of psychological variables, the most important of which is the "sense of completeness" experienced by both the patient and her partner. Adding the nipple/areola complex not only makes the breast look more natural to the patient and her spouse/lover but also makes it feel more familiar and acceptable (and more like it was). A major clue to understanding this response lies in the fact that the more a woman is likely to experience herself as "like her former self," the more likely she is to forget her differentness and the more likely she is to feel sexually attractive and get sexually aroused. This finding has far-reaching implications for understanding both the psychological adaptation of mastectomy patients and the alleged improved body image and sexual responses of breast conservation patients whose postoperative physical appearance is the closest to one's presurgical body image as is possible following an operation for breast cancer.

BREAST-CONSERVING OPERATIONS

Both medical technology and psychosocial oncology have progressed to the point where clinical trials have been instituted to evaluate the medical efficacy and wisdom of breast conservation surgery as an alternative to mastectomy.[15,50] If the two treatments do not yield differences in longevity or disease-free survival time, then the ultimate decision about choice of treatment may indeed lie in the quality-of-life findings, which are just beginning to be recorded.

In a report published in 1979, Sacks[40] acknowledged that the women he treated with breast-sparing operations felt anxious and unsupported by their social network. These women expressed the lack of approval they felt from friends and physicians at that time for choosing a breast-sparing treatment, which was viewed quite suspiciously then. Many of these patients said they experienced moderate to severe isolation for their decision. While Europe and the Netherlands had praised the value of more conservative breast cancer therapies for a number of years, the United States lagged behind in publishing outcome studies in this area which would provide confidence for the less radical approach in this country. In addition, the paucity of studies that had been published here were fraught with methodological flaws and very small numbers of patients. It was originally assumed that women who demanded breast-sparing treatment were vain and aggressive and unwilling to tolerate the degree of deformity necessary to cure their disease. In addition, there was speculation that such women might experience a "trade-off" not just in survivorship but in terms of psychological equanimity if they had to worry about the possibility of cancer growing in the breast that was preserved and conservatively treated. Unequivocal support for this procedure has been slow in mounting, but today's medical findings, combined with the description of these women's favorable adjustment, are certainly tilting the balance toward the less mutilating operations.

The first study to evaluate psychological differences between mastectomy and lumpectomy was conducted on a population referred by their physicians because they were well adjusted emotionally and had not presented any problems to their physicians.[41] The study concluded that the mastectomy patients did not differ from their lumpectomy counterparts in any significant way regarding psychological symptomatology, marital adjustment, or life activities. A significant difference, however, was found in the way each group felt about their body image. The lumpectomy patients clearly had a more positive response to their body after surgery. A caveat regarding this study is the fact that the lumpectomy patients all elected the more conservative treatment, while the mastectomy patients had been told what treatment they were to have. It is quite possible that some of the satisfaction noted and the more positive adaptation reported in the breast conservation group was due to their freedom of choice and not just their more intact physical outcome. The mastectomy patients, on the other hand, may have had difficulty adjusting both to their physical defect and the fact that they were virtually powerless in the decision about their treatment. One way to gain information about this issue is to observe the findings in a study that allowed women their choice of operation so that one might more easily isolate the factors that were related to (1) the amputation of the woman's breast, as well as (2) those related to the absence of free choice. In a research investigation where women did get to choose between treatments, the results revealed that the mastectomy patients felt their breasts were not so important to their overall self-esteem, and that they experienced that part of their body as alien. In addition, the women who chose radical surgery also expressed serious concern about the consequences of radiation therapy.[2] This type of study, which allowed women freely to select their treatment, underscored how much the therapy one selects is related to psychological factors, especially if she does not feel that the therapy will compromise her survival. Quality of life, therefore, becomes an increasingly weighty contributor to making treatment recommendations and needs to be carefully analyzed for each individual. While every patient's definition of quality of life is unique, a universal group of variables influences all breast cancer patients' decisions regarding their treatment and needs to be addressed prior to initial therapy.

Steinberg and Wise[47] factored out three major areas that could be subsumed under quality of life when they compared the psychological adaptation of 41 mastectomy patients to 21 women who had undergone lumpectomy and radiation therapy. These three areas were: (1) emotional distress, (2) life's activities, and (3) fears and concerns.

When followed for more than one year after initial treatment, the lumpectomy patients in this study maintained an overall and noticeable improvement in psychological adjustment. Specifically, they felt more attractive and feminine, and stated they did not change their pattern of undressing in front of their partners. In addition, the breast-sparing group reported there was no decrease in the amount of breast stimulation experienced before and after surgery. Furthermore, the breast conservation group also stated they experienced a higher level of social support from family and friends (in contrast to the earlier years when lumpectomy patients were spurned). The reasons for this are not clear, but it may be that some women view their breast conservation therapy as a "watered down" version of breast cancer treatment. They see it as no big deal or trauma just to have a biopsy and some radiation compared to having to have a breast amputated with the attendant deformity.[37] Today, friends of lumpectomy patients may feel not so different and more at ease to relate to them.

Fear of Recurrence After Conservative Procedures

If little or no difference between treatments is revealed in terms of global psychological symptomatology, then fear of recurrence becomes a rather critical component in the final decision to have one's cancerous breast removed versus having it spared and treated. In a controlled clinical trial at the National Institutes of Health (NIH), retrospective psychological questionnaires revealed no significant differences between lumpectomy patients and mastectomy patients in this regard.[42] However, this finding may be related to the nature of the standardized follow-up built into the protocol rather than individual psychological attributes. Such a detailed and predictable follow-up schedule may help reduce patient's anxiety about having to be vigilant to detect any symptoms necessary to report to their physicians. In addition, the clinical trials obviate the financial burden often experienced in the private sector, and this source of distress is mitigated, thereby diminishing some of the pressures created by having to pay for expensive medical care of this type. Whether the findings reported in the study emanate from an institutionally fostered sense of well-being indigenous to the NIH, or because of a real difference is not yet clear. Additional studies will be necessary to see if such findings are generalizeable.

One such study was conducted in the Netherlands by Bartelink.[4] This study concluded that the 114 women who underwent breast conservation therapy showed *less* fear of recurrence of their disease than the 58 mastectomy patients. Why this confounding variable is so, and when and why it appears, requires more studies with larger numbers of women in both randomized trials (without selection bias for their therapy) as well as study groups where the women can willfully choose their treatment. What may be operating for those women whose breast is preserved is a kind of denial process fostered by visualizing a minimally altered body. Such an intact body image reinforces a sense of well-being, which is not so easily supported when there is such a gross reminder of the disease in the form of a missing breast. Having to confront an ugly mastectomy scar, having to put an external prosthesis into one's brassiere every day, or even observing a major discrepancy between one's natural breast and a reconstructed one are contraindications for being able to block out the negative experience of breast cancer surgery and all the horrors it can connote. On the other hand, the less frequently and the less traumatically a woman has to deal with the outcome of her surgery, the less intrusive and psychologically debilitating it is likely to be. Conscious concerns can certainly be minimized by physical appearances and an "almost normal looking" breast can augur more "normal" feelings about one's body in particular and perhaps about one's life in general. Breast conservation therapy patients are not forced to make so many changes in their range of activities, style of dress, or adaptation to what they look like. Follow-up psychological evaluations will be necessary to determine if the denial that is operating is an adaptive psychological coping strategy or a maladaptive defense that could interfere with the lifelong health care vigilance required to monitor the type of chronic disease breast cancer appears to be.

The data accumulating in the psychosocial literature certainly give weight to the salutary benefits associated with breast conservation therapy. Subsequent investigators such as Kemeny (unpublished material), Lasry and Margolese (unpublished material) and de Haes[11] all seem to confirm the advantages experienced by women who undergo conservative therapy and preserve their own breast and feminine self-image. There seem to be fewer changes in all areas of psychological and behavioral functioning for lumpectomy patients and no added fear about the disease recurring. Interestingly, the psychological benefits identified are clear and consistent, and do not seem to be offset (for any demonstrable period) by radiation therapy as adjunct to lumpectomy. Lasry and Margolese (unpublished material) have found a significantly greater level of psychological distress in the lumpectomy patients who also underwent radiation therapy than those who did not. The magnitude and duration of the emotional distress in breast conservation patients (those who do and those who do not have radiation therapy) compared to mastectomy and reconstruction patients still requires much more detailed investigation under more tightly standardized conditions so that reports will not be "lumping" all breast conservation patients under just one label, but will make the distinctions based on the amount of the breast removed or distorted, and the additional stress radiation therapy seems to impose.

The findings from the studies reported here do strongly indicate that different types of primary breast surgery do differentially influence quality-of-life responses. Certain subsets of patients may now be identifiable who are at particularly high risk for emotional morbidity following certain types of breast cancer surgery. Some of this morbidity can be offset by the type of treatment that will support existing psychological defenses, preserve self-esteem, and conserve cosmesis.

The women who are likely to benefit most psychologically from breast conservation therapy are:

1. Younger women who are strongly invested in their bodies and experience their breasts as critical to their overall sexual enjoyment.
2. Older women who feel strongly that they want to preserve an intact body image and should not have to be embarrassed to admit it, especially if they lead a more traditional lifestyle.
3. Women of all ages who do not have partners (for whatever reason), and who are motivated to find a new lover or husband and will be seriously inhibited in their search without their breast.
4. Women of all ages who have had strong conflicts about their breasts and have had them reduced or enlarged, indicating earlier unresolved negative feelings about that part of their body.
5. Women who saw a loved one undergo a particularly ugly mastectomy procedure, especially if survival was not significantly extended.
6. Women who do not fear the short-term or long-term consequences of radiation therapy, either because they deny some of the realities or because they understand and are willing to assume the risk.
7. Women who know the mounting facts and have explored the possible consequences of this type of treatment, i.e., thought about what it is like to have radiation therapy, and have made a conscious decision that this treatment is the one they want to *live with*.

SUMMARY

For almost one hundred years, mastectomy was the standard of care for breast cancer. Women and the doctors who recommended this treatment accepted, with varying degrees of sadness, the physical mutilation and psychological suffering with which it was associated. Today, there are increased options for treating this disease, each with its own set of burdens and benefits (especially regarding chemotherapy). The health professional, in concert with the patient being treated, need to communicate to each other how each views the risks and rewards connected to each type of therapy. There is no longer only one major modality used in the surgical care of the breast cancer patient. Learning about the acceptable alternatives is the responsibility of the patient, and communicating it to her is the province of the doctor. The critical questions to be asked by both are:

1. What is the loss of the breast likely to mean to the individual woman being treated?
2. How negatively does she imagine her life's activities to be affected by a particular therapy?
3. What is the likelihood of that particular therapy exacerbating her fears about recurrence (separate from that which is already associated with having been diagnosed with cancer)?

Today, treatment recommendations must be made with an understanding of the biology of the disease, the psychology of the individual woman, and the emotional consequences such therapy will engender in that patient.

REFERENCES

1. Abt V: The impact of mastectomy on sexual self-image, attitudes and sexuality. J Sex Educ Therap 4:43–46, 1978 (Winter).
2. Ashcroft JJ, Leinster SJ, Slade PO: Breast cancer patient choice of treatment: Preliminary communication JR Soc Med 78:43–46, 1985.
3. Bard M, Sutherland AM: Psychological impact of cancer and its treatment. IV. Adaptation to radical mastectomy. Cancer 8:656–672, 1955.
4. Bartelink H, Van Dam F, Van Dongen J: Psychological effects of breast conserving therapy in comparison with radical mastectomy. Radiat Oncol Biol Phys 11:281–385, 1985.
5. Becker H: Psychodynamic aspects of breast cancer differences in younger and older patients. Psychotherap Psychosom 32:287–296, 1979.
6. Berger K, Bostwick J: *A Woman's Decision: Breast Care, Treatment and Reconstruction*. St. Louis, CV Mosby, 1984.
7. Bransfield DD: Breast cancer and sexual function. A review of the literature and implications for research. Int J Psychiatr Med 12:197–211, 1982–1983.
8. Clifford E: Psychological effects of the mastectomy experience, in Georgiade NG (ed): *Breast Reconstruction Following Mastectomy*. St. Louis, CV Mosby, 1979, pp 1–22.
9. Clifford E: The reconstruction experience: The search for restitution, in Georgiade NG (ed): *Breast Reconstruction Following Mastectomy*. St. Louis, CV Mosby, 1979, pp 22–35.
10. Clifford E, Clifford M, Georgiade NG: Breast reconstruction following mastectomy. II. Marital characteristics of patients seeking this procedure. Ann Plast Surg 5:343–346, 1980.
11. de Haes JC, van Knippenberg L: The quality of life of cancer patients: A review of the literature. Soc Sci Med 20:809–817, 1985.
12. Dowden RV, Blanchard JM, Greenstreet RL: Breast reconstruction; timing and local recurrence. Ann Plast Surg 10:265–269, 1983.
13. Enelow A: Psychosocial rehabilitation for cancer patients. Front Radiat Ther Oncol 10:178–182, 1975.
14. Finch D, Mettlen C: The role of stress, social support and age in survival from breast cancer. J Psychosom Res 27:177, 1983.
15. Fisher MD, Bauer PH, Margolese RM, et al.: Five-year results of a ran-

domized clinical trial comparing total mastectomy and segmental mastectomy with or without radiation in the treatment of breast cancer. N Engl J
Med 312:665–673, 1985.

16. Gerard D: Sexual functioning after mastectomy: Life vs lab. J Sex Marital
Therap 8:305–315, 1982 (Winter).

17. Goin NK, Goin JM: Psychological reactions to prophylactic mastectomy
synchronous with contralateral breast reconstruction. Plast Reconstr Surg
70:355–359, 1982.

18. Golden J: Sex and career. Dan Med Bull 30 (Suppl 2):4–7, 1983.

19. Golden M: Female sexuality and the crisis of mastectomy. Dan Med Bull
30:13–16, 1983.

20. Harris JR, Hellman S, Silen W: *Conservative Management of Breast Cancer: New Surgical and Radiotherapeutic Techniques.* Philadelphia, JB Lippincott, 1983.

21. Holland J, Roland J: Patient rehabilitation and support, in Harris J,
Helman S, Henderson C, et al. (eds): *Breast Diseases.* Philadelphia, JB
Lippincott, 1987, p 638.

22. Jamison KR, Wellisch DK, Pasnau RO: Psychosocial aspects of mastectomy. I. The woman's perspective. Am J Psychiatr 135:432–436, 1978.

23. Lester LJ: A critical viewpoint by a general surgeon toward reconstructive
surgery after mastectomy. Clin Plast Surg 16:15, 1979.

24. Levy SM, Schain WS: Psychological response to breast cancer: Direct and
indirect contributions to treatment outcome, in Lippman M, Lichter A,
Danforth D (eds): *Diagnosis and Management of Breast Cancer.* Philadelphia, WB Saunders, 1987.

25. Lewis FM, Bloom JR: Psychosocial adjustment to breast cancer: A review
of selected literature. Int J Psychiatr Med 9:1–17, 1978–1979.

26. Lieber L, Plumb MM, Gerstenzang ML, et al.: The communication of
affection between cancer patients and their spouses. Psychosom Med
38:379–389, 1976.

27. Maguire GP, Lee EG, Bevington DJ, et al.: Psychiatric problems in the
first year after mastectomy. Br Med J 1:963–965, 1978.

28. Marchant D: Would low dose estrogen/progestin be safe for this 45 year
old woman with menopausal symptoms. Case 3. Primary Care and Cancer
July, 1985.

29. Meyerowitz B, Sparks RD, Spears IK: Adjuvant chemotherapy for breast
carcinoma. Cancer 43:1613–1618, 1979.

30. Meyerowitz BE: Psychosocial correlates of breast cancer and its treatments. Psychol Bull 87:108–131, 1980.

31. Miller PJ: Mastectomy, a review of psychosocial research. Health Soc
Work 4:60–65, 1980.

32. Morris T, Greer HS, White P: Psychosocial and social adjustment to
mastectomy: A two-year follow-up. Cancer 40:2381–2387, 1977.

33. Nathan EP, Johanning HH: Enhancing marital sexuality: An evaluation
of a program for the sexual enrichment of normal couples. J Sex Marital
Therap 11:157–164, 1985.

34. Noone RB, Frazier TG, Haywood CZ, et al.: Patient acceptance of imme-

diate reconstruction following mastectomy. Plast Reconstr Surg 69:632–638.

35. Nugent P, O'Connel TY: Breast cancer and pregnancy. Arch Surg 120:1221–1224, 1985.

36. Peters MV: Wedge resections with or without radiation in early breast cancer. Int J Radiat Oncol Biol Phys 2:115–119, 1977.

37. Peters-Golden H: Breast cancer: Varied perceptions of social suport in the illness experience. Soc Sci Med 16:483–492, 1982.

38. Renneker R, Cutler M: Psychological problems of adjustment to cancer of the breast. JAMA 148:833–838, 1952.

39. Rosato FE, Horton CE, Maxwell GP: Postmastectomy breast reconstruction. Curr Prob Surg 17:590–629, 1980.

40. Sacks EL, Gerstein OG, Mann SG: Conservative surgery and radiation therapy for breast cancer. Front Radiat Ther Oncol 17:23–32, 1983.

41. Sanger CK, Resnikoff M: A comparison of the psychological effects of breast saving procedures with the modified radical mastectomy. Cancer 48:2341–2346, 1981.

42. Schain W, Edwards BK, Gorell CR, et al.: Psychosocial and physical outcome of primary breast cancer therapy: Mastectomy vs excisional biopsy and irradiation. Breast Cancer Res Treat 3:377–382, 1983.

43. Schain WS, Wellisch DK, Pasnau RO, et al.: The sooner the better: A study of psychological factors in women undergoing immediate versus delayed breast reconstruction. Am J Psychiatr 142:40–46, 1985.

44. Schain WS: Breast cancer surgeries and psychosexual sequelae: Implications for remediation. Semin Oncol Nurs 1:200–205, 1985.

45. Silva Neto JB, Fontelles JA, Assis P, et al.: Results of radical mastectomy for stage I and II breast cancer: Implications for breast reconstruction. Breast 9:20–22, 1983.

46. Stehlin JS Jr, Evans RA, Gutierrez AC, et al.: Treatment of carcinoma of the breast. Surg Gynecol Obstet 149:912–922, 1979.

47. Steinberg MD, Juliano NA, Wise L: Psychological outcome of lumpectomy versus mastectomy in the treatment of breast cancer. Am J Psychiatr 142:32–39, 1985.

48. Taylor SE, Lichtman RR, Wood J, et al.: Illness related and treatment related factors in psychological adjustment to breast cancer. Cancer 55:2506–2513, 1985.

49. Teimourian B, Adham MN: Survey of patients; responses to breast reconstruction. Ann Plast Surg 9:321–325, 1982.

50. Veronesi V, Saccozzi R, DeVecchio M, et al.: Comparing radical mastectomy with quadrantectomy, axillary dissection and radiotherapy in patients with small cancer of the breast. N Engl J Med 305:6–11, 1981.

51. Vessey MP, McPherson K, Roberts MM, et al.: Fertility in relation to the risk of breast cancer. Br J Cancer 52:625–628, 1985.

52. Wellisch DK, Jamison KR, Pasnau RO: Psychological aspects of mastectomy. II. The man's perspective. Am J Psychiatr 135:543–546, 1978.

53. Wellisch DK, Schain WS, Little JW, et al.: Psychosocial sequelae of nipple/areolar reconstruction. Plast Reconstr Surg, in press.

Index

abscess, chronic subareolar 104, 107f
adenocarcinoma 101, 102f, 211-218
adenofibroma 82, 83f, 220-221
adenosis 121, 123
adrenalectomy 171, 253, 325
advanced local disease, chemotherapy for
    167-170
Africa
  breast cancer statistics 55-56, 58t
American Academy of Family Physicians
    81
American Cancer Society 21, 35, 79-81,
    202, 233, 323, 339, 344, 358-
    359
  Breast Cancer Detection Demonstration
    Project (BCDDP) 79-80, 95
  Reach to Recovery program 358-359
American College of Obstetrics and Gyne-
    cology 81
American College of Physicians 81
American College of Radiology 81, 92, 95
American Society of Therapeutic Radiation
    Oncologists 28
amitriptyline 306
Anderson Hospital 200, 205, 239
anthracyclines 172
antidepressants 306-307
antiemetics 306, 307-308
antiestrogen *See* antineoplastic agents, hor-
    mone-specific, tamoxifen
antineoplastic agents
  alkylating agents
    chlorambucil 172t
    cyclophosphamide 158, 160, 167, 169t,
      172t, 297, 327
    L-phenylalanine mustard (L-PAM) 15-
      16, 158, 159f, 160-161
    melphalan 167, 172f
    thiotepa 158, 172t
  antibiotic antineoplastic agents
    doxorubicin 167, 169t, 171, 172t, 253
    mitomycin-C 172f

antimetabolites
  5-fluorouracil (5-FU) 15, 158, 160-
    161, 167, 172f, 327
  methotrexate 158, 160, 167, 169f, 172f,
    297, 307, 327
combinations *See also* chemotherapy; hor-
    monal synchronization
  cyclophosphamide, methotrexate, and
    5-FU (CMF) 158, 159t, 162t,
    167, 172t, 327
  cyclophosphamide, methotrexate, 5-
    FU, vincristine, and prednisone
    (CMFVP) 158, 159t, 160
  hormone-specific agents
    aminoglutethimide 163, 171, 253, 325
    megestrol acetate 163, 171
    tamoxifen (TAM) 30, 161, 163, 164f,
      165, 168, 169t, 170, 249, 254
  investigational chemotherapeutic agents
    bisantrene 172f
    mitoxantrone 172f
  vinca alkaloids
    vinblastine 172t
    vincristine 158, 160, 172t, 297
antipsychotics 63, 307-308
anxiety
  preclinical 22-26, 30
  clinical 26-32
  postclinical 32
"apical node" 12, 119
Armed Forces Institute of Pathology 239
Asia
  breast cancer statistics 55-56, 58t
aspiration cytology *See* biopsy, fine needle
    aspiration
axillary adenopathy 211
axillary dissection 14, 27, 131, 119, 149-
    151 *See also* lymph nodes, dis-
    section; mastectomy, total; mas-
    tectomy, modified radical

Bader, Judith 29

381

Breast Cancer Task Force 22
Cancer Information Service (CIS) hot-
line 29
Early Breast Cancer Trial 29
National Consortium of Breast Centers 8
National Hospice Organization 344
National Institutes of Health (NIH) 7, 25,
31, 375-376
National Intravenous Therapy Association
344
National Surgical Adjuvant Project for
Breast and Bowel Cancer
(NSABP) 8, 142, 149, 153, 157,
163, 166
B-01 158, 159t
B-04 12-14, 194, 200
B-05 16, 158, 159t
B-06 12-14, 16f, 29, 109, 132, 199, 205
B-07 158, 159t
B-08 158, 159t
B-09 249
neuroleptics *See* antipsychotics
neuropsychiatric syndromes 296-297
New Jersey law re: breast cancer treatment
49
nipples 150, 224-226, 228f *See also* breasts;
Paget's disease of
the breast
reconstruction of 188-189, 372-373
nipple discharge 73, 77t, 19f, 219
evaluation of 90
node-negative breast cancer 32, 165-167,
248
Nolvadex Adjuvant Trial Organization
(NATO) 165
nonmastectomy treatment 138-153
nonpalpable lesions 5, 86, 91, 94
nortriptyline 307
nuclear grading 121
nurses and nursing
in clinical research 267, 341-342
in coordination of care 266, 267, 269-
271
in end-stage care 344-345
in patient education 335, 336, 337t, 338-
341, 342
in symptom management 343-344
in technical procedures 336, 338, 342,
343-344
professional conferences 337, 341, 343
specialties:
medical oncology 269, 341-345

radiation oncology 269, 338-341
surgical oncology 336-338

obesity 58t, 62 *See also* diet
occult carcinoma 211-218
oncogenes 255
Oncology Nursing Society 344
One Flew Over the Cuckoo's Nest 51
one-stage procedure 26
oophorectomy 66t, 163, 164f, 170, 171,
173, 325
oral contraceptives 63
oxazepam 308

Paget, Sir James 222
Paget's disease of the breast 150, 211, 222-
227
palpable mass 4, 71, 109
Papanicolaou, George Nicolas 99
Papanicolaou method 99-100
papilloma 23, 90, 91f, 102, 106f
paraffin 116, 117
parenchymal reconstruction 113
pathologist 30, 115, 124
pathology
department of 267, 269
Pathology of Breast Lesions (symposium)
115
peer counseling 356
Pennsylvania law re: breast cancer treatment 49
Penthouse 21
personality style 298, 366-367, 369, 373-
374
Peters, Vera 139
Peters-Golden, Holly 362
*Philadelphia County Medical Society Breast
Cancer Registry* 238
physical examination 3-4 *See also* breast
self-examination
physical therapy 313, 327
for lymphedema 318-319, 321-322
posture 314
range of motion 315, 316f-320f
strength 317-318, 321f
*Planned Parenthood of Central Missouri
v Danforth* 51
Playboy 21
pneumocystography 90, 92f
postmenopausal women 24, 30, 62-65, 73,
368
preferred-provider associations (PPAs or